Advance Praise for *The Right Bite*

"*The Right Bite* hits the nail on the head—it provides a common-sense approach to weight loss. This book has all the answers!"

—COVERT BAILEY, author of *The Ultimate Fit or Fat*

"Excess sugar and processed food in our diet is causing a worldwide health crisis. The Right Bite shows people the simple path to a slim, healthy body—enjoying the foods nature intended!.."

—PAUL KIRBY, Vice President of Hodgson Mill, Inc.

"At last, an authoritative, compelling, and comprehensive synthesis of nutritional breakthroughs guaranteed to reduce waistlines, restore health and undo the damage of past fad dieting. Finally, we physicians and therapists have been given a scientific solution for the treatment of weight control problems."

—R. CRAIG DOUGAN, M.D.

"I found great hope in knowing that there is a way to change my body and the way it handles food so that I will be freed from this feeling of having to watch (and worry about!) every bite I take."

—WILLIAM A. LONG, JR., M.D.

"*The Right Bite* is packed with practical tips for breaking your weight gain triggers and achieving lasting weight loss success with proven mind-body approaches and a flexible, livable meal plan. I highly recommend this book!"

—ELIZABETH LEE VLIET, M.D.
author of *Women, Weight, and Hormones* and
*Screaming to Be Heard: Hormone Connections
Women Suspect and Doctors Ignore*

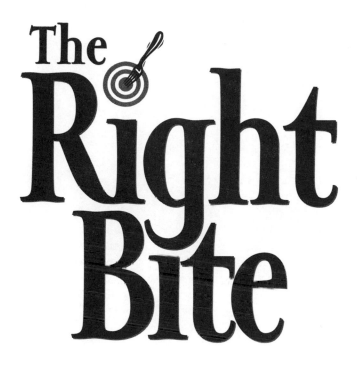

The Right Bite

Outsmart 43

SCIENTIFICALLY PROVEN FAT TRIGGERS

and Beat the Dieter's Curse

Stephanie Dalvit-McPhillips, Ph.D.

FAIR WINDS
PRESS

GLOUCESTER, MASSACHUSETTS

Text © Stephanie Dalvit-McPhillips, Ph.D.

First published in the USA in 2001 by
Fair Winds Press
33 Commercial Street
Gloucester, MA 01930

10 9 8 7 6 5 4 3 2 1

Printed and bound in the United States
Printed and bound in Canada

Cover design by Laura Shaw Design
Book design by Jill Feron/Feron Design

ISBN 1-931412-63-4

The information in this book is for educational purposes only. It is not intended to replace the advice of a physician or medical practitioner. Please see your health care provider before beginning any new health program.

Dedication

With love, I dedicate this book to my husband Tom—
my soul mate, blithe spirit, and cherished life partner.

Acknowledgments

This book took the combined efforts of many individuals and I especially wish to acknowledge the following:

Hal Zina Bennett, who brought to this book a rare combination of talents—wisdom about human nature, broad experience about the world of publishing, and the writing skills of an accomplished author. In the process of sharing the challenges of this project with me he became, and continues to be, a dedicated friend and supporter.

Pat Dalvit and Lewis Dalvit, my parents, whose steadfast belief in the importance and integrity of my research has been an endless source of encouragement and motivation.

Sean, Kristen, and Kyle, my children, for their unwavering confidence in me.

Barbara Deal, my enthusiastic and inspired literary agent. Holly Schmidt, my dedicated editor whose artistic convictions and insights helped to shape this book. Paul Kirby for his support and faith in me. Dr. William Long, physician and scientist, who helped me see that we are truly what we eat. Jacqueline Guthrie, my sister, for her generous editing contributions.

Stuart C. Irby and Belhaven College, Jackson, Mississippi, for helping to fund my early research.

And Ludwig.

Table of Contents

Foreword

This is an extraordinary book, written by a remarkable person. It is one of a kind: a book on weight control that conquers every fear, meets every objection, deals with every problem.

The information Dr. McPhillips has assembled here is both complete and scientifically accurate, yet expressed in a language everyone can understand. She has used her keen powers of observation to note every problem that people struggling with weight problems encounter. She has unearthed the causes—those based in the realities of human physiology, those rooted in people's misconceptions, and those embedded in our society's peculiar attitudes and practices surrounding food and weight. She has devised solutions to all the problems, tested them, refined them, and tested them again. In the process, she has brought to bear both enormous empathy and a fierce determination to simply not quit until she had got it right, all of it. She now has it right, and that is a monumental achievement.

The book will teach you what you need to know to conquer your weight problems and gain excellent nutritional health in the process. Its engaging humor will keep you reading long after any other serious book would put you to sleep. Its powerful motivational messages will keep you going when you embark on Dr. McPhillip's program. And then the success of the program itself will make it a permanent way of life for you. It will enhance your life, your health, and your morale.

—Eleanor N. Whitney, Ph.D.,

author of *Understanding Normal and Clinical Nutrition*

Preface:
A Quantum Leap Beyond
Fads and Quick Fixes

When I first showed this book to publishers, I typically received comments like the following: Today's dieters want books that are simplistic and nontechnical. You obviously know your business, and I have no doubt that your program works. Your idea about weight-gain triggers is intriguing and scientifically solid, as is your plan for eliminating these triggers through a multiple strategies approach. But dieters today only want books that are simplistic . . ." And so on. You can probably guess the rest.

I was indignant. I am not only a professional nutritionist but also a person who has successfully learned to manage my own weight issues. And having helped people learn to lose weight and manage it successfully for more than twenty years, I think I know what those of us who struggle with our weight want and what we are capable of. I don't consider myself a target for quick fix fad diets. Nor do most of my clients. Frankly, I felt that this publisher was speaking down not only to me but also to anyone who has ever struggled with weight problems.

I think all of us may start out believing that there must be simple solutions. As you read on, you'll discover that in my teens and twenties, and even into my thirties, I was just as guilty of that kind of thinking as anyone. But I am also certain that most of us get to a place in our lives when we know there is no magic powder, no simple strategy that is going to change us. A part of us knows, beyond a shadow of a doubt, that we have to delve deeper, and we have to take the issue of weight management seriously if we are going to achieve the weight goals we want.

I am going to share with you a note I sent back to more than one publisher before I found the wonderful publisher I have now, who not only agreed with me but also championed my cause and the cause of every person who reads this book:

"Simplistic, single strategy diets that you are looking for are ineffective. They do not take into account the varied weight-gain triggers that destabilize metabolisms, destroy diets, and cause weight gain. In many cases these fad diets and quick fixes were themselves triggers that caused way more problems than they solved. Believe me, I know. I see it every day in my practice. I see people of both genders whose health has been damaged, whose metabolisms are seriously disrupted, and whose weight has spiraled out of control. I also see so many others who are only a few pounds overweight but who cannot seem to make the latest fad diets work for them. I know this for certain, that following a single-strategy diet is not only a health threat, as we are certainly learning with the most recent backlash to high protein diets, but they fail miserably in the long run because they simply cannot address the multiple factors that are at work with every weight issue."

I got back many suggestions from publishers who still wanted me to consider writing a diet book for them: Wouldn't I please consider writing a series of books, one for each trigger? Wouldn't I consider focusing my material on high protein diets and how to improve them, since that trend is so popular these days, in spite of medical criticism? Most cynical of all was an editor who actually told me the following:

"We are not in this business because we sell diet books that *really work.*"

I practically went through the ceiling when I read these words. I was angry for weeks about this kind of callous disregard for those of us who want to get and stay thin. I wrote back a scathing and certainly not very diplomatic letter, which I will spare you the burden of having to read.

After all this, a friend reminded me that the diet industry is a $100 billion affair. Obviously, if we were to come up with a plan that really works for a lot of people it would be a threat to the national economy. Maybe so, but I am not going to simplify the truth of what I have discovered in the twenty-plus years that I have been studying these issues. I simply cannot ignore truths that have helped so many clients lose weight and manage it successfully, year after year, even as the fad diets come and go by the dozens. People's lives are changed by my multiple strategy Right Bite Program, and I want as many people as possible to share the success my clients and I have enjoyed.

Weight-Gain Triggers Are Highly Individualized

There are perhaps as many weight-gain triggers as there are individual tastes. At the same time, it is useful to know that most people are sensitive to only a handful of triggers and will identify them very quickly. In fact, some people are sensitive to only one, and once they have identified what that one trigger is they easily take charge of their weight.

I found early on that people will gain control of their weight issues only after they have identified their own unique set of triggers. There is no such thing as just giving you a list of triggers and telling you to stay away from them. Such a one-size-fits-all approach might help a few people but overall would very likely cause more problems than it would solve. In the final analysis, we can't simplify human behavior and human individuality, so we can't simplify weight issues. To achieve the goals we aspire to in this book, we've got to go beyond quick fixes and oversimplified theories.

As you learn about your own special set of weight-gain triggers, you will also understand why past diets have failed you, or why they only worked for a short time, or why losing or maintaining weight on them has been difficult or impossible for you. You will learn that you didn't fail these diets, these diets failed you! You will learn why your weight actually skyrocketed on some calorie-restricting diets that had you eating like a mouse. You'll learn why too few calories— yes, you read it right, too few calories— is one of the most powerful weight gain triggers of all for most people. Best of all, on the Right Bite Program, you will be successful at losing weight and keeping it off permanently.

Contrary to what publishers told me, my experience has been that today's dieters are aware that single-strategy diets have their limits. Rather than just trimming off a few pounds to look better in your bikini, most of you are looking for solid information that will put you in charge of your weight and your well-being for the rest of your life. So we are not just talking about getting on another treadmill of weight-loss-weight-gain. We are talking about food wisdom that will serve you forever.

Food is a source of pleasure for most of us. That's something I never forget. As you work with my program, you will discover not only that you will learn how to take charge of your weight but also that you will begin to enjoy eating more than you ever have in your life.

Is the plan I describe challenging? Will it demand a lot of you? I have to tell you the truth. Yes. It will do both. But I hasten to add that you will not feel you are starving on it. You will not have mood swings. You will not feel strange or out of sorts. You will not feel deprived. You'll have to use your intellect to take in what I am about to say, and you'll have to be especially disciplined about following the first phase of the program. However, you'll feel full. You'll enjoy a variety of foods—in fact, variety is required! And you will enjoy a new level of energy and pleasure that you will never experience with other diet programs. Beyond that, I assure you that it gets easier as you go along, and the rewards you reap will be worth their weight in gold, measured in the pounds you've lost.

Because this book contains information that you will want for later reference, I strongly recommend that you keep a personal journal, jotting down notes, observations, and insights that you might have along the way. Do this writing in your own style, as formal or as informal as you like, remembering that these journal entries are for your eyes only. From time to time, go back and read over what you have written, noting improvements, changes, places where you were challenged, and places where new doors opened up for you.

The famous Chinese philosopher Lao-Tzu is quoted as saying that a journey of a thousand miles must begin with a single step. To which I add, a journey to the peace of mind that comes with permanent weight control begins with a single bite. Make it the *right bite*!

Introduction:
A Passion for Eating Well and Staying Thin

There is no love more sincere than the love of food.
—George Bernard Shaw

While I was in the midst of writing this book, a woman who'd heard me lecture called me on the phone. She was in tears. Her physician had just told her that diets don't work. He pointed out that she'd been on one diet after another for most of her adult life and had only gained weight. His prescription was that she should learn to love her body as it was—fat or not—and stop torturing herself, because at this point her dieting had become much more of a health threat than her weight.

This poor woman was crushed. She hated the idea of being fat for the rest of her life. I quickly informed her that she did not have to accept being fat as her fate—that while the first part of her physician's statement was true (diets don't work), the second part wasn't. What's more, I was going to show her a way to get the weight off while actually improving her health. She seemed greatly relieved.

"You should be celebrating," I told her, "because you have just crossed an important threshold that I have seen so many others cross before you on their way to achieving their weight goals." As bad as she might feel right now, I assured her that this revelation about the uselessness of diets cleared the way for lasting success with the Right Bite Program.

Over the phone I had her take a little quiz, the same one that I've included for you in this introduction (see p. xix). The purpose of this quiz is to begin the process of exposing the over forty weight-gain triggers that I have found can sabotage nearly all diets. I explained to my caller that these triggers cause increased appetite or weight gain even when a person is not overeating. They are triggers that I have found in almost every single diet I have examined.

My caller and I went through the quiz and immediately exposed three very powerful weight-gain triggers that had sabotaged all of her previous efforts to lose weight. There was now not a single doubt in her mind about what had been going on for her in the past, and she instinctively knew that she could easily eliminate these newfound triggers from her diet immediately. She made an appointment and came in to see me the following week, at which time we got her started on the Right Bite Program.

Less than a year has passed since that initial phone call. That woman has long since eliminated all her weight-gain triggers and says it was so easy and painless to do that she could hardly believe it. She is happily following the Right Bite plan, has more energy than ever, and never has even a trace of the uncontrollable food cravings that once plagued her. And by the way, in four months she had already lost twenty-three pounds, she had never felt better in her life, and both she and her doctor were singing the praises of the program.

It is the stories like this that convinced me, after many years as a diet consultant, to write this book. The message must get out that you really can control your weight, and you can do it much more easily than you might have ever suspected. There is not only hope, but absolute proof that this is so. The proof is in the clients who are still enjoying success on the Right Bite Program today, even after many years. And the proof is in my own life, because I live by this program and love it, and have done so for twenty-plus years.

The program begins by identifying the weight-gain triggers in your own life. And you can start doing that immediately with the help of the self-quiz I've included in these first pages. You will then go on to learn more about how these triggers can set off rapid weight gain and food cravings that are physiological and extremely powerful, overriding even your greatest determination to stick with a diet. Once we've identified and eliminated the triggers, it's easy to follow the food plan I've laid out for you. In part this is true because you'll be doing it without the triggers that made dieting so difficult for you in the past and in part because you will be satisfied with the variety of foods and tastes you'll find here. To say nothing of the fact that you will never feel hungry!

During the nutritional part of the program, which is divided into two phases, not only will you lose weight but you will also repair damage done by past dieting and transform your metabolism from that of a fat person to that of a thin one.

The Right Bite Program includes an easy and enjoyable physical exercise plan, one that is easily adapted to your fitness level, and a mental component that teaches you how to beat the old *fattitudes* and nutritional myths that have kept you fat.

Before going further, I want everyone reading this book to know that when you hear that phrase "diets don't work," which has become so popular these days, you need to understand that dieticians are actually saying that "single-strategy or fad diets don't work." And eating differently for a few months only for the purpose of taking off a few pounds will only get you in trouble. You simply can't expect to get the weight off and keep it off by narrowing your diet to a single food item, as we see with high-protein diets, all-fruit diets, the no-fat diet, or any other program offering a quick fix, single-strategy approach. These single-strategy weight-loss diets make about as much sense as a lone warrior going into battle against an army of thousands, and with only a single arrow in his quiver. This is because fat is a multifaceted foe, and it requires a multistrategy program to defeat this enemy.

The Right Bite Program has worked so well for so many people because it honors the fact that we are all different. Recognizing your own uniqueness, you will be tailoring this plan to fit your own lifestyle, built upon the solid, multistrategy foundation that I will be providing.

Unlike single-strategy diets you may have tried in the past, the Right Bite Program does not artificially manipulate your God-given metabolic capacities for the sake of losing a few pounds, but works in full cooperation with your biochemistry to help you achieve both optimal weight and optimal health.

Early on in my career I made a discovery that is unique to my program. It has to do with the role of willpower in dieting. If you have ever dieted, and there is a pretty good chance that you have, you know exactly what I'm talking about. To successfully lose weight on a single-strategy diet you have to exercise the willpower and resolve of a saint or one of those yoga masters who sleep on beds of nails and live on a single grain of rice each day. What few dieters know is that every single-strategy diet contains what I call "weight-gain triggers" that undermine your resolve. Ironically, these diets—whether they're the latest high-protein regimens, the all-fruit diet, diets based on blood type, or any other you might think of—are their own worst enemies. Every one of them has built-in weight-gain triggers that torpedo your willpower, alter your metabolism, or cause your body to gain weight even when your caloric intake is restricted.

You will succeed with the Right Bite Program because you will disarm those weight-gain triggers long before they sink you. People succeed with this program not because they must rely on iron willpower but because the plan teaches them how to eliminate these triggers. It then offers a trigger-free food plan that satisfies their needs for taste, food variety, and that wonderful sense of well-being that comes with feeling full.

Changing Your Mind about Losing Weight

I have found that most women over the age of eighteen have already been through a whole rash of single-strategy diets. Since men are not quite as stigmatized as women, who are expected to be skinny like the super models, as a general rule the problem is somewhat less prevalent for them. By the time I turned eighteen I'd been on at least a half-dozen diets. And once we've started down that path we have created some special problems for ourselves that must be remedied before we can succeed at losing weight. If you are anything like me and a few million other women in this world who have tried single-strategy diets, the chances are pretty good that your metabolism is nearly as confused as you are about how to lose weight. The Right Bite Program corrects damaged biochemistry from these past dieting attempts and transforms your metabolism from that of a fat person to that of a thin person.

The Right Bite Program's multistrategy approach addresses your food, your body, your physical health, and your attitudes about weight. Through this plan you control or eliminate *over forty weight-gain triggers* that are to blame for the failure of most diets and for the growing problem of obesity in the modern world. You will reach your slimmest, healthiest weight by changing your metabolism, by eliminating appetite and weight-promoting foods and substances, and by reeducating and retraining your mind to reject food myths and self-defeating attitudes that precipitate and maintain obesity.

How do you begin? I've always been one of those people who like to get to the point as quickly as possible. And the best place to start the Right Bite Program is to do a little self-test that I promised I was going to give you. That's the place to start—right now! So let's find out if weight-gain triggers are responsible for the weight issues you are struggling with now or have struggled with in the past. This can be your opening to a brand new perspective and the achievement of your perfect weight.

With the following quiz most people have changed their whole way of looking at food and weight. But bear in mind that each of us has a highly individualized system. Different food tastes and combinations of food-related factors can act either individually or synergistically to trigger food cravings or biochemical imbalances contributing to weight-gain. Through the Right Bite Program, you will find out what your particular weight-gaining patterns are, and you'll begin eliminating them right away.

The following quiz covers the most common of the forty weight-gain triggers, the ones that cause most people a lot of frustration in their efforts to lose weight. As you go through the quiz, you will notice that I've inserted page numbers referring to places in the book where you can read more about that particular trigger. You will find it useful to check out the pages noted even when the specific trigger does not appear to apply to you. By doing so, you may be surprised to uncover information that relates to you and your weight-control concerns.

As you read the quiz, don't ruminate too long over your answers. Trust your first gut-level responses, the answers that first pop into your mind. These are often the best indicators of triggers to explore further. As you quiz yourself, remember that the Right Bite Program is trigger-free itself and will also accurately identify your specific triggers. The quiz is to give you a preview. Just as it has been the case for my clients before you, your answers can reveal why you have had difficulty controlling your weight in the past and what you can do to achieve your ideal weight and maintain it forever.

Weight-Gain Triggers Quiz

1. Are you eating fewer than 1200–1400 calories per day but still not losing weight—or even gaining weight?
   If yes, the weight-gain trigger affecting you may be **too few calories.** *Yes, too few calories can actually cause a number of serious symptoms, including weight gain. (See pages 15 to 28 for more information.)*

2. Do you suffer from fatigue or feelings of malaise, depression, or nervousness?
   If yes, the weight-gain trigger affecting you may be **insufficient nutrients,** *which can cause marginal malnutrition as a result of an unbalanced diet or one that lacks variety. The effects of insufficient nutrients include low blood sugar, loss of lean body mass (muscle), an actual decrease in enzymes that burn fat, and decreased production of serotonin, a natural chemical in your*

brain that affects your feelings of well-being. (See pages 30 to 44 for more information.)

3. Do you crave sweets, suffer from headaches, occasionally or even frequently binge?
    If yes, the trigger involved may be **hypoglycemia**, *which is the result of not eating often enough throughout the day, fasting, or undereating. This can cause a wide range of problems, from depression to high insulin production to chronic fatigue to hormonal imbalances. (see pages 44 to 46 for more information).*

4. Do you find yourself engaging in negative self-talk, especially about your weight, which more often than not ends up with you overeating or binging?
    If yes, the negative self-talk itself is a weight-gain trigger for you. It comes from having learned what I call **fattitudes**, *probably very early in your life. The good news is that fattitudes can be changed. (See pages 64 to 66 for more information.)*

5. Do you use food to make you feel better emotionally, though you later regret it because it causes you to gain weight?
    If yes, the weight-gain trigger may be **stress** *as a result of overworking, a recent trauma in your life, dealing with dramatic change, excessive worry, or chronic anxiety. Stress triggers biochemical events within your body that can bring on intense cravings for sweets, drain micronutrients necessary for intellectual work and physical coordination, and cause low blood sugar. (see pages 56 to 59 for more information.)*

6. Do you like salty foods or even crave them?
    If yes, the **salt** *you are using is a powerful trigger in itself. Because salt stimulates our taste buds, it encourages us to eat more and can even send our appetites spinning out of control. Naturally, with a salt craving we seek out foods such as potato chips, french fries, and salted nuts that are also high in fats. And remember, salt causes water retention, which increases body weight and feelings of bloating. (For more on this see pages 68 to 69.)*

7. Do you gravitate toward liquid foods such as yogurt, smoothies, icies, ice cream, and sweetened beverages?

If yes your weight-gain trigger may actually be **low hydration** *(thirst), created by not drinking what your body really needs— which is water. By seeking and consuming the flavored drinks and liquid foods, you take in additional calories and still don't get enough water to satisfy your thirst. (For more information, see pages 69 to 70.)*

8. Do you get hungry just seeing, smelling, or even thinking about certain foods and sometimes overeat or eat foods not on your diet?
    If yes, you may be a person whose weight-gain triggers are built-in, causing a particularly powerful reaction to the **scents and sights** *of your favorite foods. These reactions actually trigger increased insulin in your body, boosting your appetite for the foods you are envisioning. Mental exercises can actually help you combat this particularly insidious trigger. (See pages 46 to 47 and 70 to 71.)*

9. Has a physician or health adviser ever suggested that you are at risk of getting diabetes?
    If yes, your weight-gain trigger may be associated with lack of fiber in your diet, caused by eating **highly processed foods** *and food products with a lot of refined white flour. This dietary pattern not only triggers behavior that leads to obesity, it can result in a condition known as "insulin resistance," which is a precursor of certain types of diabetes. (See pages 46 to 53, 71 to 74, and 85 to 95 for more information.)*

10. Are you a very sedentary person preferring to watch TV, take the elevator rather than the stairs, or watch sports rather than play them?
    If yes, your trigger may be **lack of exercise.** *Please see pages 49 to 50 for more infomation.*

11. Do you have what is commonly called a "beer belly"?
    If yes, **alcohol** *may be your weight-gain trigger. The consumption of alcoholic beverages stimulates hunger, depletes certain micronutrients, stimulates the production of insulin, inhibits the burning of fat, and causes low blood sugar. (See pages 77 to 80 for more information.)*

12. Do you sometimes feel starved right after you have eaten a large meal?

If yes, your triggers may be **high glycemic foods and insulin,** *the "hunger hormone," which make you feel hungrier, crave sweets, and motivate you to eat more because the foods taste better. (See pages 46 to 47 and 74 to 76 for more information.)*

13. Do you lose weight rapidly, only to regain it quickly—and to a weight higher than before?
    If yes, your trigger may be the **speed at which you lose weight.** *Quick weight loss is always followed by quick weight gain. (See why by reading pages 101 to 102.)*

14. Have you noticed a change in your weight or size since taking a new medication, either a prescription or over-the-counter remedy?
    If yes, there are many **medications** *that not only cause increased appetite and weight but also make it difficult or impossible to lose weight. (See pages 111 to 118 for a list of medications that are the biggest culprits and suggestions for alternatives that may not have the same side effects.)*

15. Have you noticed that it has been more difficult to stay thin since turning thirty?
    Your trigger could be the natural processes that come with **aging.** *But this pattern of weight-gain can be reversed so that gaining weight as we grow older is no longer inevitable. (See pages 49 to 50 and 118 to 119 to learn how you can have the body you had in your youth.)*

Many fad and quick fix diets, including the high-protein regimens, are their own weight-gain triggers. If you are like many of my clients, you have come to the Right Bite Program because you have already been a victim of one of the fad diets, which adversely changed your metabolism to a fat one and initiated weight-gain triggers that you didn't have before. Harvard researcher George Blackburn, M.D., a critic of fad diets for many years, has applauded recent medical studies that found that the theory behind high-protein diets simply doesn't stand up to scientific scrutiny. The theory is that we burn more fat on these diets because we force our bodies into a state of ketosis. However, ketosis itself doesn't cause us to lose weight; rather, when our bodies go into ketosis we lose our appetites and eat fewer calories.

High-protein diets are particularly pernicious for anyone with weight concerns because (1) they are difficult to maintain, and (2) the major weight loss comes from the loss of muscle and water. As you'll be learning in the pages ahead, our muscles are the most metabolically active tissue in our bodies. Why would anyone want to get rid of fat-burning tissue? As for getting rid of water, our bodies require a certain level of hydration to function well and to feel comfortable. There's abundant research showing that, when people go back to normal eating following a high-protein diet, they quickly gain back the pounds they've lost plus some extra ones. Of course, this would naturally occur because the diet has reduced the muscle mass that once burned off those extra calories.

I do know that I have never spoken with a single person who praised the high-protein diets much beyond the first twelve or fifteen pounds they lost. To the contrary, every single person I've interviewed complained that they simply could not stay on the diet because they felt lousy while they were on it, and they gained weight with a vengeance any time they deviated from it or started eating in a more balanced way. You will find other notes about high-protein diets, their pitfalls, and their side effects throughout the book. The main point I want to make here is that quick-fix miracle diets, such as the high-protein regimens, can be the most insidious and powerful weight-gain triggers you will ever encounter. But once you have eliminated the triggers and started on the Right Bite food plan, you will reverse any damage that's been done and start reaping the benefits of my weight-control program.

Multistrategies for Complete Success

Rather than building around a single strategy, such as restricting your diet to a single food group, as high-protein diets do, the Right Bite Program applies multiple strategies, fully integrated to shift your metabolism from a fat person's to a thin person's and keep you slim forever. You will lose weight and keep it off not by counting calories and policing yourself through an extraordinary act of will but by normalizing your damaged metabolism, enabling you to burn more calories and lose fat weight easily, all the while eating more than you thought possible. Your metabolism will change, no doubt about that, but not because it is forced into an abnormal state such as ketosis. As you proceed with the program, your body will get to the point of actually resisting the retention of body fat.

This program is not just about eating particular foods. I will also be discussing facts about your own metabolism that will give you the power to make informed choices about what, when, and how to eat. You'll be gaining some real wisdom about what foods mean to you and what foods trigger eating habits or biochemical abnormalities that impede the ability to have a thin person's metabolism and a thin person's body.

If you are looking for a way to make significant changes and reap long-term and wide-ranging benefits, read on. The multistrategy Right Bite Program provides everything you will need to bring a lasting truce in your war with fat.

A Personal Quest Fully Realized

What I offer you in this book comes out of exhaustive personal and scientific research. But the Right Bite Program is much more than a scientific innovation for me. It is the program I have personally followed for over two decades, with benefits so rich and numerous that I cannot imagine life without it. It has allowed me to maintain my ideal weight within four pounds, year after year. And on rare occasions when I go off the plan, it is easy and painless to get back on track.

I've experienced nearly every eating disorder imaginable, from bulimia to gross, out-of-control obesity. So I'm no stranger to the problems others have with food and weight. In my early twenties, I thought my quest for my perfect weight would one day be answered and that would be the end of it. But it is now obvious to me that this quest was more than a personal crusade; it would carry me into a rewarding career with the pleasure of knowing I could help others achieve the healthy, attractive bodies they dreamed of.

I first became aware of weight problems when I was eleven. One morning my father rushed into the kitchen where my mother, sister, grandmother, and I were fixing breakfast. In a panic he announced that he had found a tumor growing on his chest. The night before we'd all watched a TV report saying that women were not the only victims of breast cancer. Men got it too. Dad pulled up his sweatshirt and lay down on the kitchen floor as we gathered around him, anxiously prodding the area of suspicion. We could feel a large, rounded, slightly soft moveable mass above his solar plexus . . . definitely an emergency we all decided!

Without delay we piled into the car and raced to the doctor's office. Alerted by phone, the young physician met us in the vestibule of the clinic and ushered us into his office where, after some minutes, this slim doctor turned to us with faint amusement and delivered his prognosis: "Your father's tumor is a benign lump of adipose tissue . . . in other words, just plain fat!" Though relieved that my father was OK, this was one of the most embarrassing days of my young life.

My father eventually lost weight, but the tumor scare and my embarrassment definitely put a spotlight on the issue of body weight for me. By my sophomore year in high school I knew all the statistics—how more than 200 million people wrestle constantly with frustrating weight problems. I began asking how this could be. Every time I turned on the

TV or opened a women's magazine I was bombarded with articles, ads, and TV specials concerning weight loss. My friends told me about their mothers, and sometimes their fathers, going away to spas in Arizona or Florida to lose weight. They came back from these places looking great, yet a few months later they were right back where they started, stuffing themselves into loose-fitting sweat clothes and dresses to hide their fat.

I recall a slumber party with friends when we shared stories about the bizarre things people did in their wars against body fat. We nervously joked about being pummeled, wrapped, jiggled, psychoanalyzed, and medicated and swore we'd never submit to such abuse. We talked about surgical procedures, resculpting thighs and bellies, shortening intestines, stapling offending stomachs, and liposuction. One girl's mother even had her jaw wired shut to prevent her from eating!

I became convinced that fat was Public Enemy #1. At the same time I had become aware of the importance of female beauty in the eyes not just of men but of other women. Inundated with pictures, articles, and slender TV heroines, I was convinced that I needed to be thin and sexy.

You would have thought that, given my experience, I would have been so hyperaware of the best ways to stay trim that I never would have gained an ounce beyond my ideal weight. But just the opposite happened. By twenty I had suffered through the full spectrum of weight problems, from fat to thin to anorexic to fat and back again—in dizzying, crazy circles. Try as I might during the anxiety-ridden years between twelve and twenty-something, I could never find the right map to reach my ideal weight.

Nothing I tried worked for me. Totally wrapped up in my unsuccessful dieting efforts, I didn't notice my health had perilously deteriorated. Only a near-catastrophe awakened me before I destroyed myself. For several weeks I had become increasingly depressed, and because I had been steadily losing physical strength and vitality, I had returned to my parents' home from college. Late one evening, I was trying unsuccessfully to sleep when I became aware of anguished weeping from my parents' bedroom.

Fear and concern drew me down the dark corridor where I stopped at my parents' closed door, wondering if I should knock and ask what was wrong, or not. Then I heard my father's words, which filled me with terror. He told my mother that he had learned that I could actually die from my radical dieting. He also reminded my mother of my frequent announcement that I would rather be dead than fat. Despite my parent's unending efforts to help me, he believed they could do no more for me. Something was seriously wrong, he said, and they must mentally prepare themselves for the very real possibility that, indeed, I would end up killing myself through my obsession with weight.

Trembling, I made my way back to my room and collapsed onto the bed. I knew in my heart that my father was right. There was something tremendously wrong with my body's metabolism. Through ignorance and dogged determination to lose weight I had exacerbated my condition almost to the point of annihilation.

I spent one of the most anxious nights of my life, but I had been jolted into recognizing the seriousness of my problem. Further, the painful realization that I had driven my poor parents to despair filled me with a resolve to find a solution to this quest that had so consumed me. I would never again cause my parents to suffer such sorrow. That morning at breakfast, I announced to my parents that I was finished with my crazy dieting efforts and would fight to regain my health. My parents watched with relief as I enthusiastically ate a nutritious breakfast for the first time in nearly four years. My father remarked some years later that, given the choice, they would rather have had a fat daughter than no daughter at all—but before that morning they were certain they didn't have that choice.

Soon after this vulnerable turning point in my life, I happened to read an article by a nutrition-oriented physician from Johns Hopkins University. He described many of the peculiar symptoms and weight problems I had experienced since the age of twelve. I wrote to this physician, who recommended that I see Dr. William Long, who lived in my area.

Dr. Long reaffirmed my faith in myself. Ever since that first appointment, he has remained my mentor, guide, and friend, and I will always be grateful for his unwavering confidence in me. It was through working with him, first as a patient and then as a student of his expertise, that I received my first breakthroughs about the triggering agents that would become the heart of the Right Bite Program.

During the years I was earning my Ph.D. in nutrition, I conducted a number of controlled research studies with overweight men and women. I reached an important conclusion, based on solid scientific research, that weight problems are not ordinarily the result of "lack of willpower," as seems to be the popular consensus. Rather, they are the result of damaged metabolism and biochemical imbalances created by our diets. In over twenty years of research and private practice, I have further been convinced that it is extremely rare that deep-seated neuroses or low self-esteem are strong contributing factors in obesity. I have also found very little convincing evidence that some people are just inherently predisposed to obesity.

To strengthen my hypothesis that almost all uncontrolled eating and weight gain is physically induced, I set up two controlled studies to examine the effects of diet on bulimia, which many professionals insist is emotionally based. Bulimia is characterized by uncontrollable eating binges that make gaining an excessive number of pounds a terrifying reality to its victims. In order to prevent the inevitable weight gain from these binges, stricken individuals throw up.

My research subjects ate a diet devoid of all the triggers I regarded as physical causes of their disorders, carefully avoiding any discussion of their personal problems. Overweight people in the experiment not only stopped binging, they lost pounds. These studies proved useful in the treatment of bulimia. In addition, what I discovered about triggers and uncontrolled eating with severely bulimic persons proved to helpful for people with other weight problems. Subsequently, I applied my findings in a study involving hundreds of nonbulimic subjects who, obese or slender, needed help in controlling or losing weight.

As with the bulimia study, people who were too heavy steadily dropped pounds and inches, readily achieving their weight goals, and those who were already slender, or who had trouble sustaining a normal weight, now found they could do so effortlessly.

For over two decades now I have used the trigger-free food plan of my original studies to successfully treat a wide variety of weight problems. Although I have done further research and refined parts of the program, it was through that original research that the Right Bite Core Diet was born.

The above scientific studies, as well as twenty years of clinical experience, have convinced me that most weight problems are primarily the result of weight-gain triggers. These triggers come in a wide variety of forms, as you've already begun to see, including certain foods, food additives, and even eating habits. Further research has shown me that every single fad diet I have reviewed includes weight-gain triggers that sabotage the dieter. The saddest part of this is not just that people end up gaining rather than losing weight but that they end up blaming themselves for their failures. Guess what, if you ever found yourself in that situation, you were not the problem! The diet was to blame.

You don't ever have to be victimized in that way again. As my clients have been learning for twenty-plus years, you can lose weight, and you can do it without feeling deprived or starved, or having your willpower challenged. Moreover, you can do it while feeling full and while enjoying a wide variety of delicious foods. With the Right Bite Program, you'll eliminate the weight-gain triggers that have plagued you with every diet you've ever tried, and you will achieve the weight goal that is perfect for you.

You will learn how to avoid diet-subverting triggers that can, either singly or in combination, cause exaggerated appetites or uncontrolled weight gain *even when your caloric intake is low*. You'll become aware of intertwining physical variables that cause overeating and weight gain, and you will understand why in the past you have either been unable to lose weight or have rapidly regained pounds after working so hard to lose them. What's even more important, you will never have to suffer through such experiences again.

As my father pointed out many years ago, there are worse things than being fat. But with the Right Bite Program, you really can be thin and stay thin. Imagine being able to eat as often and as much as you like while losing weight, and you can do so with the assurance that you are correcting the damage of past dieting efforts and improving your health and fitness.

Whether you are chronically obese, moderately overweight, or a normal-sized person who just wants to maintain a healthy, lean, energetic body, *The Right Bite* will help you turn your fondest weight-control dreams into an exciting reality.

Chapter One

Exposing the Hidden Saboteurs

*There must be more to life than just
eating and getting bigger.*
—Trina Paulus

She shrieked with outrage as she opened a fresh box of Raisin Bran®. Sitting at my desk, pretending to study, I braced myself, teeth clenched, and tried my best to look both surprised and innocent. It happened often. I always knew she was going to yell and carry on because, you see, I was the one responsible for her outrage.

As she poured the crisp, *raisinless* flakes into her empty bowl, I held my breath, head lowered in embarrassment, fearing that if we had eye contact I might be compelled to confess what I had done. I suspect that only those who have experienced an eating problem will fully sympathize with my embarrassment at this little drama, and you'll know I'm not exaggerating. I wanted to press my hands to my ears to block out my roommate's complaints. I held myself motionless, shoulders up around my ears, hunched over my books, praying that she would not somehow discover my secret. Would some oversight on my part provide a clue pointing to me, the guilty person?

You see, I was guilty of an unpardonable sin, not just of stealing the raisins from my roommate's cereal—that was the least of it—but of once again going off my diet. Something in my diet—actually, as it turned out, it was *something missing from my diet*—was triggering cravings I could not control. I am not sure what caused me the most shame at my lack of self-control, seeing how my behavior upset my roommate or my inability to control myself or the extent to which I would go to satisfy my craving.

While my roommate was in class, I would steal back to our room and slit open all her miniature cartons of breakfast cereal. I'm not talking about simply pouring out a large opened box, picking out the raisins and dumping the flakes back. I'm talking about opening an entire cardboard tray of those small cartons of individual helpings, you know, the kind that you get for camping trips or that your mother sends you when you're in college. And in order to do this so that I wouldn't be detected, I'd perform this deed with all the care of a brain surgeon, resealing each carton so that I left no evidence. I'd eat every single raisin, twelve little boxes worth when possible, before shrewdly and craftily pouring back the cereal flakes and resealing the tops with glue.

I was unstoppable. Every time my roommate came home with a fresh supply of her favorite cereal, I was at it again, picking out all the raisins to satisfy my hunger for sweets. And every time, I could count on her shrill protestations. She simply could not figure out what was happening. I always resealed each box with such care that only a microscope and a trained eye could have detected my deed.

Why didn't I just go to the market and buy myself a box of raisins, or cereal with raisins in it, so that I could raid my own stash of food? Because I was on a diet. Most of the time I stuck to my meager meals of dry toast, salads, and water—or whatever my diet of the month happened to be. I prided myself on my ability to stay on my diet, as I watched all the young women around me binging and dieting and constantly weighing themselves. I wouldn't have been seen dead purchasing fattening foods for myself. Besides, if I actually walked into a grocery store and purchased a box of raisins, or some other sweets, I would have to admit that I had a problem and that I really wasn't sticking to my rigid diet at all.

Though I can laugh at my pitiful behavior now, and even have fun telling people in my workshops about my devious past, at the time it was happening I was mortified and ashamed. I was certain I was the only person in the world who ever did such bizarre things. I was equally certain that few people in the world would be able to sympathize with my behavior or my feelings about my weight. And by the way, I never did tell my roommate what I'd done. Until this book, the fate of those tasty morsels has remained an unsolved mystery. After all, how could I have told this lovely Japanese exchange student that she had fallen victim to a raisin thief! I imagined that in the polite society from which she had come raisin thieves were the lowest of the low. Surely she would have considered me mad if I'd confessed that I'd plundered every stash of raisin bran flakes that she ever brought to our room, not just one little box at a time but an entire tray of twelve whenever the opportunity arose. Were she to find out, would she laugh at my ridiculous obsession or would she insist on having her room changed and then tell everyone in the dorm about me? And so, with the fruits of my labors feeling like a lead weight in my belly, I presented myself as the very essence of innocence. My secret must not be revealed.

This true story might seem farfetched if you've never been on a diet. But in my workshops and at my lectures, participants not only find humor and truth in my tale but telling it frees them to share similar experiences that they have had in their efforts to control their body weight.

I hope you don't get the impression from this that I think our struggles about weight loss are a laughing matter. They are anything but. Yet, I also know that if we are to find lasting solutions, we absolutely must take the time to be truthful with ourselves and own up to even our most bizarre behavior. Sometimes, a little humor can help us stand back and observe ourselves with a more objective eye, which brings us closer to a truce in our war with weight.

One year, in despair, I even tried psychoanalysis. After three months of poking around inside my psyche, I realized that my psychiatrist was ferreting out problems that didn't exist.

"OK," I told my psychiatrist one day. "So what if I do overeat because my mom is pushy? I can assure you, she will always be pushy — and that's her most endearing quality! Besides, I'm convinced that mothers are supposed to be pushy. I wouldn't have mine any other way!"

My analyst responded by exhaling a lung full of pipe smoke in my direction. He sighed, wearily shifted his spectacles onto the top of his head, and announced that my time was up. I didn't go back.

To find new answers I started asking different kinds of questions, and I asked a question that nobody had ever asked before: Objectively, losing weight was a simple matter of eating fewer calories, so why was it so difficult to do that? Wasn't there something very essential that we were all missing here? Millions of people wanted to lose weight more than anything in their lives. So what was it that drove them to abandon perfectly good plans to accomplish that? What I began to explore was the possibility that the answer was not psychological but physical, and what's more, I was convinced that I would find the culprit in the diets themselves.

What were the inner mechanisms, the biochemistry, that converted food to fat instead of energy? What causes a person who is hardly eating anything to suddenly gain weight rapidly? And, on a deeply personal level, what went wrong when I was dieting that I would steal raisins from my roommate's stash of raisin bran flakes and continue eating them long after my stomach cried out for me to stop?

What makes us gulp down a meal so rapidly that we neither taste it or even remember eating? And what is it that causes an otherwise serious-minded, determined, steadfast, and sensible person to lose so much self-control that she will try to stuff the entire contents of a refrigerator into her mouth!

After twenty-plus years of hearing my clients' success stories I knew I had to write this book, to share what my clients and I have learned. I have discovered that virtually everyone I have ever treated, from those who are only a few pounds overweight to those who are grossly obese, suffers from exposure to insidious *weight-gain triggers—usually caused by their past or present diets or by a food or food-related substance in their lives!* These triggers not only perpetuate uncontrolled eating, they do so through physiological means. What's more they can induce weight gain even when your caloric intake is low.

But the best part of all? We can liberate ourselves from the tyranny of these weight-gain triggers and achieve our ideal weights.

What Are Triggers?

A trigger, as the word suggests, is the starting point of an action—often an action with rather significant consequences. Pull the trigger of a gun and somebody is liable to get injured or die. Pull a weight-gain trigger and you're going to have changes within your body that will produce uncontrollable cravings, gnawing feelings of hunger, and disruptions of your normal functioning that will cause you to get fatter even when you are starving yourself. Some weight-gain *triggers* are nonfood components, including a certain way of thinking about yourself and your weight that sets off your appetite. Soon after these triggers are pulled, you are off and running, gobbling down the very foods that you know you shouldn't be eating and have been diligently trying to avoid. Some triggers compel you to gorge yourself or binge. Others work in a more insidious way, causing you to gain weight even when you are not overeating. Some weight-gain triggers do all of the above. However you wish to define them, all you really have to remember is this: *Triggers fire off your appetites with a big bang, causing you to overeat, gorge yourself, or binge. They cause accelerated weight gain, even when you are not overeating.*

The answer that everyone was seeking to this dilemma was right there before our eyes all along: Identify and eliminate weight-gain triggers that send our appetites and weights sailing out of control, and we no longer have to fight the cravings and biochemistry that have been undermining us. How do we do that? (1) By supporting the physiological processes we were born with for maintaining our ideal weight, instead of manipulating them, and thus damaging or impairing them; (2) by eating in a way that corrects our abused metabolism and builds optimal health; and (3) by choosing wholesome foods that do all of the above while meeting our needs for taste and variety and satisfying fullness.

The Right Bite Program stops the havoc that weight-gain triggers produce but that extends beyond fat into issues of lowered self-esteem and self-doubt. These emotional side effects of being fat are also weight-gain triggers that can undermine your will and often manifest themselves as gnawing hunger that will hound you until you are convinced that the only way to stop the hunger pangs is to eat. Other weight-gain triggers come in the form of too few of the right kinds of calories, which means that you are sacrificing the pleasure of food yet still gaining weight rather than losing it.

With the Right Bite Program, you will conquer your weight-gain triggers, reduce your weight, and in the process enjoy increased self-esteem and dignity as your confidence about losing weight builds. What you will achieve in this program is not just the added assurance you get from looking great and feeling great but something more: You will experience a big sigh of relief to discover that weight-gain triggers, not a weak constitution, are responsible for your loss of control around food. To really understand the ruinous power of weight-gain triggers, and then to learn how you can eradicate them, is nothing short of life-changing. I've seen it with hundreds of clients following the Right Bite Program, and it guides my own eating behavior every day of my life. I know it can work for you.

How to Know If You Are Presently a Victim of Weight-Gain Triggers

It's a rare person in this world who is immune to the effects of weight-gain triggers. I've seen highly conditioned athletes and dancers who, in spite of being disciplined in every other way, had one or more weight-gain triggers that threw them off their training time and again. I've seen people who, though they didn't have weight problems, nevertheless had triggers that corrupted their diets, making them feel bloated, lethargic, and fuzzy-minded. But how do you know if these triggers affect you? You've already done a short self-quiz in the introduction to this book. This quiz is different, and it is important to answer these questions with the knowledge that the answers you get will help you identify and retire your own weight gain triggers forever.

TWENTY QUESTIONS: YOUR FIRST STEPS TOWARD FREEDOM FROM WEIGHT-GAIN TRIGGERS

1. Are you convinced that just looking at food causes you to gain weight?
2. Do you gain weight even when you go on a low-calorie diet?
3. Do you constantly battle to lose weight?
4. Do you find it impossible to stay on a diet even when you are determined to succeed?
5. Do you ever have occasions when you binge or overeat?
6. Are there certain foods you just can't stop eating once you start?
7. Do you drink caffeinated beverages?
8. Are you slender but maintaining your weight at the level you want is a constant battle?
9. Do you have a strong craving for certain foods or seasonings?
10. Do you ever feel abnormally hungry, even after you have just eaten?
11. Do you ever skip meals or fast, sometimes just to make up for a dietary indiscretion earlier in the day or because you didn't like what the bathroom scale told you?
12. Do you frequently experiment with one diet or another?
13. Do you smoke or do you live with or work around people who smoke?
14. Do you drink alcoholic beverages?
15. Are you a female? (Yes, due to radical hormone changes every month, we women harbor triggers just being ourselves!)
16. Are you obese or moderately overweight?
17. Do you take appetite suppressants?
18. Does your weight on the scale remain too high even though you exercise a lot and believe you are eating a healthy diet?
19. Are you an exercise dropout?
20. Do you sometimes eat until your stomach feels uncomfortable and bloated?

What's your score? If you answered yes to two or more of these questions, you are vulnerable to weight-gain triggers that are presently preventing you from attaining your weight-loss goals. The good news is that you will soon have in your possession the keys for unlocking the door to a life free of cravings and filled with energy, even as you are dropping the pounds.

A Case in Point

I want to introduce you to Debra, who was a client of mine several years ago. Her story is particularly illustrative since it shows how identifying and eliminating weight-gain triggers can change your life. Her failures at losing weight caused her to suffer low self-esteem. As she eliminated her weight-gain triggers and got down to her ideal weight, her insecurities were transformed into confidence and glowing self-regard. It wasn't just knowing that she looked great that changed her, though, it was having the absolute proof that she had conquered her weight problems and that her past failures were not a character defect but were due to a lack of knowledge. Debra's life was literally transformed as she identified her triggers, erased them from her life, and lost weight. Here's her story:

Although she'd been slightly overweight most of her life, Debra never dieted seriously until high school. Like many teenagers, her idea of dieting was to skip breakfast and lunch, subsisting on diet cola drinks during the day. By dinner time, she was ravenous, however, and to satisfy her appetite she not only ate dinner but also sweets and other junk food.

In spite of what Debra saw as her sincerest efforts to lose weight, she gained it. High school kids being what they are, she was ridiculed about her weight, and to escape humiliation she spent most of her lunch break in the bathroom.

When her efforts to lose weight by skipping meals failed, she turned to diets that were currently popular with young people. One was a high-protein diet. Another was an all-fruit diet. But her weight remained the same, and she felt miserably hungry all the time.

Debra graduated from high school and went on to college. There she gained even more weight, which is not unusual, even for people who have always been thin. In this new setting, Debra went back to her old pattern of skipping meals and drinking diet colas. But it became increasingly difficult to abstain from eating. Students in the dorm were always eating snacks and sharing pizza. And if that wasn't temptation enough, there was a vending machine with tantalizing snacks on every floor.

Soon after graduating from college, she got a job in an insurance firm, where she met Dale. At first he was quite charming, and they were married within a couple months after they met. Then, before a year had passed, her new husband, who was also overweight, started belittling Debra for her weight problem. One would have thought that, being overweight himself, he would have sympathized with her struggles with weight, but this was not the case. What was worse, he usually belittled her in front of other people.

With a sedentary job, and increasing tensions in her marriage, Debra's weight snowballed. In spite of eating like a bird, she was barely able to maintain her weight, much less slim down. When she ate what others would consider a *normal* meal, she gained weight. If she overate at even a single meal, she ballooned.

She came to me seeking a consultation following an incident that occurred on New Year's Eve. Several of Debra's friends planned to attend a dinner dance at the country club, and Debra and her husband were invited to join the party. Wanting to celebrate her first New Year's Eve with her new husband, she bought a flaming red dress, had her hair curled, and even had an extension added. She had never splurged on herself like this before, but it was a special event for her, and she wanted to look beautiful.

The party met at Debra's house before going over to the country club. While her husband played host, fixing their guests drinks, Debra finished getting ready. When at last she came down the stairs to join her guests, all eyes turned to her. Most people though her quite radiant. But her husband, who had already had too much to drink, exclaimed, "Good god, you look like an overcooked bratwurst!" Then, as if to prove that it was all in good fun, he put his arms around her and gave her a peck on the cheek, turning to the others to say, "Isn't she a great sport?"

Debra, of course, was devastated. She had never seen this side of Dale, which apparently came out whenever he drank. In deference to the others, however, she put up a good front so as not to ruin the party.

At dinner, Dale continued to make fat jokes, and the more he drank, the crueler his jokes. He was too insensitive to notice that nobody was laughing. Meanwhile Debra became increasingly withdrawn.

During the evening, Dale refused to take Debra to the dance floor. He loudly proclaimed that he was afraid that she'd step on someone's foot and they'd be sued. Debra burst into tears, excused herself, and went racing off to the bathroom.

Several days later, she told me what happened next. The bathroom had a lounge area that was beautifully decorated. There were chaises and beautiful chairs, scented sachets, flowers, lovely wallpaper, and even a lady attendant.

Debra sat down in one of the chairs, not only hurt by the cruel fat jokes, but stunned to discover this side of her new husband. As she sat down, the leg of the chair broke and she tumbled to the floor in a heap. In the process of getting up, her heel caught in her panty hose, running them badly. As if that wasn't enough, during her fall her hairpiece caught between the chair and the wall and was yanked loose.

At this point her friend Tanya came in to see what was taking Debra so long. She found Debra in tears, totally devastated. Tanya comforted her and helped her put herself back together as best she could. As the two women talked, Tanya, a former patient of mine, told Debra about her work with me. That is how Debra found her way to my office the next day.

I worked with Debra to explore her weight history. By the end of two long interviews, we had identified her key weight-gain triggers. As you read over the following paragraphs about what we discovered, you may recognize one or two of your own triggers. The most important weight gain trigger, however, came as a real surprise to Debra and may come as a surprise to you. (Hint: Just read Trigger #1.)

Trigger #1 *Insufficient Calories*

In her effort to control her weight, Debra had nearly starved herself, consuming only 800 calories a day. The most immediate problem this created was a ravenous appetite and a metabolism ill-equipped to handle the junk food she frequently binged on to quell the dreadful cravings that gnawed at her belly.

Trigger #2 *Malnutrition*

This second trigger is related to the first. Even if you complement an 800-calorie diet with the best vitamin-mineral supplements, you will still be nutrient deficient. The average person needs a minimum of 1400 calories per day and a high-quality vitamin-mineral supplement. Without this, your glucose-starved brain will be scavenging every bit of protein and carbohydrate it can find, and converting these to the precious glucose it needs. As this occurs, it sets off chain reactions within your body that signal you to eat more, to consume calories to replace what your system believes is a crisis in the food supply. For those of you who want to know more about these biological mechanisms, we'll be exploring this trigger in greater depth in later chapters.

Trigger #3 *Lack of Physical Exercise*

Debra had never been physically active, not even as a child. She spent most of her time at work behind a desk, and as tensions escalated at home, she abandoned all her efforts to exercise. As a result, the quality and quantity of her muscles decreased, as did her ability to burn calories, so whatever Debra ate went straight to fat storage.

Trigger #4 *Frequency and Size of Meals*

Debra usually ate one large meal a day. Studies have shown that when you consume most of your calories in a large, single meal each day, your body reacts as if it is facing a famine. Like a hibernating animal anticipating the long winter fast, it takes the opportunity of the large single meal to store extra calories in fat. We may experience this as a ravenous appetite, urging us to eat more, even when we know we are violating all our best intentions to watch our calories.

Trigger #5 Lack of Fiber

Debra complained of being constipated, usually a sure sign among dieters that they are not getting enough fiber in their diets. High fiber is not only necessary for regularity it is important in weight loss. When I explained this to Debra, she became annoyed, insisting that she knew all that and was careful about getting her fiber. Further probing revealed that her idea of "high fiber" in her diet was eating one prune per day. We need twenty to thirty-five grams of fiber from a variety of sources to be healthy.

Trigger #6 Caffeine

Caffeine stimulates the adrenal glands, producing hormones associated with the so-called "fight-or-flight" response. This response gives us an illusion of energy because we have forced stored glucose into service and activated the sympathetic nervous system, which makes us feel more energetic. When glucose is depleted, however, which happens quickly, we feel ravenous and overeat. Debra had been drinking coffee and caffeinated soft drinks all day long. In fact, her consumption of caffeine was equivalent to about eight cups of strong coffee per day.

Trigger #7 Sugary Foods

Whenever she went off her diet, which happened every few days, she craved sugar. To extinguish these cravings, she ate foods such as white bread with jelly, sugared cereals straight from the box, candy-coated popcorn, and Oreo cookies. All of these high-glycemic foods caused her body to produce excess insulin, which lowers blood sugar, causing the rapid depositing of fat. These high insulin levels also made her feel hungry.

Trigger #8 Nutritional and Personal Misconceptions

In our initial interviews, Debra told me she believed she overate because she had low self-esteem. In time, however, she learned differently. She was actually overeating because of the truly formidable triggers in her diet. These triggers destabilized her metabolism, affecting many of her vital processes. Her body had a desperate need for food. Debra's belief that she should be able to control her eating—even with impossible-to-ignore biochemical events such as those we've described above, was a false assumption. It was her body's internal alarm signals that caused her to overeat. Blaming it on her lack of willpower or low self-esteem was a misconception that only compounded her eating problem.

Of course, most overweight people suffer from negative self-talk. In a society that idolizes the anorexic look, as ours does, we can't help but pick up on other people's judgments of us. So Debra viewed herself as not only fat and ugly, but a total failure—a worthless human being—because she was never able to stay on a diet.

When we have a perception of ourselves as a failure, as Debra did, it tends to act as a self-fulfilling prophecy. Even her choices of relationships had mirrored this fact. We indeed fail, or make self-defeating choices, even when we are given the skills, knowledge, and opportunities to be successful. But bear in mind that all these issues can be side effects of weight-gain triggers. To help Debra move past her sense of failure, I prescribed a program of what I call "mental sit-ups." These were mental affirmations that she repeated to herself several times a day, reminding herself that she was not a failure.

The truth was that her weight loss efforts had been laced with the poison of diet-sabotaging triggers that made it virtually impossible for her, or anyone else in her position, to succeed. Now that these triggers were removed, she could not only succeed at losing weight but would also develop a completely positive view of her capacities. Without these affirmations to override false perceptions of herself, Debra would have embarked upon the Right Bite Program convinced that she was a failure and so would have made only a half-hearted attempt, resulting in exactly what she feared: failure. Then she could have said, "See, I told you I couldn't stay on a diet!"

Also, Debra erroneously believed that feeling tired was a sign that her body was burning fat. Unless she felt lousy on a diet, she believed she was not losing weight. She equated feeling energetic with overeating. It was important to have her understand that on this program, she would feel energetic while losing weight. Without this understanding, she would reject the diet, cheat by cutting calories, or lose control and start eating sugary foods that would make her feel the way she was accustomed to feeling—awful! Then the whole cycle of starving herself and having her appetite spiral out of control would start again.

I explained to her that this kind of malaise is caused by low blood sugar. When prolonged, this condition begins to break down muscle tissue—not fat! Nobody could feel good, mentally or physically, under these debilitating circumstances.

It is interesting that after Debra normalized her eating, I once again asked her what she believed caused her to overeat. She replied, unequivocally, "Weight-gain triggers." Her negative self-talk about low self-esteem and being fat and ugly were the symptoms—not the cause!

While Debra would discover other weight-gain triggers in her diet as she worked with me, these eight were the big ones. The food program I prescribed for her was entirely trigger-free, consisting of three regular meals per day, with two or more snacks, and no fewer than 1400 calories. In addition, she took a special vitamin-mineral supplement to make certain that she was getting the nutrients her body required. She was amazed to observe that her food cravings ceased immediately on the Right Bite Program and that she could lose weight so effortlessly.

We added trigger-free physical exercise to her program gradually since this was new to her. Because her husband ridiculed her when she tried to exercise at home, she used her two fifteen-minute coffee breaks to walk around the long hallways in the office building where she worked. In addition, she used thirty minutes of her hour-long lunch break to take a brisk walk. The more she walked, the more she got to enjoy the exercise, until she was finally seeking extra activities, such as bowling with friends once a week. She later joined a health club.

By eating three trigger-free meals plus two or more trigger-free snacks a day, she keeps her blood sugar levels stable, prevents hunger, and controls weight. She has stopped drinking caffeinated beverages entirely, which was difficult for her at first. She tested caffeine many times before she was absolutely convinced that it triggered hunger pangs for her that too often caused her to binge.

As her eating patterns smoothed out, she found that she no longer craved sugary foods. Although she occasionally missed these treats, she weighed the satisfaction of "just one cookie" against how much better she felt now that she had her weight down and her diet under control. Given the benefits of this new way of life, saying no to sweets came easily.

The more progress she made with losing weight, the more Debra recognized that she truly could control how she ate. Her achievement empowered her in ways she had never before experienced. The ongoing program built on her rising self-esteem through mental calisthenics that provided positive self-talk.

Debra checked in with me on a regular basis until she had gotten her weight down to a svelte 130 pounds. She had lost 41 pounds and was absolutely delighted not only with how she looked but with how she felt. She had more energy than she'd ever had in her life. She wore clothes she had always dreamed of wearing but never could because of her weight. She thoroughly enjoyed regular workouts at the gym, and the walks during her coffee breaks and lunch hour not only helped her keep off the weight but also gave her a chance to unwind from the pressures of her job.

About six months after she stopped working with me, Debra surprised me with a phone call. "I have just lost an additional 250 pounds of ugly fat!" she exclaimed. I was speechless. What could she mean by that? And then she filled me in: She had divorced Dale. Though I ordinarily avoid commenting on my clients' domestic problems, this time I remembered how cruel Dale had been about Debra's weight. My words of congratulations were out of my mouth before I could stop myself.

Triggering Success Instead of Weight Gain

Although specific details vary, Debra's story is not at all unusual. It illustrates how weight-gain triggers can dramatically sabotage our best efforts to lose weight, even when we are nearly starving ourselves. Her story reveals the hidden health hazards of improper dieting and how it is frequently the very thing we do to lose weight that puts it on.

We also see from Debra's story how our weight and our well-being are not just about the food we put in our stomachs but also about the thoughts and feelings we put in our minds. Weight-gain triggers come in many different forms, and the more you learn about them, the more this knowledge will enable you to change your life, just as Debra did hers.

In the coming chapters, you will discover how to identify your own unique triggers, how to eliminate them, how to exercise, and even how to change your thinking to eliminate the weight-gain triggers that up to now have been undermining your will and your finest efforts to manage your weight. This scientifically proven program will help you quickly and comfortably achieve permanent control of all the factors that cause you to gain weight. By tailoring the plan to your own unique metabolism, you'll find out how easy it is to enjoy vibrant health while maintaining exactly the weight you want.

Of course, if you are going to lose weight and keep it off, you do have to think about calories. But calorie counters beware! What was once thought to be the single incontestable truth about dieting—that we have to consume fewer calories—may well be the most destructive trigger of all. I'll tell you why and what you can do about it in the next chapter.

Chapter Two

Enemy #1—
Insufficient Calories

*If we mammals don't get something to eat every
day or two, our temperature drops, all our vital signs
fall off, and we begin to starve. Living at biological red alert,
it's not surprising how obsessed we are with food; I'm just
amazed we don't pace and fret about it all the time.*
—Diane Ackerman

If you get nothing else from reading this book, I would hope and pray
that you get this message: TOO FEW CALORIES—NOT TOO
MANY—may well be the most important weight-gain trigger in your
life! Millions of people the world over unnecessarily starve themselves
to lose weight, and in the long term the only thing they gain is more
weight. If you are one of these people, stop.

"Now that's a switch!" you are probably saying. "How can you, a professional nutrition expert, tell dieters that one of our biggest problems
could be that we are consuming too few calories? It doesn't make sense.
Surely you know that extra calories turn into fat!"

Yes, of course. I do know that any calories you don't burn in your
daily activities are going to turn into fat. But too few calories can create
a metabolism that encourages obesity and resists the burning of fat. The
problems that too few calories can create are so extensive that I make
this issue Enemy #1 on my weight-gain trigger list. One of my clients

even suggested that we call it the "T-rex" of weight-gain triggers. I like that image!

This tyrannosaurus of triggers claws its way, tooth and nail, into almost every weight-loss diet I have ever researched. However, eliminating it from our lives is far easier than you might imagine, so there is no reason why you ever have to starve yourself again. Your liberation from this T-rex of weight-gain triggers starts with knowing that it affects several key metabolic systems in your body.

The bottom line? In the long run, if you drastically cut calories, sooner or later you will overeat, while simultaneously initiating internal changes that will make and keep you fat. Stop your little dance with T-rex, and you will also free yourself of the fat person's metabolism that this dietary practice has imposed on you, and you'll shift instead to a thin person's metabolism to lose weight and keep it off.

To understand what happens when you cut back on calories to lose weight, here's what you have to deal with: The human body contains a complex system for monitoring itself and making all kinds of adjustments to stay healthy. One of these systems is the body's inherent ability to regulate calories. When you go without food for a period of days or you radically reduce your caloric intake to far less than you are burning in your daily activities, your body notices this. Boy, does it notice! It decides that you are starving and throws the panic switch. All the built-in systems that are designed to protect your health when you are faced with starvation go into action. Your body doesn't realize that you have plenty of food stashed in the pantry and that you have a supermarket nearby where you can buy whatever food you want or need. The end result is that your body decides that you must be living in the midst of a famine, so it puts out the order to start squirreling away any sources of energy it can find, and of course this is stored as fat. Your body is very good at doing this, and it certainly doesn't check out your pantry and refrigerator before doing what it believes it must do to keep you from starving to death.

How do you know if you are cutting calories to the point that your body has gone into this save-everything mode? There's a pretty good chance that you can pick up the clues from how you are feeling physically, from your mood, and from reactions that you are getting from the people around you. If you've ever been on a very low-calorie diet, you and the people around you probably noticed mood swings. Maybe you get downright out of sorts, jittery, or irritable, or walk around with a sense of free-floating anxiety.

That vague or not-so-vague physical discomfort and anxiety you experience during such times is not just in your head. It is biochemical. Your body is warning you that something is wrong, and it will flip the panic button and set all survival systems into action if you deprive it of its basic nutritional requirements.

The good news is that you have a choice. You can choose to promise your body that you will never starve it again for as long as you live. Eliminating this single trigger means no more skipping meals, fasting, or wiring your jaw shut so that you won't eat. And it means knowing that one of the best ways to lose weight, if you have been drastically slashing calories and are still overweight, is to moderately increase your intake of calories so that your body can function optimally.

Here's another nutritional tip that can help free you once and for all from this weight-gain trigger: One of your body's first orders of business is to obtain crucial calories to feed your brain. If it doesn't feel it has enough available calories for that, it will make the assumption that you have absolutely lost every last speck of good sense that you ever possessed, and it will try its best to compel you to overeat or binge. And the chances are that when nobody is looking—and you can catch your better self off guard—you're going to do just that!

So what happens if you bite the bullet, exert superhuman will, and continue to starve yourself? Your body will start transforming itself into an ever more efficient fat-storing machine.

At this point, at least seven physiological processes swing into action. The message goes streaming out to every cell in your body: *Waste nothing! Turn everything that even resembles food into fat! If you don't need it right now, store it.*

What are you creating here? I'll tell you what you're creating. You are becoming an organism that is extremely good at storing fat and at resisting the burning of it. As in the quote by Diane Ackerman at the beginning of this chapter, your body has started *"living at biological red alert."*

But why put yourself through all that when it is so unnecessary for achieving your ultimate goal—control of your weight.

The T-Rex Complex

The idea that eating too little can make you fat challenges the stereotypes about weight-loss. So, it's important to understand how and why this could be. What is it that happens in our bodies to make this possible? There are seven key factors to consider when you undereat. These are:

1. Blood sugar levels.
2. Serotonin levels.
3. Muscle protein.
4. Metabolic rate.
5. Lipoprotein lipase.
6. Malnutrition or borderline malnutrition.
7. Poststarvation hyperphagia.

Each of the above items involves a different set of functions within your body, and each one operates in a different way. The following pages explain all you need to know about them to strike the perfect balance between too few and too many calories.

1. Low Blood Sugar

Most people first notice low blood sugar as mental and physical symptoms, with varying degrees of severity. For example, you might feel mild hunger that increases in intensity as food is withheld, causing a further drop in blood sugar levels. Then you might feel a little disoriented—lethargic, depressed or just *out of it*. After a while, you might start acting erratically, or feeling emotionally upset at small things. You might feel shaky, dizzy, headachy, or confused. You might be surprised to learn that insomnia can be a symptom of low blood sugar. Along with these symptoms, you will usually experience an intense craving for sweets and carbohydrates.

What's happening is this: Your body's top priority is to meet its vital energy needs. When you eat, your body converts the natural sugars in your food to *glucose* (blood sugar), which circulates throughout your blood stream, carrying this immediately available *fuel* to your brain and to muscle cells in your vital organs and musculoskeletal system. Any glucose that you don't use immediately is stored in your liver and muscle cells as *glycogen*, and any excess is stored in fat cells. Between meals, only glycogen from your liver—and not from the muscles—replenishes the glucose in your blood, while your brain cells, and other cells, keep drawing from it to meet their own energy needs.

Now, the problem is that ordinarily your brain and nervous system can only make use of blood glucose that you get either from the food you eat or that your liver has made available. In fact, your brain is quite a glucose hog. When you are not exercising or doing any kind of physical labor, your brain, which weighs less than two pounds, uses two-thirds of your circulating glucose supply. Whatever is left over after that, your muscles can scoop up for their use. Your muscle cells store their own glycogen, but they are not much into sharing, hoarding most of it for themselves. When your blood sugar drops as the result of dieting, or between meals, your muscles draw upon the glycogen reserves in their own cells and from fat cells for energy. Meanwhile, your brain and nervous system are gobbling up whatever glucose your liver has available.

Before long, you've simply drained whatever stores of glycogen you may have had in your liver. Ordinarily, you would be able to boost the available blood sugar by eating something—preferably some carbohydrates. But if you are being a really determined dieter, that's not going to happen. Your body—muscles, organs, nervous system, and brain—is by now running on empty.

You will experience this glucose deficiency as low blood sugar, which is characterized by intense cravings for sweets. Your body will demand that you eat. Unless you happen to be a devout masochist, there's an awfully good chance that you are going to cry uncle and give in to your cravings. That's when you abandon all of your best intentions and dive into the chocolate chip cookies. Binge time!

As soon as you turn to the sweets, your blood glucose rapidly rises. This stimulates the islets of Langerhans, which are the insulin-producing parts of your pancreas, releasing insulin into your blood stream. The insulin then goes to work, stimulating the uptake of glucose into your cells and storing glycogen in your liver and muscles. The insulin also helps to convert any excess glucose into fat and store it away on your body. And believe me, if you are a person who has ever binged on sugary foods after experiencing low blood sugar, you have plenty of excess sugar calories to store!

It's easy to understand why diets with insufficient calories are so often abandoned. You are hungry all the time because your body is suffering from low blood sugar. Every dieter should learn to recognize the symptoms of low blood sugar for what they are. They are potent reminders that your diet is dangerously low in calories. If prolonged, low blood sugar can result in serious damage to the body and nervous system, which you will understand momentarily.

2. DECREASED SEROTONIN LEVELS

Serotonin is an important brain chemical, a hormone that normally produces a sense of well-being during our waking hours. It is one of the brain's neurotransmitters. Its presence in our brain affects our mood, food cravings, sensations, and ability to sleep. Reduced levels of serotonin have been shown to produce a lowered tolerance for pain. Diminished concentrations can also result in our feeling depressed, which in turn triggers a craving for carbohydrates. Ironically, to do its job well serotonin must have carbohydrates—foods that most diets restrict.

To produce this serotonin, there have to be ample carbohydrates in your diet, along with some protein. When you go into starvation mode, your body is not receiving enough of the proper nutrients to make serotonin. As you might guess, serotonin production plummets—and naturally, so does your sense of well-being!

Research has shown that as serotonin levels decline, its depletion creates *carbohydrate hunger*, even in those who suffer no depression. You begin to crave sweets, the very foods you are trying to avoid! These cravings can become so intense that they ravage the efforts of even the most disciplined dieters. If you have ever found yourself binging maniacally after a couple days on a low-calorie diet, don't blame it on your lack of will. Blame it on the carbohydrate hunger and the depletion of serotonin in your system. Blame it on this T-rex of weight-gain triggers.

3. MUSCLE PROTEIN

We've already discussed the importance of glucose in your body—the fuel that keeps the engines running. When you are severely restricting calories, it becomes your body's top priority to distribute its fuel sources to the areas that most need them. Remember that a third of your body's available glycogen reserves are in your liver, but these are limited to about 1200 to 1800 calories and will be depleted in several hours, depending on your level of activity.

Once the glycogen reserves of your liver run out, your body starts turning to its other sources of fuel. This is your body's dilemma at this point: Does it let your brain cells die for lack of glucose or does it start calling upon your lean body mass to make sacrifices to save those aforementioned cells? To safeguard your brain from sugar shortage you body begins to cannibalize its own body protein for making new blood glucose. So next time you're on a diet, feeling out-of-sorts, and somebody asks what's eating you, you can honestly tell them it's yourself!

When glycogen stores are severely depleted your body can also find a way to use fat as fuel for your brain. It does this through a series of chemical events whose end result is an alternate source of energy known as "ketone bodies." Normally produced and used in only small quantities, ketones can be used by some, but not all, brain cells. Many areas of the brain continue to rely exclusively on glucose, so your body protein continues to be sacrificed for that purpose. To extract this glucose, the entire protein molecule has to be pulled apart. The result? Muscle cells are destroyed and your muscle masses begin to shrink.

While your body is shifting to the use of ketone bodies for energy, it will simultaneously reduce its energy output, trying to conserve both its fat and lean tissue. As the lean (protein containing) organ tissues shrink in mass, they perform less metabolic work, reducing energy expenditures. As your muscles waste away, they do less work and demand less energy, reducing expenditures even further. Hormones released at this time also slow down your metabolism in an effort to conserve your lean body mass as long as possible. Because of the slow metabolism, fat loss falls to a bare minimum—less in fact than would be lost on a moderately low calorie diet.

"What's the big deal?" you might ask. "Does it matter if my muscles get smaller?"

If you do anything physical in your life—and this can include activities as ordinary as running to catch the bus or shopping at the supermarket—it matters very much. You simply can't perform well without healthy muscles. But in terms of weight-loss, there's another consideration: As your body starts breaking down muscle protein, you are losing lean body mass, which burns more calories than fat cells do. So the more muscle tissue you lose, the fewer calories you burn, and the more calories you will store as fat. That's when the pounds start accumulating—in spite of the fact that you are barely eating anything. Even if you manage to lose a little weight while radically reducing calories, your fat loss will slow down or even stop so that whatever weight you do lose will be predominantly your lean body mass—muscle!

If your main purpose for dieting is to lose unwanted fat, embarking on a very low-calorie diet is not going to produce the long-term results you want. In fact, it will produce just the opposite. Your fat loss will dwindle, your fat stores will increase, your cravings will increase, and healthy, calorie-burning muscle tissue will be compromised or just plain destroyed.

4. METABOLIC RATE

Keep in mind that your body doesn't know the difference between starvation and a deliberate choice to cut back on calories for the purpose of losing weight. As soon as you start eating a great deal less than you regularly do, your body will respond by going into its conservation mode, doing everything it can to forestall the time when it will have to start cannibalizing its lean body mass for glucose. This manner of operating includes a slower metabolic rate, temporarily reducing the rate at which your body burns calories and fat. Not only will you find it increasingly difficult to lose body fat on a very low-cal diet, your body fat will increase more rapidly than ever when you go back to eating normally.

While this automatic metabolic adjustment is a life-saving response in the normal course of our lives, it triggers a vicious cycle for the dieter. For the moment, suppose that sticking to this low-cal diet just becomes too much for you. And let's say you finally give up the struggle and go back to eating normally. Bear in mind that, even if you begin eating as you ordinarily would, your body is still in starvation mode with a sluggish metabolism. Because you've triggered its survival mechanisms with the low-cal diet, your body interprets your more normal eating pattern as excessive. Since your body is still reacting as though it were in the midst of a famine, it won't burn as many calories as you are taking in. Your shrunken muscle cells can't use the stuff. And your slowed metabolism is overwhelmed. So now you have created the perfect climate for weight gain. What's a body to do but convert these extra calories into fat? What's going to happen next? You can probably guess. Good sense, the bathroom scale, and the fact that you can't get your jeans on, all tell you that you need to cut back on your food intake. So you ease back into your diet again. Seems logical enough, doesn't it? Maybe to you it does, but your body is following a very different logic. Pretty soon it can't figure out what the heck you are doing! You get heavier and heavier even as you limit your caloric intake more and more. At this point, it is safe to say that you have lost control—even when you are heroically trying to stick to your low-cal diet.

Unfortunately, T-rex has not yet finished with his dirty work. There's more to come. Having once begun the process of breaking down available protein in muscle cells to make glucose for the brain and slowing your metabolism further, your body will begin to feel the effects of protein deficiency. Under normal circumstances, proteins from meat, eggs, dairy products, and legumes are used for growth and repair. If protein isn't available for this purpose, these important jobs fail to get done. Well, on a severely low-cal diet your body converts most food to energy to fuel your brain, and will do so even with protein foods. Even if you go on a high protein diet, your body will grab those protein molecules, convert them to glucose, and feed them to your brain cells first. Reparation and growth take a back seat to your hungry brain cells' needs. Obviously, the longer you stay on a very low-cal diet the longer your body will put off the job of reparation and growth.

Let's assume that you carry this very low-cal regime to extremes. Here's what will eventually happen: As your brain utilizes protein to make glucose, you may very well notice significant changes in your health. For example, you may notice that you are more prone to infection and that you have difficulty recovering from even minor illnesses. Your hair and skin may begin to look dull and dry, taking on an unhealthy appearance. Maybe your face starts to look drawn, with circles under your eyes. This is a worst-case scenario, of course, but if you have ever seen photos of people who were starving, you will have seen all of these symptoms in the extreme. In my work, I have seen people suffering all of the effects of protein deficiency, some of which have even been life-threatening.

Protein deprivation of the kind that we experience on low-calorie diets can also affect our mental capacities since brain chemistry has been disturbed. You would experience this as mental problems such as depression, emotional instability, and lack of concentration. These symptoms go away within hours or days as you start eating in a more balanced way.

5. LIPOPROTEIN LIPASE

Have you ever wondered how, in just a few days, you can gain back all the weight it took you weeks or even months to lose? Blame it on the complex alchemy of a few hundred thousand years of evolution on this planet and the human body's capacity for surviving famines. To be more specific, blame it on an enzyme called "lipoprotein lipase."

The role of this enzyme is to pluck fat from any food sources it can and store it away in fat cells. Lipoprotein lipase is like the squirrels of the forest, gathering nuts and burying them in secret places as insurance against droughts or a long winter. In the case of the dieter, your lipoprotein lipase is anticipating the long winter of your next low-cal diet siege.

Every time you drastically undereat, you are triggering the increased production of these enzymes. You actually encourage their proliferation. They can, in fact, become so bounteous that practically everything you eat turns to fat! Over the years, I have worked with people who complained that they would regain in one or two moderate meals all the weight they had lost in six months of rigid dieting. It is a heartbreaking, frustrating, and morale-destroying experience, leading more than one dieter to draw the conclusion that achieving their ideal weight was impossible.

Just so we don't end on a despairing note, I want to assure you that the program I describe in this book does address this problem. What's more, dieters who follow my program will regain control and achieve their ideal weights.

6. MALNUTRITION AND MARGINAL MALNUTRITION

When we think of "malnutrition," many of us will recall a poignant photo of a starved child with skinny legs and a bloated belly, staring out at us from a CARE fund raising poster. But malnutrition isn't limited to victims of drought and famine. As a nutritional consultant, I've found it in a surprising number of people with weight disorders, particularly with those who are caught up in the out-of-control cycles triggered by very low-calorie diets.

Gross malnutrition is rare among dieters but *marginal malnutrition* is far more prevalent than you might imagine. The latter refers to a deficiency in nutrients or an imbalance of the same. Laboratory tests and obvious clinical symptoms make gross malnutrition easy to detect. However, the person with marginal malnutrition is harder to recognize. They may feel *OK* but *not totally up to par*, while routine blood tests fail to reveal any alarming abnormalities.

Most dieters I encounter in my practice are marginally malnourished. They may complain of being listless or depressed and anxious. They may find it difficult to perform mental tasks that once were easy for them. They might be having a difficult time recovering from a cold, the flu, or some other illness that they ordinarily get over quickly. Perhaps they find it difficult to concentrate for long periods of time, or they feel distracted and slightly disoriented. And they may confess to me that a spouse or other family member has told them they are being "too emotional" or "forgetful." Fatigue, apathy, depression, malaise, hormonal imbalances, and water retention plague the dieter with marginal malnutrition. Water retention is particularly hazardous because it is easy to interpret it as weight gain, triggering a more ardent effort to lose weight, which only compounds the problem.

One of the most frequently overlooked deficits for marginally malnourished dieters is iron deficiency, which, if prolonged, leads to a condition characterized by small, pale, red blood cells, which most of us know as anemia. However, we can feel the serious effects of iron depletion long before it can be diagnosed as anemia. The symptoms of mild iron deficiency include irritability, fatigue, weakness, pallor, and heart palpitations.

Although there are no standard laboratory values to define marginal malnutrition, I am convinced that it is one of the most insidious and underrecognized health problems that dieters face. When people begin eating nutritious diets and they get their weight under control, malnutrition symptoms disappear. Energy levels return to normal. Mental concentration increases. Peoples' emotional lives become more balanced. Sleep and exercise patterns even out, and they begin to enjoy a sense of well-being they hadn't experienced since they first started dieting.

If you are on a diet that contains insufficient calories, you will become marginally malnourished even if you take a vitamin-mineral supplement. One reason for this is that your system will have difficulty assimilating what it needs to stay healthy. In addition, no supplement contains all the vitamins and minerals we need. Food also contains thousands of phytochemicals, compounds in plant-derived foods that make important biological contributions to our health and well-being. These phytochemicals are neither vitamins nor minerals but are absolutely essential. Nor can we get essential amounts of calories in the form of protein, carbohydrates, and fats from vitamin-mineral supplements. This is why it is so important to eat ample amounts of nutritious foods as well as taking supplements.

Any low-calorie dieter taking medication, whether over-the-counter or prescription drugs, and any such dieter who has an illness, should be particularly alert to the problems of marginal malnutrition. Many medications disrupt your body's capacity to absorb sufficient nutrients, and illness can inhibit the absorption capacity as well. Always be aware that this combination of being sick, being on medication, and being on a diet can be catastrophic. You may have already had the experience of getting a series of illnesses, of infections escalating, or of getting increasingly depressed or low at such times.

When we are on diets with insufficient calories and insufficient nutrients, the compulsion to overeat and binge becomes a gargantuan trigger. You'd need the fortitude of a knight to slay this dragon! And after following the diet, when you've finally determined that you've either lost enough or *had* enough, you're going to need to consume two to three times the calories of a well-nourished person to get healthy again. Your body's cravings to satisfy nutritional needs your head can't always identify will promote appetites that will inevitably undo all you've sacrificed to achieve.

7. POSTSTARVATION HYPERPHAGIA

After you've spent a number of weeks on a diet with insufficient calories, you are going to discover a little demon within you. That demon comes in the form of biochemical changes in your body that scream at you, "Eat! Eat! Eat!" Remember, your body thinks you were cutting back on your food because you were faced with a famine. It doesn't know about the diets you imposed on yourself in the name of a trim figure.

Following the dictates of survivalist tactics that have ensured human survival for these thousands of years, your body is going to urgently insist that you eat to replace all the fat stores and lean body mass you lost during what it still believes was a period of starvation. This phenomenon is known as poststarvation hyperphagia.

The term *poststarvation hyperphagia* refers to the extreme sensation of hunger we experience after a period of starving our bodies. As I described earlier in this chapter, you can experience similar sensations at the end of a day when you have gone without breakfast and lunch. But now we are talking about what it's like to maintain a starvation diet over a period of many days or weeks with no reprieve, no binging or days off the diet to eat in a more balanced way. If the hunger pangs you felt during the day was a 3 on a scale of 10, we are now be talking about hunger pangs rated at a 10.

Unlike our natural mealtime desire for food, hyperphagia's hot, gnawing sensations of hunger unleash appetites that are virtually impossible to ignore. *Poststarvation hyperphagia* can last from a few days up to many weeks.

Poststarvation hyperphagia is based on the body's four biochemical perceptions:

1. Its glycogen reserves were depleted for a prolonged period of time.
2. Its serotonin levels were in short supply.

3. It had to break down muscle proteins to fuel the brain.
4. It had to slow your metabolic rates to a minimum to conserve the small energy supplies that were available. It quickly increased the production of lipoprotein lipase—and those higher levels are still being maintained—in order to store whatever fats come through the system.

All of these contribute to the symptoms of hunger that you experience during and even after you've stopped dieting and you have started eating normally.

There's plenty of solid research in the medical journals showing that the more fat and lean tissue we lose during a diet, the greater will be our craving for food to replace it. It is a rare person who fails to answer this call. Sadly, however, even after your biochemistry normalizes, you don't end up with the same weight you were before you dieted—you weigh more. Here's why:

✓ Our bodies store fat first, and they store it more quickly and easily than they restore lean body mass. This means that even after you've responded to the poststarvation hyperphagic instincts that are triggered by the diet, your body continues to overload with excess fat during the slower rebuilding of its lean body protein.

✓ Thermogenesis: During weight loss, your body burns less energy. That reduction in the use of energy continues through the postdieting, hyperphagic period. Your body burns fewer calories to assist and accelerate the process of restoring fat to your body.

As unfair as it may seem to you as a person trying to lose weight, keep in mind that these weight-gain triggers are based on survival instincts that are intended to save your life. Given the history of our planet and human migration patterns, none of us would have survived this long without these inborn drives. Remember the history of the Donner party during the migration to California in 1846. Trapped in a Sierra snowstorm, their food provisions soon ran out. Already exhausted and gaunt from their long trek across the continent, fellow members began to die at an alarming rate. The story was made famous because at one point, driven by their own desire to survive, some members decided to eat the flesh of some of those who had died. In the end, only the members who had higher levels of body fat survived; those with lower levels of body fat perished.

It All Comes Down to This

As simple as it might look on the surface, severe calorie slashing never lets you lose pounds and afterwards maintain a healthy weight. On the contrary, this T-rex of triggers will eventually carry you further and further down the path to being chronically overweight—ounce by agonizing ounce.

Now that you understand all this, and hopefully have vowed never to starve yourself again in the name of losing a few pounds, it's time to take a close look at how The Right Bite Program can help you. This program was designed with a deep understanding of what happens when a person goes on a calorie-deficient diet, and what becomes necessary to get back on track with a nutritional program that is both healthy and slimming. The program allows you to:

✓ Lose pounds while eating at a high-calorie level;

✓ Maintain liver glycogen reserves, thereby stabilizing blood sugar levels;

✓ Maintain adequate levels of serotonin in the brain;

✓ Lose only unwanted fat as you build lean muscle tissue;

✓ Increase your body's metabolic rate, thus burning more calories than ever before;

✓ Reduce levels of lipoprotein lipase, nature's fat depositer;

✓ Eliminate uncomfortable mental and emotional symptoms that accompany low-cal diets;

✓ Lose weight without having to fight a T-rex hunger campaign.

As you move forward to eliminate this weight-gain trigger from your life, using the Right Bite Program, take a moment to reflect on this: We all regret certain things we have done in the past, and starving yourself might be one of them. But whatever you do, don't blame yourself for not being able to reach and maintain your dieting goals through starvation types of diets. Succeeding with such programs never was a matter of your having enough willpower. If you have been trying to make these diets work for you, realize that it is your body's own natural drive for survival that you must work with. As soon as you learn to complement and cooperate with your natural drive, your extra pounds will fall away, you'll feel better than you have felt in years, and you will be able to maintain your ideal weight. Stop fighting with the healthy survival systems that your body has evolved since the dawn of time. It's not a battle you can or even *should* win.

The good news is that your body's survival mechanisms ultimately become valuable assets in your quest for the perfect weight. Through the Right Bite Program, you can lose weight comfortably and safely. You can do so even though you have disrupted your body chemistry with low-cal diets. In fact, through the Right Bite Program you'll repair the damage that past diets have inflicted and reestablish your optimal capacity for easily burning fat—in the healthy way that nature has always intended.

Chapter Three

The Seven Deadly Sins, Plus Four

Fake food—I mean those patented substances
chemically flavored and mechanically bulked out to kill
the appetite and deceive the gut—is unnatural, almost
immoral, a bane to good eating and good cooking.
—Julia Child

Some weight-gain triggers sneak up on us. They can seem harmless at first. But they move in swiftly, annihilating any progress we might have made in stabilizing our diets. These triggers are easy to overlook or underrate but, by knowing what they are ahead of time, you can catch them long before they inflict their damage. Your best defense where they are concerned is a good offense, liberating yourself from their influence even before they can affect you. That's what this chapter is about—exposing the eleven most deadly triggers so that you can eliminate them from your life forever.

DT(Deadly Trigger) Number One:
The Empty Swallow—Insufficient Nutrients

When I was in graduate school, longer ago than I like to remember, one of our classroom lectures began with the teacher encouraging us to share dieting horror stories. One story in particular sticks in my mind: Beth, who was about twenty pounds overweight, raised her hand. Considering herself knowledgeable about nutrition, she had designed her own diet about five years before. It consisted of nothing but eating huge amounts of broccoli, which is considered one of the most nutritious vegetables we can eat. Beth's weight loss was spectacular the first week, but she said she started feeling weaker and weaker. She also felt depressed and had difficulty concentrating. During the eighth week of her diet she woke up and found most of her hair on her pillow, caused by the absence of protein in her diet. She leapt from bed, ran to her mirror and found to her horror that she was almost entirely bald. Needless to say, her exclusively broccoli diet ended that day, and as she added more nutritious foods her hair began growing back.

No matter how healthy a single food may be, you'll reap its greatest nutritional value when you combine it with others in ample quantities. In fact, a nutritious diet must have five characteristics:

✓ The foods must be adequate, that is, they must provide sufficient quantities of all the essential vitamins, minerals, and energy-yielding nutrients, plus fiber necessary for maintaining health and body weight.

✓ The diet must be balanced, that is, one nutrient must not be overemphasized to the exclusion or expense of another. For example, although most fruits are rich in vitamin C, they are not good sources of B vitamins and protein. Since our bodies need a wide variety of nutrients, it would be a mistake to limit your choices to foods that only contained a few of the necessary nutrients.

✓ Foods must be nutrient dense and calorie sparse. That is, they must deliver the most nutrients for the fewest calories.

✓ The foods must not provide excess fat, salt, sugar, or other unwanted items. This doesn't mean that you have to totally avoid these foods but that you definitely practice moderation with them.

✓ The foods chosen must provide a variety of tastes, textures, and eating experiences. If you stick to the same selection of foods day after day, you are probably going to feel bored very soon and start eyeing foods that excite your taste buds.

For optimal health and to best control your weight, your body requires six classes of *nutrients*—carbohydrates, proteins, fats, vitamins, minerals, and water. These food components are essential for your body to function. The forty-odd nutrients scattered throughout these six classes have many functions that range from providing energy to serving as building material, to maintaining or repairing the body, to supporting growth. By understanding the roles they play in your life you'll be able to make food choices that provide you with maximum vital energy and nutrients without weight gain.

Carbohydrates and fats are the most important energy-yielding nutrients. Although protein can yield energy when the other nutrients are deficient, its major use is to provide materials that form structures and working parts of body tissues.

Vitamins and minerals provide no energy. All vitamins and minerals act as regulators—that is, they are substances that assist in all body processes, from digesting food to building new cells to fighting infection to healing wounds.

Water, the sixth nutrient is especially important because it is constantly lost from our body and must be constantly replaced. I will discuss water further later.

Some of our nutrients, called "essential nutrients," must be obtained from food if we're to avoid deficiencies such as the ones Beth encountered on her all-broccoli diet. Essential nutrients are found in all six classes of nutrients.

Here's an important fact to remember when thinking about any diet: No matter how advanced the study of human nutrition may be, scientists have never been able to concoct a formula diet or supplement that provides the perfect balance of nutrients to support optimal growth and health. Also, there is no food that in and of itself is perfect, that provides everything we need to stay healthy. Foods are chemically complex, giving us much more than nutrients. The potato, for example, contains more than 100 known compounds. For this reason, it is easy to understand how important it is to satisfy the five requirements of a nutritious diet. Eating just one food, even if you take a multiple-vitamin-mineral supplement, can be a dietary disaster.

What happens when we are deficient in any of the nutrients? Although the information available about each nutrient could fill a set of encyclopedias, I will focus mainly on the symptoms of nutrient deficiencies that affect your ability to control your weight and appetite. I'll also focus on major nutrient deficiencies that affect you psychologically since these are deficiencies that act as triggers.

THE IMPORTANCE OF CARBOHYDRATES

Carbohydrates have two major functions: (1) they provide our bodies with energy and (2) they spare our bodies' protein from being broken down and used for energy. In fact, carbohydrates provide us with the main "fuel" that allows us to function.

Carbohydrates are present in all plant foods and in only one food taken from animals—milk, which contains milk sugar, known as lactose. Our bodies will convert carbohydrates, regardless of where they come from or how complex they are, into "blood sugar," which is properly termed "glucose." Every cell in your body depends on glucose, and under normal circumstances the cells of your brain and nervous system depend solely on glucose.

It is particularly important that your diet be sufficient in carbohydrates. Why? Because while your reserves of body fat can be utilized to fuel your muscle cells, as well as internal organs, they can never be converted to glucose to feed your brain adequately. Maintaining a healthy intake of carbohydrates is your insurance against many weight-gain triggers. When your body is suffering from a carbohydrate deficit, it is forced to turn to protein reserves and convert them to glucose, thus diverting protein from critically important functions. The role of protein is so vital in our bodies that we cannot afford to shortchange ourselves on it. We can protect our protein by having adequate carbohydrates available at all times, ensuring that we don't have to turn to our protein for energy.

Also, believe it or nor, to efficiently burn body fat you need adequate carbohydrates. Without carbohydrates, your body goes into "ketosis," which, by the way, is a state recommended in high-protein diets. When your body goes into ketosis, unusual byproducts created by the breakdown of less efficient burning of fats start accumulating in your blood. While we don't know all the side effects of these byproducts, we do know that ketosis must be avoided during pregnancy because it has been shown to cause irreversible brain damage in the unborn child. We can speculate that if ketosis produces a state in the mother's body that is detrimental to the unborn child's development, it may have similarly negative effects on our own bodies that have yet to be determined.

Let's talk more about ketosis since it ultimately involves weight-gain triggers. You may recall our discussion from Chapter 2, that not only does your body break down protein to feed your brain, but it also finds a way to use its stored fat to fuel your nervous system. It combines acetyl CoA fragments, derived from fatty acids, to produce ketone bodies that in turn fuel some, but not all, of your brain cells. Within this long chain of biochemical events, body protein is continually sacrificed to produce glucose to keep your brain and nervous system functioning properly.

In the past few years, thousands of people have been attracted to high-protein, low-carbohydrate diets because they result in dramatic weight loss. No matter how much protein you eat on these diets, protein is still taken from body tissue—and that means sacrificing lean body tissue, which itself reduces your ability to burn fat. Yes, you might be able to boast that you've just lost eight pounds in two days on your high-protein diet, but here's the downside: at best you have lost a single pound of fat, while losing six to seven pounds of lean body tissue, water, and minerals. So what happens when you go back to eating a more balanced diet? Anyone who has been through this routine knows the answer only too well. Your body will gobble up and retain the nutrients that it now finds in the carbohydrates, and you will zoom back to the weight you were before you went on this diet. And if that's not a weight-gain trigger I don't know what is.

One client, Victor, came to me for dietary counseling after his cardiologist advised him to stop his high-protein diet and eat in a more balanced way. Three months after going back on a nutritious diet, Victor had ballooned up to twelve pounds more than he weighed when he started the high-protein diet. This in spite of the fact that he was eating reasonable helpings and staying away from deserts and greasy foods. His physician had become alarmed but after putting him through many expensive medical tests could find nothing wrong, and so Victor had ended up in my office, seeking answers.

To understand how and why diets that are low or devoid of carbohydrates end up being weight-gain triggers, consider for a moment how your body obtains energy from the food you eat. Remember that in order to move your muscles you need to burn a combination of fat and glucose. Covert Bailey uses the metaphor of a fire to make this point. He asks us to imagine that the body is a fireplace in which you are attempting to build a fire. Toss in a nice big oak log, then hold a match under it. Nothing happens except that the match burns down and goes out. But if you put some crumpled up newspaper and some nice dry kindling under the log, then set a match to it, you soon have the log burning nicely and the room warming up.

In the biochemistry of your body, glucose is like the crumpled newspaper and dry kindling in our analogy. Fat is like the log. It won't burn unless you light a smaller fire—glucose—under it first. When your muscle cells can't get glucose to fuel them, they'll turn to body fat for energy. The trouble is that in the absence of glucose your muscle cells do a poor job of burning the fat. In the process they put out a lot of half-burned waste products known as "ketones." To use another analogy, ketones might be compared to the smoke given off by a smoldering fire; just as smoke goes up the chimney, ketones go out in the urine. One popular high-protein diet claims that ketones in the urine indicate that lots of fat is burning up. Covert Bailey disagrees. He asks instead what it means when lots of smoke is coming out of the chimney. Does lots of smoke always indicate a hot fire burning inside? Unfortunately, it only indicates a weak fire producing lots of smoke. So you can only deduce one thing for sure when ketones show up in your urine: poor combustion of fat, rather than fat burning at an efficient rate.

But wait, there's more! If you eat a high-protein, low- or no-carbohydrate meal, you will lose lean body mass because your body can use the dietary protein to make glucose for only two hours after eating. After that, there isn't any more dietary protein available, and despite the fact that you had a big protein-rich meal, you will have to fulfill further protein needs by getting it from body tissue. What's your brain going to do when it needs glucose? It will turn to the one place it knows it can get glucose—your muscle tissue. Now you are right back to the whole problem of losing lean body mass—a weight-gain trigger to be avoided, since it greatly reduces your body's natural ability to burn fat!

What happens if you eat too much protein? There's a point when you simply can't use all the protein you're taking in. The excess protein, accompanied by excess fat you've consumed with the protein, is sent to your liver, where it is deaminated (amino groups removed). This is a stressful process, pushing your system to its limits. During deamination, nitrogen is released from the protein and converted to ammonia, which is toxic to your body. The ammonia is converted to urea, which is also toxic but much less so than ammonia. High-protein diets warn that you must drink large quantities of water to make certain that you rid your body of urea. But many people find it difficult or uncomfortable to drink as much water as they should. So their bodies will take the water from their own healthy tissue. All this water and urea taxes their poor kidneys, which work overtime in a valiant effort to rid them of the toxic urea.

In the final analysis, we human beings are not very good carnivores, and when you try to force your metabolism to work like a lion's, your effort ends up being its own weight-gain trigger. While it is true that your digestive system can adjust and make use of an exclusively protein diet for short periods of time, depriving yourself of carbohydrates over a prolonged period will place impossible burdens on your body. Not only will you be endangering your health, but you'll also end up creating a powerful weight-gain trigger that you otherwise would never have had to contend with. While the Right Bite diet corrects metabolisms that have been damaged by high-protein diets, the better approach is to avoid creating this trigger in the first place by making certain that you have a diet with the appropriate ratios of protein and carbohydrates. With weight-gain triggers as with your general health, the same old adage holds true—an ounce of prevention is worth a pound of cure.

Last, I have to ask why so many of the people promoting high-protein diets, and who claim to have been on them for years, are overweight themselves. Could it be that they are, as the popular song says, "just talking loud and saying nothing"?

Over time, people on low-carbohydrate diets also begin to experience two types of hypoglycemia or low blood sugar, resulting in dramatic drops in energy and, in many cases, severe mood shifts. I will discuss these issues in more detail in a subsequent trigger heading. Suffice it to say that if you maintain a low carbohydrate diet, it will wreak havoc with your energy levels, your mental and emotional capacities, and your weight.

Were all this not enough to convince you, diets with insufficient carbohydrate also cause a decreased synthesis of serotonin. You will recall from the last chapter that the hormone serotonin inhibits carbohydrate hunger. Without it, we crave sweets and binge. Once you give in to the urge to eat abundant carbohydrates—usually in the form of sweets— you will experience rapid weight gain because your low carbohydrate diet has become its own weight-gain trigger.

INSUFFICIENT PROTEIN

Insufficient protein has devastating effects on your body and your brain because of the major role it plays in growth and repair. Protein is essential for maintaining our fluid balance and our acid-base balance. It is important for the formation of antibodies in our immune system, which protect us from infections, and for producing hormones. Insufficient dietary protein wreaks havoc with our bodies and our attempts at weight control because of its adverse effects on our lean body mass, nervous system, strength, and vigor. Therefore, make certain that any diet you embark on has adequate supplies of this essential nutrient in a healthy ratio with other essential nutrients.

Here are three key tips and reminders concerning your protein intake:

1. **Get sufficient calories**: Make certain you eat a diet with sufficient calories (Don't forget the T-rex of weight-gain triggers). Remember, that even if your *entire* diet were nothing but protein, your body would convert your body's own protein to glucose if calories were otherwise unavailable.

2. **Get enough protein**: If you eat a diet that is either devoid of proteins or consists of poor protein sources, you will be depriving your body of the nutrients you need for rebuilding damaged tissue or building new cells. For example, remember what happened to Beth on her all broccoli diet, a diet that supplied only minuscule traces of protein.

3. **Don't forget the "kindling"**: Be sure your diet supplies adequate carbohydrates and fat—even if you are eating sufficient calories in the form of high-protein foods.

When you become protein deficient, antibodies that fight infection and help to fight cancer cells in our bodies are degraded. Your hair and skin cease to be maintained. And basal metabolic rates decrease as your muscles atrophy, which will cause you to gain weight easily when you do eat normally.

Another trigger related to insufficient protein comes into play when your blood protein drops and your hormonal balances are disturbed by too little protein in your diet. What happens is this: with protein deficiency, fluid leaks out of the blood vessels into the body tissues and spaces, causing edema, that is, swelling. We all know the edema associated with protein deficiency; it's called "bloating." When you experience bloating you tend to mistake it for fat, and the usual response is to say, "Uh, oh, time to get serious about dieting!" You cut back on the calories, but you don't get thinner. On the contrary, you get bigger, and you put on more weight. The weight, however, is not fat; it is further bloating, triggered by the very thing you are doing to lose weight.

When your body's protein sources are depleted, you must eat two to three times more protein food to regain what you've lost in essential amino acids. This need is comparable to the protein needs associated with growth in our formative years. Unfortunately, although your adult protein needs may be enormous, your caloric needs are not, so along with regaining the necessary amino acids, you also start storing new reserves of fat.

A final reminder: protein deficiency creates depression and behavioral problems that become weight-gain triggers themselves, reinforcing incorrect dieting patterns that can lead to an ever-increasing collection of weight-gain triggers.

The Right Bite Program will keep you on track to prevent this all too common, vicious circle of the chronic dieter. Not only will the program prevent this destructive spiral of events from occurring in the first place, it will repair any damage to your metabolism, liberate you from any holds weight-gain triggers may have on you, and set you off on the right path.

INSUFFICIENT FAT

You would think that with the high-fat American diet, fat deficiency would be rare. However, many weight-conscious people eat such bizarre diets that this is not the case. They try to avoid fat in any form, and in the process fall victim to weight-gain triggers they would never suspect.

I first became aware of fat deficiency acting as a weight gain trigger when a client came to me complaining that she was overeating fats—not just foods with fats—fats and oils! Dolores would diet for a while, lose some weight, and then get such a craving for fats that she would drink vegetable oil right out of the bottle, just as one might take a swig out of a bottle of soda. Just the thought of doing this practically made me gag, but not Dolores. She confessed that she sometimes took bread, soaked it in a little dish of olive oil until the whole thing was soggy, and then spooned it up as if it were the world's most wonderful delicacy.

Dolores' favorite dip for potato chips was a scoop of butter and peanut butter on each chip. Was she fat? Yes, Dolores was huge.

I sat down with Dolores, and we went over her entire diet in great detail. I discovered that she had a very strict weight-loss regimen that she stuck to whenever she wasn't binging. And the first thing that popped out at me was that it was absolutely devoid of oils and fats. When I saw that I immediately looked her in the eye and announced that she had to add oils to her daily diet. I thought she was going to fall off her chair! She could not believe I was suggesting that she add to her diet the food item that she had seen as the source of her problems. However, after I explained to her that her diet contributed to a deficiency in essential fats and oils, and that this was actually triggering the craving that spiraled out of control, consumption of fats and oils, she settled down. I had her add three to six teaspoons of oil to her daily diet, and within four days she had stopped her cravings for oil and was already losing weight.

After my success with Dolores, I became particularly aware of how diets too low in fats can trigger bizarre dietary behaviors, and I've found that an extraordinary number of dieters crave greasy or oily foods and even go on fat binges. Yes, make no mistake, insufficient fat in your diet can become a weight-gain trigger. You might not be soaking slices of bread in olive oil, as Dolores did, but maybe you stop off at the fast food drive-in now and then for "just a small bag of French fries." And did you know that in that small bag of French fries you'll be consuming nearly as much fat as Dolores did when she treated herself to bread dipped in olive oil?

Some nutritionists maintain that we need only two teaspoons of oil a day in order to get all the essential fats that our body cannot produce.

Based upon my experience with my clients, I disagree with this finding and believe that the amount of oil and other nutrients a person needs per day is highly individualized. If there are no easy standards to follow, how do you determine what your own intake of essential fats might be? When you get to the Right Bite Core Diet, which I discuss in later chapters, you'll find out exactly how to do this. In the meantime, suffice it to say that there is a way to determine your own individual needs not just for oils but for all other nutrients as well. The Right Bite Program is, in fact, designed to fully respect your individual body chemistry, tastes, and needs, and help you identify exactly what these are.

Are there some fats and oils that are better than others? Yes, and these are:

✓ **Canola oil:** Rich in monounsaturated and omega 3 fatty acids (and low in saturated and polyunsaturated fats, which are shown to suppress the immune system)

✓ **Flax seed oil:** Rich in the omega-3 essential fatty acids crucial in regulating the immune system

✓ **Olive oil:** Over 80 percent monounsaturated, which is neutral to immune function and may also be beneficial in preventing heart disease

INSUFFICIENT VITAMINS AND MINERALS

Dieters are usually deficient in one or more vitamins and minerals, and any of these deficiencies can become a weight-gain trigger. I will provide you with some of the deficiency symptoms associated with them. These are not complete lists of deficiency symptoms, however. To provide complete lists and discussions of each vitamin and mineral would not be practical for the purposes of this book. Also, these lists are not meant for self-diagnosis because many deficiency symptoms of vitamins and minerals overlap one another, and can mimic disease states. The purpose of these lists is simply to alert you to the importance of satisfying the five characteristic, of a nutritious diet—adequacy, variety, balance, moderation, and calorie control—and the deleterious consequences that may result when you do not. When we have a deficiency in any area, we may consciously or unconsciously start seeking ways to satisfy that deficiency—a search that can lead us right into the grips of another weight-gain trigger if we're not careful.

The vitamin-mineral lists I provide can give you important insights into your own nutritional deficiencies. This can help you pinpoint why your dietary habits are not getting the results you would like.

As you read these lists you may find yourself saying, "Yes, I feel that way," or "I have that symptom." But try to avoid the temptation to self-diagnose and begin taking megadoses of the vitamins and/or minerals you believe you need. To do so could produce just the opposite result from that you are seeking.

In the Core Diet of the Right Bite Program you'll be learning exactly what your individual nutritional needs are and how best to guarantee that these needs are being met. In the meantime, anyone who has been dieting should be alerted to at least the more serious symptoms of being deficient in vitamins and minerals.

Symptoms Associated with Dietary Deficiencies of Micronutrients

> ### *Vitamin A*
> night blindness
> diarrhea
> infections
> painful joints
> depression of immune reactions
> anemia

> ### *Vitamin D*
> rickets
> deformities of limbs, spine, thorax, and pelvis
> pain in pelvis, lower back, and legs
> bone fractures
> decreased calcium and/or phosphorus in your blood
> muscle spasms

> ### *Vitamin E*
> premature bursting of red blood cells
> fibrocystic breast disease

> ### *Vitamin K*
> hemorrhaging
> prolonged clotting time

Note: Vitamins A, D, E, and K are fat soluble. They are found in the fat and oily parts of foods and they can be stored in liver and fat tissue. Because they can be stored you can go for longer periods of time without eating food sources rich in these vitamins, therefore the risk of toxicity is greater than a deficiency, especially if you take large supplements of these vitamins. If you take in more fat soluble vitamins than your body can use, they tend to move into the liver and fatty tissue in your body and remain there rather than being excreted. An example of this would be the symptoms of vitamin A toxicity, which include jaundice, spleen enlargement, diarrhea, and kidney stones.

Vitamin B1: Thiamin
fatigue
enlarged heart, abnormal heart rhythms, heart failure
low morale
wasting
difficulty walking
mental confusion

Vitamin B2: Riboflavin
fatigue
cracks at the corners of the mouth, magenta tongue
skin rash
light sensitivity

Vitamin B3: Niacin
fatigue
irritability
mental confusion
dizziness
diarrhea

Vitamin B6
fatigue
irritability
weakness
insomnia
kidney stones

Folate
depression
anemia
suppression of the immune system—
infections
fatigue
apathy
weakness
confusion

Vitamin B12

anemia
fatigue
irritability
constipation
palpitations
degeneration of peripheral nerves

Pantothenic Acid

vomiting
gastrointestinal distress
insomnia
fatigue

Biotin

loss of hair
depression
lassitude
muscle pains
anorexia
nausea
abnormal heart action
insomnia

Vitamin C

scurvy
anemia
fatigue
depression
frequent infections
emotional shakiness or hysteria
physical weakness
bleeding around teeth and gums
muscle degeneration
rough, brown, dry, scaly skin
slow wound healing
ends of long bones become softened,
malformed, and painful
fractures
loose teeth

Calcium
stunted growth in children
weak bones and teeth
muscle cramps
osteoporosis
nerve and muscle irritability

Magnesium
weakness
confusion
lack of muscle coordination

Sodium
mental apathy
muscle cramps

Chloride
muscle cramps
mental apathy

Potassium
muscle weakness
palpitations
lightheaded feeling
confusion

Iron
reduced work productivity
reduced tolerance of work
weakness
fatigue
reduced resistance to cold
inability to regulate body temperature
itching of skin
pale nail beds, eye membranes, palm creases
craving to eat clay or ice (believe it or not,
this is well documented!)
lactose intolerance and possibly intolerance
to other sugars
impaired wound healing
impaired cognitive function
reduced learning ability
impaired visual discrimination

Iron (continued)
increased distractibility
headaches
pallor
listlessness
irritability
dependency on glucose metabolism
(thus one becomes hungrier sooner)
decreased ability to burn calories

Note: It is critical to understand that iron deficiency, even when you are not anemic, can be responsible for destructive effects on your metabolism. All of the symptoms above may be experienced before anemia manifests itself and is discovered in the routine blood test given to diagnose anemia. Routine blood tests do not always reveal iron deficiency.

Zinc
mental lethargy
irritability
loss of taste
poor wound healing
diarrhea (which increases the need for all nutrients)
increased infections
impairment of central nervous
system and brain functioning
interference with folacin absorption and
vitamin A metabolism, so symptoms of
these vitamin deficiencies often occur
alteration in thyroid function and metabolic rate
alteration in taste, causing loss of appetite
growth retardation
abnormal glucose tolerance
mental lethargy
irritability
generalized hair loss
emotional disorders

Copper
Anemia

Iodine
sluggishness
weight gain

> **Chromium**
> adult-onset diabetes
> growth failure
> impaired carbohydrate metabolism

> **Selenium**
> heart failure
> enlarged heart

Inadequate protein, carbohydrate, fat, vitamin and/or mineral intake causes a multitude of problems ranging from physical to emotional. Deficiencies overlap each other, mimic each other, and act cumulatively. They all affect your ability to control your eating and your weight by producing weight-gain triggers that send your appetite and your metabolism into tailspins. The Right Bite Core Diet satisfies all five requirements of a nutritious diet, ensuring that you will not suffer from any nutrient deficiencies.

Two: The BS (Blood Sugar) Trigger— Transient Hypogycemia

As you read along you will note that blood glucose and its regulation are associated with a variety of weight-gain triggers. However, low blood sugar, or hypoglycemia, deserves to be highlighted in its own right to fully understand its role in creating weight-control problems.

We hear a lot about hypoglycemia these days. Since it is usually self-diagnosed, it is overdiagnosed to the point where it has become a catch-all for every discomfort, erratic behavior, and lack of motivation in our society. Additionally, hypoglycemia is perhaps one of the most controversial, maligned, and misunderstood malfunctions in medical history, in part because it manifests itself in a wide diversity of symptoms. It does not show up on routine laboratory tests, and the one test that can detect it, the glucose tolerance test (GTT), is not part of the standard physical exam. Then there is the problem with the diagnosis. Some doctors feel that the GTT is a reliable diagnostic tool, and some do not. To complicate matters further, many people never develop the classic hypoglycemic symptoms, even when their blood sugar levels are low enough to cause the kinds of dietary problems we've been discussing.

One person may get along nicely with a blood sugar level of 70 mg, whereas another person may need 90 mg to function normally. Each person is born with a certain genetic background that makes his or her nutritional needs entirely different from those of any other. Still, it would be rare to find healthy nondieting men or women who are suffering from hypoglycemia. Chronic dieters and people with eating disorders are another matter, however: they consistently show up with one or both of the two kinds of hypoglycemia—fasting and postprandial. Both affect weight control and the sense of well-being, and both types need to be examined in the roles they play as weight-gain triggers.

FASTING HYPOGLYCEMIA

Fasting hypoglycemia occurs whenever most of the available glucose is used up in your system; it is prevalent any time you skip meals or exercise to excess. You may have noticed this form of hypoglycemia in the morning—after all, when you first awaken you haven't eaten for several hours. You've no doubt also experienced it anytime you were on a low carbohydrate diet. Dieters are notorious for skipping breakfast and even lunch and subsisting on caffeinated drinks. They start suffering symptoms because their brains lack adequate fuel in the form of glucose. Symptoms include a craving for sweets, headache, mental dullness, fatigue, depression, difficulty concentrating, and confusion.

In an effort to jolt their sluggish heads into a state of alertness and assuage their cravings for sweets, dieters often consume large quantities of fattening carbohydrates and beverages loaded with caffeine and/or sugar. Once sweets and other carbohydrates are eaten—and they most certainly are—fasting hypoglycemia can turn into reactive, or *postprandial*, hypoglycemia, which is a fancy way of saying that low blood sugar occurs after eating. Only the iron-willed anorexic can usually resist fasting hypoglycemia. Although she will experience and repress sugar cravings, she is nonetheless a victim of fasting hypoglycemia, limping zombielike through her day as her body continues to cannibalize whatever healthy tissue remains.

POSTPRANDIAL OR REACTIVE HYPOGLYCEMIA

There are two processes in your body that maintain normal blood glucose. First, when blood glucose gets too high, your body produces insulin, which converts the excess glucose to glycogen or fat. Second, when blood glucose gets too low, and you fail to eat food to replenish it, your body draws glucose from your liver. This process is normally neatly balanced, but many diets knock this balance awry. When you follow a carbohydrate-restricted, or very low-calorie diet, then binge on sweets, postprandial, or reactive, hypoglycemia results. After you gorge on sugar-laden foods, your blood glucose levels shoot up too high and too rapidly. The insulin your body produces in response to this sugary load is often way out of proportion to the amount of sugar reaching the blood. In effect, your whole system for handling sugar goes a little crazy. With this excessive insulin, your blood sugar nosedives, leaving you with only a fraction of the glucose you need to function normally. That's the point at which you experience fatigue, irritability, weakness, a rapid heartbeat, anxiety, sweating, hunger, and headaches.

Most of my clients have experienced this kind of reaction at some time in their lives. Furthermore, most people with *normal* glucose regulation can develop the symptoms of reactive hypoglycemia just by devouring a large dose of simple sugar after three days of following a low-carbohydrate, high-protein diet. Any time you end a low-carbohydrate diet by overeating sweets, you're making yourself a candidate for this form of hypoglycemia.

Could you be a victim of this low blood sugar, weight-gain trigger from time to time? Do you fast, skip meals, or eat insufficient calories or carbohydrates? Are you following one of the popular high-protein diets? When you break your diet do you overeat sweets? If you are like most of us, you probably do. The weight-gain triggers caused by fasting and postprandial hypoglycemia may be experienced by anyone. The behaviors and foods causing these temporary conditions are very easy to encounter. The Right Bite Program presents a plan that eliminates hypoglycemia.

Three: The Hunger Hormone—Insulin

Insulin's nickname is the "Hunger Hormone," and therein lies its power as a weight-gain trigger. High levels of insulin cause you to feel hungry, to eat more, and to enjoy sweets more. Insulin also promotes *lipogenesis*—which literally means "the making of fat." When insulin levels in the blood go up, this stimulates the synthesis of fats and fat storage in your body. The basic job of this hormone is to help remove excess glucose from your blood and store it as glycogen in your liver and muscles and as fat in your fat cells. And guess what? Insulin is best at packing the fat cells because there is always more room in our fat cells—they just get bigger and bigger—while glycogen stores are limited.

Insulin is also important for maintaining and stimulating the activity of *lipoprotein lipase*. This is the enzyme that facilitates fat deposition (discussed in "Insufficient Calories"). As the result of the increased activity of lipoprotein lipase, the transport of fat into your fat cells is accelerated.

And lastly—but so important—insulin inhibits the breakdown of fat.

Research has shown that such symptoms of postprandial hypoglycemia are not due just to low blood sugar but to the presence of the insulin itself. In fact, it has been found that with high levels of insulin present, we will experience many of the symptoms associated with low blood sugar, even when blood sugar levels are actually normal.

Insulin can have a devastating effect on our brains. Too much insulin can cause our brain cells to absorb more than their usual number of electrolytes (ions that circulate in the blood) and then swell with water. This condition is known as "hyperosmolarity," and has symptoms that are a lot like hypoglycemia. This can help to explain why there is little agreement among doctors on establishing diagnostic standards for what constitutes low blood sugar. Apparently, many people are suffering not from hypoglycemia but from hyperosmolarity. The good news is that the Right Bite Program can help to correct both conditions and normalize your system.

Finally, if you happen to be a person who consumes large amounts of refined carbohydrates (sugary beverages or foods), you are causing your pancreas to constantly produce insulin. This may lead to a dangerous condition called "insulin resistance." If you have this condition, your fat cells resist insulin, making it harder for excess glucose to enter their cells. This can lead to type II diabetes. I will discuss this more fully under the trigger heading *Fat*.

Be assured that in addition to enjoying a variety of tasty foods on the Right Bite Core Diet, you'll also be protected from hypoglycemia and any of the other deficiencies that turn into weight-gain triggers.

Four: Sugar

People in the modern world now consume an average of fifty pounds of sugar per person every year—roughly a pound a week. Twenty years ago the average was less than half that, and most of that came from whole food sources. The main reason for this has been the explosion of the fast food and convenience food industries, which cater to the needs of our rapid-paced society. These industries find that their products sell far better with the addition of sugar. There are many who believe that sugar does not contribute to obesity. My own research and experience with people trying to lose weight suggests a different stance. Here's why:

✓ Sugar makes it possible to consume huge amounts of calories quickly because it is concentrated, lacks fiber, and is not filling.

✓ Because it is easy to consume large amounts of sweets at once, some people produce too much insulin in response to this onslaught. As you will recall, insulin is known as the hunger hormone, and there is simply no way to dispute the fact that it is a major weight-gain trigger for that reason. In fact, it is a double weight-gain trigger since it produces low blood sugar, which also elevates the appetite. Whether because of the hunger hormone factor or low blood sugar, a sugary diet sets up a vicious cycle of ravenous hunger, overeating sweets, and oversecreting insulin. People who complain of being painfully full yet starving are victims of this cycle.

✓ Lipogenesis—the making of fat—is influenced by the rate of glucose metabolism. Therefore, a high sugar intake and subsequent chronically high insulin level promotes obesity.

✓ When people eat sweets, they may tend to eat fatty foods at the same time, since so many desserts include not just sugar but high levels of fat. For instance, chocolate candy is also high in fat. An ice cream sundae or a piece of pie may also include whipped cream. A person with a sweet tooth also seeks out cakes, cookies, and pastries that are not only high in refined sugar but also high in fat. If you take all of these factors into account, it is safe to say that the sweetness of sugary foods itself is a weight-gain trigger, one that makes more sweet food just that more enticing.

✓ Many people's obesity has its roots in their overeating of sugary foods at one time or another in their lives, or of getting into a pattern of eating snacks high in sugar throughout the day. In addition, there is considerable evidence that carbohydrate binging is a *prominent* behavior among people who eventually become obese.

✓ Sweetness is definitely a preferred taste for most humans. In research studies people have been offered foods that have been sweetened and those that have not been. In every instance, the sweetened food was preferred above the other. Even newborns preferentially consume more of a sugar solution than an unsweetened one.

✓ When we try to trace why we all seem to love the taste of sugar so much, we discover that eating anything sweet releases endorphins for most people. And while beta-endorphins, produced within our brains, make us feel calm, and even euphoric, they also stimulate our appetites. And when we eat more, we want more. The more sugar you eat the more beta-endorphins are released, ad infinitum. And people who are compulsive eaters of sugary foods are found to have a higher level of beta endorphins than those who don't eat as many sweets. These findings certainly provide us with some strong evidence for why sweet foods act as weight-gain triggers, and why food manufacturers would want to put sugar in their products.

✓ Some researchers have also observed that when sugar is eaten in high concentrations over time, endorphin receptors increase. This mimics the same mechanism seen with drug addictions particularly with opium-based addictions, although different nerves are involved. Sugar increases the number of opiate receptors in our brains, at the same time increasing our sensitivity to these substances. If you have been addicted to sweets in this way, you will actually experience "withdrawal symptoms" when you stop eating sugar. So if you ever hear yourself saying, "I'm addicted to cherry cheesecake," take heed. You may not be joking.

✓ Because it displaces nutrients, sugar can cause nutritional deficiencies, which are magnified when we are already following a calorie-restricted diet. This type of marginal malnutrition is hard to diagnose and almost impossible to believe because the person suffering from the deficiencies is often overweight or obese from the overconsumption of sweets. People who are obese look like they are suffering from an overabundance of nutrients, when in reality just the opposite is often true—they are overeating sweets and undereating nutritious foods. Such a person could be said to be under the influence of at least three weight-gain triggers: malnutrition, the overproduction of insulin, and the capacity of sugar to stimulate the production of endorphins.

Five: Lack of Exercise

A friend once told me, "I'm a thin fat person." Baffled, I asked her what she meant. She replied that, as long as she dressed in long skirts or pants and long-sleeved shirts, she gave the illusion of being very slender, but in shorts or a bathing suit she was flabby and fat. She said that she weighed the same as she did when she was nineteen (she was forty-two at the time of this conversation) and couldn't understand why she was so pudgy.

As we get older, our metabolisms slow down, and if we fail to maintain a good exercise regimen there is a decrease of about one-third of a pound of muscle tissue per year, starting in our thirties. The normal decrease in energy expenditure that comes for most of us as we age, combined with the loss of muscle mass, causes us to burn fewer and fewer calories. Gradually, body composition shifts so that muscle tissue is replaced by fat, resulting in the "thin fat person"—assuming that you weigh the same as you did in your youth, which most of us don't! The good news is that if you pay attention to this—nature's own weight-gain trigger—you need not end up as my friend did.

Many of my clients ask why we are so sedentary. One reason is that our lives revolve around labor-saving and energy-conserving devices, and our leisure time has been reduced to gazing at a television or computer screen. In fact, television watching is by far the most popular spare-time activity in our nation—all too often accompanied by munching away at fat- and sugar-laden snacks!

More than two-thirds of American adults are completely inactive or irregularly active, and most people who are trying to lose weight, or maintain a present weight, find it a great challenge to do so without physical exercise. According to the Centers for Disease Control, of more than 73,000 overweight people surveyed, only 28 percent exercised even the minimum amount recommended for health. In fact, lack of exercise is one of the most important contributors to weight problems in our country.

In Chapter 10, I will discuss physical exercise in more detail. That discussion will cover the benefits of exercise, anaerobic and aerobic exercise, types of exercise, fueling exercise, and finally developing your individualized exercise program. In the meantime, consider a sedentary lifestyle a major weight-gain trigger, one that you will be eliminating with the Right Bite Program.

Six: Fat

The consumption of fatty foods presents a special physiological challenge for anyone trying to control his or her weight, and for that reason requires special attention as a weight-gain trigger. In an interesting study by Wayne Miller, M.D., two groups of rats were placed on diets with exactly the same number of total calories. However, one group ate foods with over 40 percent of the calories coming from fat. This diet, by the way, is close to the fat ratios of the typical diet in the United States, which tends to center around eating red meat. The second group of rats ate foods with only 11 percent of the calories coming from fat.

After eight weeks, the rats on the high-fat diet weighed 32 percent more than the rats on the low-fat diets. In addition, the high-fat group had more body fat—51 percent versus the low fat group's 30 percent, which is considered normal in healthy rats. Dr. Miller believes that fat has the same pound-promoting effects in humans as it does in rats—and guess what, he's right!

FATTENING FACTS ABOUT FAT—
THE FAT WE EAT AND THE FAT ON OUR BODIES

When you have a diet high in fat, it will show up both in your body image when you look in the mirror and in physiological changes in your metabolism. Your percentage of body fat with a high-fat diet will be higher than that of a person with a low-fat diet, even when your total caloric intake is moderate. If you want to lower the percentage of body fat that you are carrying, eat more simple carbohydrates and fewer fatty foods, while keeping your caloric intake moderate. Put simply, the more fat calories in your diet, the more fat on your body and the fewer calories it will take for you to gain the same amount of weight as your counterpart eating a high-carbohydrate diet.

J.P. Flat, M.D., at the University of Massachusetts Medical School, has done considerable work in this area. He has stated that our bodies have no inherent mechanism to regulate fat balance, though it does have such mechanisms for protein and carbohydrates; therefore you must regulate the intake of fat yourself. In Dr. Flat's own research, he had volunteers eat two similar breakfasts, with the same total calories, except that one had 375 of those calories in fat. He found that in both cases the carbohydrate and protein calories were burned as quickly as they were taken in; most of the fat calories were not burned off but were stored in fat cells. So even though the two groups of people ate the same number of calories, the group eating the fat gained weight, and the other did not. Evidently our bodies are biologically programmed to burn about as many protein and carbohydrate calories as we consume, but not so with fat. It seems our bodies are determined to store fat calories, making fat an especially important weight-gain trigger.

One reason your body finds it easier to store dietary fat as body fat than to store carbohydrates as body fat is because it takes less energy to do so. To store dietary fat requires only about 3 percent of your ingested caloric intake, whereas the storage of carbohydrates as body fat requires 23 percent. As we eat more carbohydrates, the energy required to digest, absorb, transport, metabolize, and store them also increases. This energy is referred to as the "thermic effect" of food.

A high fat diet causes people to overeat for several reasons:

✓ Fats make foods taste delicious. For example, how many calories in French fries or potato chips can you eat versus how many plain boiled potatoes?

✓ Fat has very little bulk, making it easy to overeat. Two teaspoons of fat, for example, have 80 calories, whereas a 4-ounce potato has also 80 calories. Which food form would be most likely to fill you up?

✓ We need carbohydrates in our diet to feel completely full and satisfied. What this boils down to is that you could eat a 500-calorie helping of fatty meat and still not feel full or satisfied. Your body still wants carbohydrates, and to satisfy the signals your body is sending out, you eat another 400 calories in carbohydrates, at which point you finally experience satiety.

When told to eat until fullness, people who sat down to a high-fat meal ate 1350 calories, and those given only low-fat, high-carbohydrate foods to choose from felt stuffed after eating just 680 calories. In addition, those who had the high-fat meal were more likely to overeat the following day.

When you become overweight, and your fat cells enlarge, those cells become sluggish in response to insulin. You will recall that when blood glucose levels are too high, it is insulin that facilitates the transformation and storage of glucose to glycogen, which your body has a limited capacity to store. Insulin also facilitates the entry of excess glucose into fat cells, which have an unlimited storage capability, where glucose is stored as fat. As fat cells enlarge, becoming more resistant to insulin, excess glucose remains in your blood longer than normal and rises still higher. The excess glucose stimulates your overstressed pancreas into producing even more insulin—much more than is needed under normal circumstances, bringing your soaring blood glucose levels back down to normal. Then, when your fat cells finally respond, a veritable tidal wave of glucose floods into your fat cells. All this has been triggered by the exaggerated level of insulin. Keep in mind that insulin resistance causes this and is one of the metabolic consequences of obesity: as body fat increases, insulin resistance increases. The personal repercussions are pretty obvious to you as well as to the rest of the world: you wear them on your body as bigger bulges and pouches.

There is growing evidence that the longer you eat a high-fat diet, the more your body actually begins to shift toward storing fat instead of burning it for energy. So, once again, if you are going to reach weight goals that you can comfortably and happily maintain over time, it is essential that you learn to strike a happy balance with your fat intake. And that is a key function of the Right Bite Core Diet.

Seven: The Dieter's False Friend—Caffeine

In spite of the fact that people turn to caffeinated beverages for "energy" when they are dieting, these drinks are one of our worst enemies. Why? Because they camouflage our bodies' physical signals and artificially stress the body. With caffeine, we don't know when we're hungry, full, tired, rested, or alert. Caffeine is bad not only for the dieter but also for the nondieter, because the pick-up we experience with it is temporary and earned at a huge physiological price.

Many dieters drink coffee and other caffeine-containing beverages because they feel such drinks aid them in their efforts to diet. Subsisting on a low number of calories, they associate caffeine with a badly needed surge of energy and with the suppression of appetite. Although beverages containing caffeine initially inhibit hunger, the effect is only temporary, and in time those who are sensitive to caffeine's effects will ultimately overeat. So here is a "diet aid" whose initial help turns into a hindrance—a weight-gain trigger in the guise of a helper.

How does caffeine work? If you really want to impress someone with your knowledge of biochemistry, just drop the name *phosphodiesterase*. This is the name of an important enzyme produced in our bodies. I will call it PDE for short. Enzymes normally facilitate your body's metabolic reactions, but when caffeine is introduced into your system it inhibits PDE's ability to function. A complex series of events then unfolds, resulting in your body increasing its production of epinephrine, more commonly known as the "fight-or-flight" hormone. Epinephrine is normally produced when you are under stress or in danger, such as having a near collision while driving on the freeway. Studies have shown that the level of epinephrine is 76 to 158 percent higher after caffeine is consumed, compared to a placebo.

Caffeine evokes an artificial stress environment in your body. Now why in the world would we want to go and do that when we all have quite enough stress to deal with already? To better understand why you do not want to create an artificial stress situation in your body, you need to know what happens during real stress.

When our bodies are subjected to actual stress, such as a hungry lion leaping over its fence at a zoo and chasing us to the safety of the nearest rest room, we need a tremendous amount of fuel to cope with the emergency of trying to save ourselves. In this case, we will need a lot of fuel to make us run *really fast*. The body has devised a way to do just that. A rise in epinephrine elicited by the perceived danger causes glucose to be mobilized from the liver, while triggering the production of new glucose (gluconeogenesis) from our protein reserves (muscles). This rapid rise in blood glucose explains why we do not feel hungry when we are confronted by a major stressor—or for that matter after drinking a beverage containing caffeine. There's a significant rise in blood glucose levels, which signals our brain that we are not hungry. Think about it this way: it would not be in our evolutionary interest to have to stop and eat while being chased by wild, man-eating animals.

When most of us consume caffeine, we are not in such dire circumstances, and even if we were, we would not need caffeine to produce extra fuel for energy—when danger threatens, our bodies mobilize fuel all by themselves. We don't need caffeine to escape from a burning building either, or to leap out of the path of a coming train, or to whisk our child away from the wheels of a speeding car.

Fine, you may be saying, but what could this possibly have to do with weight control? Plenty!

There are several scenarios that illustrate how caffeine exerts its toxic weight-gain trigger effects:

The Well-Fed Dieter: Many dieters consume caffeine-laden beverages with their meals. Not everyone is sensitive to caffeine, but if you are a person who is, the caffeine-induced rapid rise in blood glucose levels will stimulate your pancreas to release insulin in an attempt to bring your blood sugar down to normal. As a result, too much sugar may be removed from your blood, precipitating low blood sugar and its accompanying symptoms of hunger and a craving for sweets. You can get into a vicious cycle when caffeine repeatedly stimulates a rise in blood sugar while at the same time insulin is fighting to lower it. Dieters perceive this drop in blood sugar as uncontrollable hunger and a craving for sweets and other carbohydrates. Caffeine-sensitive dieters will feel hungry sooner after eating a meal accompanied by caffeine—a meal that without caffeine would have prevented hunger longer without ravaging blood sugar levels.

The Unfed Dieter: Let's say you are dieting and you are already experiencing real hunger because your blood sugar levels have dropped and your glycogen stores are becoming depleted. You may then turn to beverages containing caffeine (coffee, tea, cola or even some noncola drinks) in an effort to blunt your feelings of hunger so that you won't be tempted to eat. The caffeine-stimulated rise in blood sugar will camouflage true hunger so that you will not eat at a time when it is critical to do so. This phenomenon makes the black coffee or cola drink, so loved by dieters, a poor choice because its temporary effect of depressing appetite is really based on its action of pushing sugar into the blood stream. Instead of eating and digesting new food, which is the normal thing to do, your body will burn the glucose, which has been forced from glycogen stores and muscle proteins. Although this will temporarily inhibit hunger, glycogen stores are soon depleted, and gluconeogenesis cannot keep pace with your body's utilization of glucose, so you once again experience low blood sugar and gnawing hunger.

Your body's vital need for glucose will eventually force you to overeat sweets and other carbohydrates. Because so much time has elapsed between the first hunger pangs and the caffeine-induced rise, followed by a drop in your blood sugar, the hunger you now experience can be particularly extreme.

CAFFEINE AND SUGAR—A DOUBLE WHAMMY

The combination of caffeine and sugar is particularly lethal. You will recall that eating sugary foods and other carbohydrates will stimulate the release of insulin in order to bring high blood glucose levels down. However, caffeine attacks by another route—your adrenals—stimulating the release of epinephrine. Epinephrine then stimulates your liver to break down its stored glycogen, thereby releasing glucose into your blood. It also initiates the making of new glucose. This sugar, of course, goes into the blood stream combining with the sugar in the caffeine containing beverage. To the pancreas, the source of the sugar makes no difference: it will produce insulin whether the sweet is coming from a candy bar or the reserves stored in the liver. In this case, you have sugar from two major sources—the beverage and your own glycogen reserves.

So here, you have a very confusing situation for your body. On one hand you have insulin working frantically to bring blood sugar down, and on the other hand you have the caffeine-induced rise in epinephrine working just as arduously to raise blood sugar. Eventually, your blood sugar level will drop as your glycogen stores become exhausted, with catastrophic results—overeating.

Caffeine adversely affects your efforts at weight control in still another important way. Caffeine causes your brain to use a lot more blood glucose than normal at a time when blood flow to your brain is decreased. Don't forget that the fight-or-flight syndrome, triggered by caffeine, originally evolved for human survival. It carefully maps out where blood should go in order to meet the threat or run from physical danger. So your heart, lungs, and large muscles are given top priority since they are more necessary than your brain for fighting or running. So now you have reduced blood flow to your brain while your brain is demanding more blood glucose than usual. This is like dripping gasoline into your empty tank when your engine is accelerating. Because of the speed with which your brain is using blood glucose, you may experience uncomfortable hypoglycemic symptoms at a glucose level that is not usually associated with being hypoglycemic. It only takes two to three cups of coffee to cause this rapid and sustained reduction in cerebral blood flow with increased glucose utilization by the brain—and yes, you will feel hungry.

Caffeine is addictive. Sudden abstinence from the drug—and technically it is a drug—after long use, even if that use has been moderate, causes a characteristic withdrawal reaction. The most common withdrawal reaction is a headache. Other symptoms include lethargy, fatigue, muscle pain or stiffness, mood changes, nausea, and vomiting. The symptoms of withdrawal usually begin twelve hours after your last caffeine fix, peaking at somewhere between twenty and forty-eight hours later, and lasting approximately one week.

And, yes, you guessed it—the Right Bite Core Diet eliminates this weight-gain trigger, because it is caffeine free.

Eight: Stress and Strain Cause Weight Gain

In college, I first became acquainted with stress-induced eating when I encountered my first big stressor—and it was really, really big. I had been friends with a young married couple, Bob and Carol, for about six months. We were very close and did everything together, from studying to attending movies. One day I was invited to dinner at their home, to which I had never been. When I arrived punctually at seven, I was startled by Carol greeting me at the door clad only in her underwear and bra. She explained that the air conditioning was out and hoped I did not mind roughing it with the fans. Bob appeared shirtless and dressed in boxer shorts. I suddenly felt over dressed in my flowered halter-top dress.

Dinner was lovely, and after we finished Carol asked if I would like to see the rest of the apartment. I acquiesced and Carol led the way, ending the tour in their master bedroom. The bedroom was beautiful with a king-sized bed, flower arrangements, thick carpeting, and a lush bathroom adjoining, complete with a large Jacuzzi®.

I needed to use the restroom and also wanted to freshen up, because it was frightfully hot in the apartment, so I excused myself momentarily. When I finished and had begun to open the door a horrifying spectacle greeted my eyes. Bob and Carol had shed their scant clothing and were involved in very energetic sexual activities on their bed, romping around quite vigorously. For a moment I just stood there paralyzed, aware that they knew I was watching, then shut the bathroom door and waited. When I heard the bed stop squeaking and the muffled gasps and sighs cease, I thought it safe to venture out. I peeked out the door and saw Bob sitting on a chair pulled up to the front of the bed as though he were about to watch a movie and thank goodness back in his shorts.

However, Carol continued to recline in the buff on her bed. It finally dawned on me that I was in trouble.

I remembered thinking of the crippled Apollo 13's distress call when the captain said, "Houston, we have a problem!" I knew I could not stay in the bathroom forever and wanted desperately to escape. I quickly scanned the bathroom and noted two large windows. After silently hoisting the window open I leaned my head out hoping to find a way to exit my uncomfortable situation. I was seemingly trapped on the second floor of this apartment. Frantically, I began to open cabinets and closets and found the linens. With trembling fingers, I rapidly tied together several sheets and secured one end to the plumbing under the sink. Pulling the sheets tightly to make sure they were secure I slid out the window, legs first and shimmied down my makeshift rope, aware and not caring that my dress had slid up almost over my head.

As I ran to my car I looked over my shoulder just in time to see Carol and Bob looking out the window beckoning and calling me. I would have sooner returned to Bluebeard's castle! No one could have moved faster than I that night, and within minutes I was safely back in my dorm room—where I ate and ate and ate, and ate some more.

For some, stress is a potent appetite trigger. Why some of us overeat in response to stress and others cannot eat at all remains a mystery.

Virtually any agent can produce the stress response. While we ordinarily associate stress with danger, it can also be associated with very pleasant events. For example, a passionate kiss can cause stress and not be dangerous. The only way to avoid stress is to die, for we are all always under some degree of stress.

For the present discussion, however, we will be concerned with an excess of stress—anything that interferes with the body's normal balance in a damaging way and anything that you experience as a threat to your equilibrium. It can be *physical*, such as fatigue, disease, overwork, and dietary abuse, or it can be *psychological* such as divorce, death of a loved one, changing schools, or even an unexpected event at a friend's home. According to a study conducted at Emory University Medical School, when we're excessively tired, we eat more and we eat more often. Research has shown that sleep-deprived individuals increase their calories by more than 10–15 percent per day.

When your brain perceives that something is a threat to your equilibrium—and remember, in most cases this is a highly individualized perception—the stress response begins and is mediated by both hormones and your nervous system to bring about a state of readiness to meet the "emergency." You'll recall that this response, which we previously discussed in our section on caffeine, is better known as the "fight-or-flight response," and is an inborn response for dealing with physical danger. Although many, if not most of our dangers today are psychological, consisting of stressors such as deadlines at work, traffic on the freeway, or problems at home—your nervous system and hormones will respond as if the threat were physical. The pupils of your eyes will widen, enabling you to see better. Muscles will tense, breathing will speed up, bringing more oxygen to your lungs, and your heart will start beating more rapidly. Blood vessels in muscles expand, enabling them to receive nutrients more quickly. Meanwhile blood vessels in your gastrointestinal tract slow down. After all, it would not be to your advantage to have to stop and go to the bathroom when you are fleeing from danger.

To conserve fluid, less blood flows to your kidneys in times of stress. And to minimize blood loss at possible wound sites, less blood flows to your skin. You hear better and feel pain less. Your brain produces substances that dull the sensation of pain that could distract you from dealing adequately with the emergency. Even your hairs stand on end as the tiny muscles around them contract.

This total stress response is effective for short-term situations, but if the stress is prolonged, and if the body cannot respond to the stress physically (you cannot fight or flee from your enemy), your body will become weakened and drained of its energy reserves.

During stress, your body needs extra fuel, and all three fuels are taken from the body's various stores: glucose from the limited stores of glycogen in your liver, then protein primarily from muscle tissue, and then fat. Calcium and other electrolytes are also lost during stress. In addition, most of us have no desire to eat during the initial presentation of the stress, so there is a further depletion of nutrients in our system. This initial lack of appetite is created by the fact that fuels are flooding your blood stream from other sources.

Stress is a weight-gain trigger and its effects are especially severe on those who are dieting as opposed to those who are better nourished:

1. Incorrect dieting itself is a stress with all the added repercussions associated with insufficient nutrients and calories.
2. Any added stress itself robs the body of additional valuable nutrients, the deficiencies of which exacerbate overeating.
3. Prolonged stress rapidly depletes your glycogen reserves, causing low blood sugar so that once the stress is over you will crave and overeat sweets and carbohydrates.
4. Short-term stress can also induce overeating for some people. Let's say you get stopped for speeding and you get a ticket—a stressful and frustrating situation for most people. During this stress, under the influence of epinephrine, glucose is drawn from liver glycogen stores, raising blood glucose levels. Your body is

flooded with glucose that it will probably not be able to burn off by physical exertion in this situation, and so stores it as fat, as we know. Glycogen stores are then depleted even though no glucose has been used for energy. Blood glucose falls an hour or two earlier than it would have, and you get hungry and eat sooner.

5. Many people find that just the act of eating relieves stress. For many people it is a substitute for comfort that they are unable to get in other ways. A friend who works in a day care center recently told me about a mother who always brought her four-year-old son a jelly donut, dripping with powdered sugar, when she came to pick him up. "Sweets for my sweetie," she always crooned as she handed it to him. On the few occasions when she failed to bring the jelly donut, or when she brought a substitute treat, the little boy sulked and told his mother he didn't want to go home. Teachers at the center noted that whenever the little guy was stressed or lonely—which was often—he asked for candy or something sweet to eat. He was also considerably overweight for his age. This is an excellent example of how many people learn to substitute food for love.

6. Stress lowers our body's *serotonin* levels, which can cause you to overconsume sweets and carbohydrates in an effort to produce more of this important *neurotransmitter* (a hormone in our brain) that has a soothing quality.

7. Eating can augment the production of substances in our brains that act like opiates such as morphine. Stress uses up these opiates, and eating helps to restore them to levels that relieve the stress.

8. Stress increases cortisol levels. This is another hormone that, when high enough, causes the body to deposit more fat around your midsection.

9. Stress temporarily boosts your blood sugar and insulin levels, which suppress your fat burning processes.

10. Stress can also affect your thyroid hormones, making them less effective at controlling your weight.

Although we can't totally eliminate stress in our daily lives, there are things that we can do to minimize it, as well as be prepared for it. The Right Bite Program addresses how to control this weight-gain trigger so that you can continue to reap its benefits without being unduly affected by its penalties.

Nine: Your Primitive Brain

Have you ever seen a dog shaking and foaming at the mouth in fear during a thunderstorm? All the soothing and stroking in the world will not take the dog's terror away. If the dog would just understand that thunder is nothing more than a sound, perhaps it would not be frightened. Since dogs cannot understand, we either let them shake and dig holes in our carpet or we tranquilize them and hope that the next time it storms they won't be so scared.

Most animals have largely primitive brains. Their reactions arise primarily from an area of the brain called the *limbic system*, specifically the *amygdala*. The area of the brain that enables humans to reason, plan, learn, and remember is called the *neocortex*. To illustrate the difference between these two areas of the brain, it's sometimes helpful to remember that love arises from the neocortex and lust from the limbic system. Animals such as reptiles have no neocortex. Baby snakes must hide from their parents to avoid being eaten because snakes do not experience maternal love.

People, like animals, have fears. Some are rational like the fear of poisonous snakes and insects. However, many of our fears and thoughts are not rational, and we react like dogs to thunder when we think of them or are exposed to them. In other words, we allow our emotions, or thoughts we hold in our mind, to drive our actions before our intellect gets a chance to intervene. In these situations, our primitive emotional brain completely overrides our cognitive brain.

Without these emotional responses we would scarcely be able to function, and we should be grateful for that because these responses have thus far ensured our survival. To illustrate how the primitive brain has ensured our survival, think of the times that you have put your foot or hand into water that was too hot and pulled it out with rapid-fire reflexes. Or the times when you spotted danger while you were driving and acted to avert a terrible wreck. Your neocortex gets the message after the amygdala does. However, had you waited to intellectually process the fact that the water was too hot or the highway danger was the result of a careless driver, you might have been severely scalded or ended up sitting trapped in a mangled car. Also, think about the times that you may have blinked to protect your eye from a swooping insect or ducked to miss a flying object. We respond in these ways so frequently that most of the time we think nothing of it. You can thank your amygdala for these life-saving and injury-preventing responses.

Dieters are notorious for having thoughts, fears and behaviors that are fueled and reinforced by the primitive brain. Used incorrectly, the primitive brain is one of the dieter's worst weight-gain triggers.

For some chronic dieters the feeling of fullness literally frightens them after a binge—they equate fullness with fatness. And they fear fatness. They have told themselves so many thousands of times "fullness is fatness" that whenever they are full they feel as terrified as a dog at thunder. They will go to any extent to escape the feeling of fullness, even fast or drink nothing but water and caffeinated beverages. One of the first things I teach people who have this fear is that fullness is never fatness on the Right Bite Core Diet. In fact, they quickly learn to associate that fullness with losing rather than gaining weight.

Changing the fear reaction to feelings of fullness can be a major challenge and ultimately a triumph of the neocortex over the primitive signals of fear sent out by the amagydala. You can see from this that your primitive brain can be one of your most challenging weight-gain triggers, causing you to react in ways that are far from being healthy.

Your brain, with its learned fears and misperceptions, can function in other ways as a weight-gain trigger, perpetuating unhealthy dieting and eating behavior, enforcing erroneous negative thinking and emotions, misconceptions, distortions, and nutritional myths and misrepresentations. Following its lead, you may continue impulsive behavior that will ultimately damage your body or your mind, or will cause you to overeat.

How do you undo the potent signals sent out by your primitive brain? *Self-awareness* is your biggest ally here since it allows you to learn and exercise some self-control. Self-awareness starts with being smart about what you feel—knowing when the *thunder* poses a real danger and when it does not. That kind of awareness makes it possible to tame and harness your primitive brain. After an emotional response comes into your awareness and you process it intellectually through your neocortex, your chances for handling it improve. To accomplish this awareness, you need to be able to step back and recognize what you are feeling or thinking. Once you've begun to master this ability, you have the power to change the inner programs that once filled your mind with thoughts and feelings that promoted weight-gaining behaviors. If all this sounds like a challenge, rest assured that it is much easier to do than you might imagine. Chapter 11 will show you how to liberate yourself from deceptive signals from your primitive brain.

Ten: Chocolate and Other Food "Addictions"

What better way to start this section than with the confessions of a true chocolate addict? The following are the reflections of my friend Leslie Cabarga:

> *It all starts with a Tootsie Roll®. You know, the small-change kind at the convenience store counter. Just one won't hurt. How could it? I unwrap the little treat and as I put it in my mouth and start to chew, I can't for the life of me recall what would*

have ever possessed me to go on that no-chocolate diet. The inno-
cent chocolate roll is delicious, but certainly not a threat by any
stretch of the imagination.

Time passes. It's about 11:00 p.m. Granted, it's snowing out-
side, but for some reason I really want a chocolate ice cream bar.
Now! So I'm thinking, Ben and Jerry's is such a cool company, and
they use only natural milk (no hormones) in their ice cream bars.
And don't they donate 1 percent of their profits for peace? Surely
they deserve my support. Tonight, it's not about no-chocolate diets!
Nay, tonight it is about me taking a stand, striking a blow
against totalitarianism. I feel emboldened.

I must confess that it briefly occurs to me that I might be back-
sliding into my chocolate habit. But after a few moments of seri-
ous contemplation I still can't remember what I could have
thought was so evil about chocolate in the first place. So in the
interest of supporting Ben and Jerry's admirable company, I
decide I'll purchase and eat just one of their ice cream bars.

The next day I'm in the checkout line at the health food store,
slipping into a state of hypnotic reverie. My breath momentarily
catches, the way it does when I step out of a warm shower into a
cold room as I reach for a towel, hoping to suppress all sensations.
Of its own volition—I swear it's true—my hand edges mysteri-
ously toward an organic chocolate bar. Good wholesome food. It
says so on the package. I'm reminding myself that I am very for-
tunate, taking a moment to silently acknowledge my gratitude
that heroin is not the object of my affection.

I resolve at this moment to allow myself to have chocolate
only once a week—every Friday— as a sort of weekend treat.
Surely that won't be overdoing it!

Then on Saturday I attend a party, and there are chocolate
desserts . . . and they're free. It would be a crime to pass up
FREE CHOCOLATE! No one in their right mind could possi-
bly argue with that. Besides, the generous hostess has worked
hard to make these delicacies. It would be the height of rudeness
to not partake of her efforts.

And then on Sunday they're giving out samples of chocolate
at the Farmers Market. It was a market test. How could I turn
them down? This is not just about chocolate. It's a responsibility
to my community.

The Quest picks up steam. I throw all caution to the winds.
My drive in pursuit of chocolate is stuck on cruise control, and
I'm racing down the freeway at breakneck speed. Where is the
driver in all this? An imaginary finger in the sky points in my

direction. Me? Not me. I'm not driving. Can't tell you who it might be.

Every day—usually at the same time as the day before—The Quest announces itself. Every ounce of my creative intellect is summoned in pursuit of its cause. At every suggestion of a family outing, a digital readout flashes before my mind's eye like the Terminator scanning the scorched terrain for signs of danger. We're going to the Beach. Ah, Ben and Jerry's is right there. We're going to the Mall. Godiva chocolates! We're going downtown. Yeah, great, there's that little bakery on Third Street. And so it goes.

The Quest can endow an ordinary person like me with superhuman powers. Like on my honeymoon trip to Switzerland. Some four years earlier, friends had led me to a particularly fine konfiture shop nestled somewhere in the heart of bustling downtown Zurich. Now, with my bride's hand firmly in mine, and with my nose pointed upward like a bloodhound's, I lead her unerringly up this narrow street and down that one, around this corner—no, I think it was that corner—and right to the doorstep of that chocolate shop where colored marzipan is cleverly formed into every conceivable shape and where the chocolate is so fine the recipe could only have been passed down from God's mother.

I know I'm not alone in my chocolate addiction. Once my second wife and I had a fight. I went straight for my usual chocolate consolation. Moments later I discovered her munching chocolate too. Next time I'll just marry a Hershey bar and eliminate the middle ma'am!

I resolve to go cold turkey and kick the killer cocoa bean. I'll lose weight, have great digestion, a glowing complexion, tons more energy, and a clear mind! My wife scoffs as I hang a sign on the bedroom door—"Five days without chocolate." For three weeks I tick off the days. Three whole weeks, fifteen days!

Then it all starts with a Tootsie Roll®...

There are many theories about chocolate and other food addictions and how they work as weight-gain triggers. It has been suggested that our cravings for certain foods have a biological basis associated with the *neurotransmitters* of our brains, specifically *serotonin* and *endorphins*, and the menstrual cycle, as well as with the actual psychopharmacological effects of these substances. It all comes down to this: our attraction to chocolate is not all in the taste, and it's not all in our heads. It affects us on a profound physiological level, through our brain chemistry, our hormones, and our nervous systems.

Chocolate contains several biologically active ingredients (methylxanthines, biogenic amines, and cannabinoid-like fatty acids), all of which potentially can cause abnormal behavior and psychological sensations similar to those of addictive substances such as marijuana, antidepressants, and analgesics. Also, it has been found that some people use chocolate as a form of self-medication to calm themselves down, to reduce anxiety, and to seek a feeling of well-being. It is a craving that becomes stronger when they have a deficiency in magnesium.

We've spoken briefly of endorphins, which are morphine-like compounds that are normally produced in our brains. We signal their production through many different channels, including eating, meditating, relaxing, and even sex. It is believed that these natural painkillers are produced at lower than normal levels in food addicts, predisposing them to greater intolerance to pain and discomfort. Therefore, anything that gives them comfort, such as eating a particular food, that raises the endorphin level, is sought out whenever they are distressed. An equally plausible explanation is that a particular food has a highly preferred taste and smell.

The majority of self-defined addicts (about 76 percent) maintain that they are either unable to moderate their consumption of their particular addictive food or they cannot stop eating it once they have started. As one addict stated, "Some days a whole cow looks like a normal portion." Chocolate addicts report that boxes of chocolates are particularly irresistible. Once the lid is removed, they could never have just a few chocolates; they would not stop until the whole box was empty. One woman told me that her husband keeps chocolate locked in a safe in their house to keep her from devouring it. Other addicts report extreme means to obtain the food they crave, such as looking through neighbors garbage cans after a party.

One of my clients described the helplessness she felt when confronted by her favorite food: "After one bite I cannot stop eating chocolate. The only thing that causes me to stop eating is if I run out of it and cannot find any more. Nothing short of a gun held point blank against my head could stop a chocolate binge once it starts, and even then I am not sure I wouldn't choose death before stopping."

The Right Bite Program offers solutions to control and eliminate addiction to certain foods in Chapter 8.

Eleven: Fattitudes

Musical composition is a hobby of mine. Several years ago I bought an electronic keyboard that I wanted to connect to my computer so that I could hear music that I composed. Unable to make my keyboard work, a musician friend with the same keyboard sent a nineteen-year-old computer whiz to my home to diagnose my problem and get my computer system up and working. Brad came to my home for several evenings in a row and tinkered with my system. He was massively obese, and although he would ask for sugary drinks and fattening food for snacks during his work, I always offered him healthy options.

Despite spending hours at my home, Brad never charged me for any visit or for making my computer system operational. In gratitude, I offered him my assistance in helping him lose weight. Each time I offered he declined, although he acknowledged that he wanted to lose weight. He had a list of excuses: "I've tried every diet and they don't work," "I don't like to exercise," "I am too busy," and finally he just said emphatically, "I live at home and my mom cooks for me and I don't think she would like it if I did not eat what she cooks."

All such excuses are what I call "fattitudes."

Sheila, a friend of mine, was also obese. She was an attractive, very energetic woman despite her size. One day I asked her why she allowed herself to be so overweight. Her response, "I cannot afford to buy all the healthy food that you need on a good diet." She explained that her husband gave her $400 a month with which to buy food for her family of five. I told her that was not a problem, took out my calculator, and designed a menu on the spot for her and her family—all of whom were also obese, by the way. After staring at the piece of paper, she offered several more flimsy excuses that I easily rebutted.

"Well," I replied, "you just don't want to lose weight badly enough, because I have offered you a diet that is affordable and that removes all the reasons for your past failures. Right now, you are the only obstacle to weight-loss success."

Two weeks later when I saw her, she looked less bloated, and she had a healthy glow. I commented that she looked especially nice, and she told me that she and her husband had started my diet and exercise plan and that they had each lost seven pounds. She was thrilled. After one year she has lost sixty-five pounds, and her husband has reduced his waistline to twenty-nine inches from forty-five.

On her first anniversary of starting the Right Bite Program, she confided to me that she had cried all the way home the day I first confronted her about her weight. When I apologized for making her upset she said, "No, I am glad you approached me. If you had not confronted me about my weight and my excuses, my husband and I would have done nothing about our eating and exercise." She said I gave her a reality check that propelled her to do something once and for all about her weight. She effectively got rid of all her "fattitudes."

Fattitudes are excuses that give you permission to be and stay fat. They are self-defeating attitudes. They constitute a mindset that is not firmly committed to losing weight, even though you may insist that you want to lose it and lie awake nights condemning yourself for being fat.

Fattitudes are convincing saboteurs of our best efforts because when we are in the throes of them we firmly believe they are true. Once established in our minds, fattitudes are indeed difficult to dislodge, but this can be done, and more easily than you think. I have worked with dozens of people who seemed to be trapped by their fattitudes. The Right Bite Core Diet and the exercise and mental preparation programs that go with it, will help you dissolve these old beliefs along with your fat.

Fattitudes isolate people who are concerned about their weight. They cause us to believe that we are alone in our problems and that there is no hope for change. Once isolated in this way, it is easy to fall into self-pity and a why-bother-to-even-try attitude. Have faith. If you are reading this it means that you are still motivated and ready to liberate yourself from the cruel fattitudes that are holding you back. The bottom line is that you *can* and *will* lose weight on the Right Bite Diet because the triggering obstacles to your past weight loss failures have been removed.

And yes, it even includes a plan for ridding yourself of these pesky fattitudes.

Chapter Four

Common Triggers That Almost Sneak by Unnoticed

A mariner must have his eye upon rocks and sands,
as well as upon the North Star.
—Thomas Fuller, M.D., *Gnomologia* (1732)

Some weight-gain triggers almost slip by unnoticed, mostly because they are so commonplace and familiar that you don't even think about them. In fact, it's their very familiarity that can cause you to overlook them. Overlooking them can set into motion a chain reaction that soon has your eating, and your weight spiraling out of control. The more you are aware of these, the better you are able to avoid them and thus eliminate a whole new set of triggers from your life and start dropping the pounds.

Ironically, many of my clients instinctively know what kinds of foods or behaviors trigger their eating binges. For one it might be heavily salted foods. For another, it might be going too long between meals. But instead of simply accepting what they already know and eliminating that weight-gain trigger, they start searching for all kinds of other reasons for their binges. When we finally settle ourselves down and get honest with ourselves, we find that the solution was really pretty simple. What you'll discover is that the weight-gain triggers I list here are far easier to give up than the food cravings, hunger, and overeating that result when you don't.

One: Halt the Salt

I once had a moderately overweight client whose major complaint was sudden inexplicable weekly binges that she blamed for her inability to lose weight. The binges always occurred on Friday night after eating at her favorite Japanese restaurant, a place where the food was prepared by a chef right before their eyes. My client always ordered the same dish, chicken with vegetables and steamed white rice. I suggested that she ask the chef to hold the MSG, a known flavor enhancer and appetite stimulant, and bring her brown rice instead of white. The next Friday evening, Jena and her friends went to the Japanese restaurant, and she did as I had suggested.

Jena ate her meal and, as usual, she became ravenous. Once she'd gotten home she binged. Perplexed, I decided to go the restaurant myself, where I ordered the same meal and like Jena brought my own brown rice. I carefully watched the chef prepare the chicken and vegetables. I was astonished to see that on every single slice and dice, he tossed a salt shaker up in the air that rained salt down on the chicken and vegetables. He must have tossed it twenty-five times, each time quite expertly, I might add. Although it was very entertaining to see this juggling act of flying salt shakers and knives, I instantly realized that this awe-inspiring demonstration was also the source of poor Jena's binging. She was consuming way too much salt, a potent appetite stimulant, especially for her. Unlike so many women who binge on sweets, Jena always binged on salty foods.

Since this revelation, Jena has requested that her Japanese meal be prepared without salt. Her binges have ceased, and she has reached her goal weight. Also, Jena has continued to be vigilant about her consumption of salt, using a salt substitute or using nothing at all. It took her a while to get accustomed to these changes, but now she is quite content to do without her salt.

Scientists have observed what they refer to as "sodium appetite" in healthy individuals who are not deficient in sodium. People who have developed a sodium appetite experience salt cravings and consume foods upon which salt is sprinkled in amounts far greater than their bodies actually need. Researchers believe this appetite is almost like a drug and is not a reflection of biochemical or physiological need.

We do not know exactly why or how salt increases the appetite. Some researchers suggest it is simply because it makes food taste better, so we seek greater pleasure by eating more. Others say that it actually triggers hormonal changes in our bodies, altering the balance between estrogen and testosterone, for example. Other researchers say that sodium affects the sympathetic nervous system. It is safe to say that the mechanisms of how salt can disrupt our bodily functions, our brains and our appetites are indeed very complex and probably affect every one of us.

Even if you are not hypersensitive to salt, salty foods will make you eat more simply because we all tend to seek the pleasure of eating what tastes good to us. I once served two kinds of pretzels and nuts at a party, salted and unsalted. Within less than an hour the salted pretzels and nuts had disappeared, while the unsalted ones had barely been touched. The guests who consumed the nuts had already eaten dinner and couldn't have still been hungry, so it would be safe to assume, I think, that my experiment revealed the powerful salt trigger at work.

Two: Thirst

No discussion of salt would be complete without a discussion of thirst, of course. However, one does not need an overload of salt to experience thirst. How then is thirst a weight-gain trigger? Let me share an anecdote from my own family to illustrate this:

My father, a symphony conductor, frequently gave formal dinner parties for his guest artists. On one such occasion, my parents were entertaining a beautiful soprano at our home. I sat mesmerized by her lovely face and figure and listened star struck to everything she said. Eventually, the conversation turned to how she was able to maintain such a slim figure when she had to travel and eat out so often. "Easy," she said. "I just make sure that whenever I am thirsty, I only drink water, tea, or other beverages with no calories. If I drank juice or a soda every time I was thirsty, I would be huge!"

It didn't take a mathematical genius to see the wisdom in what she was saying. Even healthy juices—to say nothing of soft drinks—can be rich in calories. Now I only drink no-calorie beverages to satisfy my thirst.

Thirst is a potent weight-gain trigger. We can easily consume twice our daily caloric requirement in order to satisfy it. Just one twelve-ounce soda has approximately 150 calories. Some are as high as 250 calories! I am always astonished at the size of drinks served at movies, fairs, and carnivals. Cups are so large they look like wastebaskets. Beer is served in pitchers or glasses the size of bowling pins.

Thirst is also tricky because it often makes us think we are hungry when all we really need to feel satisfied is a glass of water. On a hot humid day, how many times have you turned to ice cream, slushies, popsicles, watermelon, or other liquidy foods? These all add unnecessary calories, when a simple glass of iced water would more than suffice, without the weight-gain triggers contained in the more tempting treats.

Drinking plenty of water can help you control your appetite by quenching your thirst and making you feel fuller. In addition to satisfying some of our needs for simple oral pleasure, it replenishes the watery environment within your body, which carries nutrients to your cells and wastes away from them. Without proper hydration, your body temperature would be unstable, and you would lack the solvents that make it possible for your body to make use of the vitamins, minerals, amino acids, glucose, and other micronutrients that maintain our quality of life.

Three: How Dieters Are Led Around by Their Noses

Although it is common for many of us to experience temporary low periods during the holiday season, no one is more miserable at these times than those with weight-control problems. To these folks, already uneasy about eating, festive occasions can be a source of sheer dread. If you are among this group, you may be quite aware of your apprehension accelerating in intensity as newscasters, retailers, and children start counting down the days to the big holidays.

Thanksgiving, Hanukah, Christmas, and New Year's—all these should be pleasurable to contemplate, but are not for those who worry about controlling their food intake. For them, these impending days of celebration are certain to bring anxiety and a sense of being challenged to exercise superhuman will power. And if that willpower fails to keep them away from all that delicious holiday food, they can fall into patterns of self-incrimination for not being able to control themselves. If they do bow to the pressures of family and friends and summon up the courage to attend a party, it isn't long before they are overcome by an abnormal compulsion to eat—and eat and eat! Not a sugary carbohydrate escapes their salivating attention, and after taking a first bite, it is seemingly impossible for them to stop gorging.

Sometimes, as "mortification insurance," these afflicted souls stuff themselves with healthy snacks or entire meals prior to attending holiday feasts, hoping their turgid stomachs will discourage gluttony. This ploy is often futile. Even if they temporarily succeed in feeling full, their appetites begin to increase rapidly at the sight and smell of food. In just moments, a once-dignified person is transformed into a Jekyll-and-Hyde monster, elbowing aside more mannerly diners in a ravenous campaign to commandeer the dessert table.

Eventually some people become so intimidated by their impulsive eating behavior that they dare not attend any celebrations at all. I have had clients—just nomal people like you and me—confess that the thought of sitting down to bountiful feasts prepared by relatives so challenged them that they adamantly refused to accompany their families anywhere during the holidays. And these are not people who had serious food problems. They are simply people who know their limitations when it comes to being around too much tempting food. Instead, they spend holidays entirely alone. Not only were these vulnerable individuals ashamed to admit that they had uncontrollable eating problems, but their fear was so extreme that they could not express, even to themselves, the enormity of its influence on their lives.

SUBTLE APPETITE CUES

There is a strong connection between hunger and appetite cues, cues that are especially seductive and prevalent around the holidays. We know our bodies are influenced by what we eat, but to gain weight by thinking about food, seeing it, listening to it cook, and smelling it, is a mind-boggling concept! Those of you who insist you get fatter just being around food may be absolutely right. You could indeed be a person who is able to maintain a diet only until you hear the rustle of a potato chip bag.

There's a remarkable study that was conducted at Yale University by Dr. Judith Rodin. She showed that the mere thought of food can start the fat deposition process. In experiments, people were instructed not to eat for eighteen hours. At the end of this time period, blood samples were drawn from people in the study as they were being told they could soon eat the juicy mouth-watering steaks charcoal-broiling before them. Results of these blood tests revealed that in all cases insulin levels skyrocketed, causing blood sugar to be stored as fat and glycogen well before our famished subjects had taken a first bite.

As you may recall, insulin not only makes you feel hungry but can increase your weight by accelerating the conversion of sugar in the blood to fat. Also, the resulting drop in blood sugar accentuates our hunger. Dr. Rodin's experiments are important to all of us because they prove that our bodies are quite capable of pumping out insulin at the mere sight, smell, or thought of food. This rise in insulin and increase in appetite and weight gain from external cues is more pronounced in people who are overweight because of their high body fat.

If you suspect that you are vulnerable to external appetite cues, the Right Bite Core Diet provides easy and effective body-fooling strategies to prevent your pancreas from going crazy whenever an enticing hors d'oeuvre tray passes under your nose.

Four: Lack of Fiber Makes You Wider

In a study published in Lancet, ten people ate three different meals based on apples that each contained sixty grams of available carbohydrates. The meals were apple juice, apple puree, and whole apples. The people reported that they found juice alone to be less satisfying than puree, and puree less satisfying than the fresh, whole apple. From this the authors concluded that "the removal of fiber from food and also its physical disruption can result in easier ingestion, decreased satiety, and disturbed glucose homeostasis which is probably due to inappropriate insulin release." In plain words, the raw whole apple, with fiber intact, was not only more satisfying, it also helped to balance insulin and maintain healthy blood sugar levels.

This study helps us to understand why a low-fiber diet is an appetite trigger. We tend to think of fiber as bran, which is the woody part of grains that is separated from the seed portion of wheat, oats, and other grains and that is valued for its fiber, or "roughage," as it is sometimes called. Fiber is a valuable portion of our diets because it aids in the movement of food through the digestive process.

Bran, such as we get in certain breakfast cereals, is not the only source of fiber, however. We also get it from different parts of nearly every plant: the plant walls, the cereal fibers around grains, pectin (common in citrus fruits and apples), gums and mucilage (gums secreted by a branch of a tree when cut), and lignin (the woody parts of vegetables and small seeds of fruits such as strawberries).

How can high fiber curb your appetite and aid in weight control?

First of all, fiber-rich foods will fill you up much more quickly than low-fiber foods. They slow down the rate at which foods leave your stomach, and they draw water into your gastrointestinal tract, adding to your feelings of fullness. Why does all this affect our appetites? The answer may be simpler than you might think. One factor is found in our stomach's stretch receptors. When our tummies are full, these minute sense organs send their messages to our central nervous systems, our brains. If the stretch receptors are not being stretched enough, even if we have taken in sufficient calories to sustain the body, they protest. The bottom line is that our stomachs must expand to a certain point before stretch receptors will send "NOT HUNGRY" signals to our brains.

Let's take a moment to examine this idea in terms of the humble potato, since it is the most popular vegetable in the United States. Can you chomp down six ounces of chips at a sitting, about nine or ten large handfuls, totaling approximately 900 calories? I know I would not have any problem doing that. In fact, I might be tempted to finish the whole bag! But could you eat, or would you even want to eat, nine five-ounce boiled potatoes, or four and a half ten-ounce potatoes, the caloric equivalent of six ounces of chips? Not only could my stomach not hold that many whole potatoes, but it would also be repulsed at the prospect. I would be far too full. I am sure that after the first boiled potato my stretch receptors would have alerted by brain that I was no longer hungry.

Because my Right Bite Core Diet is high in fiber and nutrients, the stomach can expand until the stretch receptors are happy while calories are kept at a healthy minimum. Having said this, it is very important to emphasize that ingesting bulky, high-fiber foods just to placate stretch receptors will not take away hunger for very long unless that food contains adequate calories and nutrients as well. If the high-fiber food is nutritionless or too low in calories, you will temporarily feel full without really satisfying true hunger and you will soon be experiencing cravings again.

There's a popular belief that if we want to feel full all we have to do is eat large quantities of raw or steamed vegetables, which are high in bulk but low in calories. But every year I see clients who continue to experience hunger with this practice, because the vegetables they were eating failed to provide the nutrients and, yes, sufficient calories to satisfy the body's needs. Replacing a nutritious, high-fiber meal with a head of iceberg lettuce washed down with lots of water makes just about as much sense as gobbling down a handful of grass cuttings to give yourself a feeling of fullness.

Hunger has many faces, and it is important to acknowledge all of them. The Core Diet will teach you what foods to eat to stretch your stomach receptors in a manner that will prevent overeating but will also assuage your body's healthy and legitimate hunger.

There is another way that fiber aids in weight control. Foods high in fiber, such as wheat bran and fresh, steamed broccoli are usually low in fat and simple sugars. So eating them means you are taking in fewer calories per filling bite. In this way, we have the satisfaction of eating what may seem like a large quantity without a lot of calories. One of my favorite high-bulk, low-calorie breakfasts is a delicious bowl of oatmeal and sliced fruit.

A third way that high-fiber foods can help you control your weight is by slowing down your absorption of glucose. The benefit here is that by lowering the rate of glucose absorption you reduce the production of insulin and thus experience only a moderate rise in blood glucose. And as we previously discussed, this means that fat storage is decreased, and our appetites are kept in check.

Finally, fiber speeds up transit time through your digestive tract so that your body absorbs fewer calories. If you think of the food you eat as a train and calories as passengers, it is much easier for passengers to jump off a slow moving train than one going at faster speeds.

To reap all the benefits of fiber, it is important to choose from a variety of whole foods and not rely on processed forms of fiber, such as those you might buy in the form of pills or drinks. A variety of whole foods is important because with them you will be supplying your body with essential nutrients. Also, different fibers have different functions. For example, oat bran, barley, and legumes lower cholesterol, while the cellulose of wheat bran is an effective stool softener. My Core Diet is a high-fiber diet with a wide variety of fiber-rich foods from which to select.

Five and Six: The Glycemic Index and the Satisfaction Index

The Glycemic Index, or "GI," for short, is a system for classifying foods according to their glucose-raising potential. It provides an index for measuring how fast a particular food will raise your blood sugar level. Foods that are low on the glycemic index are the slowest to raise glucose levels. As a result, the corresponding insulin response is reduced, thus improving overall blood glucose concentrations. As you recall from Chapter 3, when your glucose level rises precipitously, your body responds by producing increased insulin—the "hunger hormone" that stimulates the appetite and increases your body's ability to store fat. By lowering the GI of your meals to a healthier level, you should be able to control your appetite and weight more easily. Sounds simple, right? Well, maybe not. In fact, if you just gobble up any food that has a low GI, thinking it will help you control your appetite and lose weight, you just might get exactly the opposite results you are looking for.

Because of the close relationship between the Glycemic Index and the Satiety Index, I have placed them together in this section. In this way you can more readily understand how the two are related.

The GI charts are based on foods consumed alone. But a single food is rarely consumed alone. If you combine foods—which is usually the case—we change their GI values. Beginning to sound complicated? Lucky for you, I've taken all of this into account in the Core Diet, but knowing what's there and why it works is also important, so stay with me here.

There are other factors that affect the glycemic index of nearly every food. These include how thoroughly the food is cooked, the presence of other components, such as seasonings and sweeteners, and the amounts and kinds of fat, sugar, and fiber in the food. As if this weren't complicated enough, there are often wide variations in the GI of the same food. For example, hot, whole grain cereals can range from a low GI rating of 42 to a high of 75. The reasons for these variations has a lot to do with how cooking and processing affects the molecular and physical characteristics of the food, such as particle size. As particle size breaks down, and thus decreases with cooking, the GI increases. Other factors that affect GI are interactions of the starch with the protein in the food and the presence of other components such as molecules that bind starch. The best example of this is the fact that the GI of a potato can be increased by 25 percent just by mashing it.

You may have noticed that some of the bestselling diet books really come down hard on the poor potato, whose GI ranges from 56 to as high as 90 depending on the type of potato and how it is cooked. But Dr. Wolever points out that despite the potato causing one of the highest glucose and insulin responses it also has the highest "satiety value." This means that calorie for calorie the potato is one of the most satisfying foods we can eat. Most people find it at least three times more satisfying than the same number of calories consumed in bread, and up to two times more satisfying than the same number of calories worth of eggs, fish, cheese, or steak.

So what should you do if you want to control your weight? Are you to eat only low-glycemic foods and avoid potatoes and carrots and other nutritious foods that have a higher GI? No, especially because there are low-GI foods that have a high fat content (chocolate and peanuts) and because there are some high-GI foods that may be good choices because they are low in calories and high in nutrition (e.g., carrots). The point is that we don't have to eliminate from our diets all foods that have a high GI. My Core Diet carefully balances GI factors by including healthier, reduced-fat and no-sugar low-GI foods that lower the GI of the *total* meal.

In putting together my Core Diet, I focused particular attention on the satiety value of foods. As any veteran dieter knows only too well, it's no great challenge to figure out which foods contain the lowest calories and eat only them. But then we end up feeling deprived, plagued by cravings that too easily turn to binging. So the real challenge is putting together a diet that is as satisfying as it is slimming. By combining information from the Glycemic Index and the Satiety Index, my Core Diet gives food-conscious people the healthiest options.

Some of the very best research on the satiety values of foods has been done by Susanne Holt, Ph.D. She developed the Satiety Index, a system for measuring different foods' ability to satisfy hunger two to three hours after eating. Dr. Holt found that foods high in fat had the lowest satiety rating on her index. This is because fat increases the palatability of food, and anything that makes food taste better stimulates our appetite. According to Holt, the more fiber, protein, or water a food contains, the longer it will satisfy. The early satiating capacity of a food strongly influences how much we will eat at the next meal or within the next few hours. Holt's Satiety Index (SI) is based on the satiety responses to white bread, that food being rated at 100. With this as our base point, the satiety index for ice cream was found to be 96 percent, or nearly the same as the SI of white bread. Contrast that with the SI of our beloved potato, which is 325 percent, or more than three times the rating of white bread. While baked potatoes can be quite satisfying, the SI rating drops precipitously when they are mashed or fried. That's because in doing so we change the fibrous structure of the potato. So, next time you are hungry, go for the potato, without butter, naturally, if you really want to satisfy your appetite.

CHOOSING FOODS WITH A HIGH SATIETY INDEX

The more satisfying a food feels to you as you are eating it, the more effective it will be in controlling your appetite. Bread, baked goods, and other highly refined foods are consistently the least satisfying foods with the highest insulin responses, whereas fruits, which are high in water content and fiber-entrapped natural sugars will fill you the most.

Holt's SI list includes findings such as the following: brown pasta is more satisfying than white pasta; whole meal and grain bread are more satisfying than white bread; oatmeal and All-Bran® are more satisfying than the other breakfast cereals. In general, simple whole foods, such as fruits, potatoes, legumes (particularly beans and lentils) were the most satisfying of all foods tested. And among meat dishes, fish was found to have a very high SI as well.

Holt found that fatty foods were not satisfying for long, and the covert addition of up to fifty grams of fat to a standard meal failed to increase satiety or stimulate an appropriate decrease in subsequent energy intake. Holt believes this is because our bodies see fat as fuel that should be used only in emergencies, storing it in cells instead of breaking it down for immediate use.

In my Core Diet, I combine the information from the Glycemic Index and the Satiety Index so that you won't have to walk around with charts and a calculator to figure out what you should or should not be eating. You are guaranteed to feel full and satisfied between meals.

Seven: 7 Calories per Gram . . . but Who's Counting?

There is a devil in every berry of the grape.
—The Koran

Alcohol

"Come on, just one little drink won't hurt," urges a thin friend. "How can you get fat by having just one?" Unable or unwilling to resist peer pressure, particularly when her friend's logic is so appealing, dieting Donna sociably consumes a Singapore Sling, and several hours later finds herself wolfing down half a gallon of ice cream and suffering intense hunger. The time-lapse between her consumption of alcohol and the uncontrolled eating episode obscures the causative connection between the two, leaving Donna puzzled and depressed by her seemingly inexplicable behavior.

Alcohol affects everyone a little differently. There are slender people who drink and stay thin and there are overweight people who drink and get fatter. There are also people who lose control of their eating habits when they drink and must struggle to diet away the pounds gained during periods of alcoholic consumption. Why is alcohol a weight-gain trigger for the latter two groups? There are four key reasons:

1. ALCOHOL IS FATTENING

It contains seven calories per gram, making it almost twice as high in calories as protein and carbohydrates, which only contain four calories per gram. Only fat, at nine calories per gram, exceeds the calories found in alcohol. Drink three beers a day, and you have gained an extra 450 calories!

Also, your body reacts to alcohol in a way very similar to what it does when you are eating foods with a high fat content. What happens is that, while your body is burning the alcohol for energy, it is preventing you from burning body fat. Thus, not only does the fat stay on your body, but any calories in the alcohol that you don't burn for energy will be stored as fat. In effect you get a double shipment of fat to send into storage on your body.

2. ALCOHOL IS NUTRITIONLESS

It provides nothing but calories—empty nutritionless calories.

3. ALCOHOL CONTRIBUTES TO MALNUTRITION

Alcohol displaces nutritious food. The more alcohol you drink the less likely you will eat enough food to provide adequate nutrients. Also, alcohol contributes to malnutrition by interfering with your body's use of nutrients, essentially making them ineffective, even when you are eating healthy foods. The vitamins and minerals most dramatically affected by alcohol include: the B vitamins, vitamin D, magnesium, calcium, potassium, and zinc.

Niacin and thiamine (B vitamins) are needed to metabolize alcohol. As a result the available supply of niacin and thiamine is soon depleted because: (a) Thiamine and niacin are water soluble, meaning the body does not store them. You must consume these vitamins daily in an amount needed by your body. Because alcohol accelerates the use of these vitamins, a deficiency would be easy to produce even in well-fed individuals. (b) People who are eating less than optimal diets already have reduced stores of these vitamins in their bodies, so any deficiency of these vitamins occurs quite rapidly.

Thiamine and niacin deficiencies have a profound effect on every cell in your body. Although there may be abundant glucose going past the cells to provide energy for their work, without sufficient niacin and thiamine your cells can't make use of that glucose. Brain cells are especially susceptible to niacin and thiamine deficiencies because they rely solely on glucose for energy. If most or all of the body's niacin and thiamine is tied up in alcohol metabolism, then no energy will be produced, even if there is plenty of glucose.

4. Alcohol Can Cause Low Blood Sugar

There are two ways that alcohol can cause low blood sugar:

1. *Alcohol-induced fasting hypoglycemia:* In my nutritional practice, I have observed, time and time again, that most dieters are chronically malnourished. This is the result of going on and off low calorie diets that fail to provide all the essential nutrients. This condition is further aggravated when alcohol is added to the mix, since it triggers a low blood sugar reaction within six to thirty-six hours after drinking even a moderate amount. In this type of low blood sugar, the alcohol prevents your body from making new blood glucose. The technical reason for this is that alcohol oxidation reduces the levels of blood glucose precursors that are available. So anyone who is on a low-carbohydrate diet or any sort of inadequate diet, is unduly sensitive to the hypoglycemic effects of alcohol. The current popularity of high-protein diets makes alcohol consumption particularly lethal, threatening ones health and one's waistline.

2. *Alcohol-induced reactive hypoglycemia:* This low blood sugar reaction occurs when alcohol is mixed with sugar—namely when soft drinks are

used to dilute alcohol—then consumed on a relatively empty stomach. In this case, the combination of sugar and alcohol *enhances* the body's insulin response to carbohydrates. Essentially, the alcohol fools the body into thinking it has received additional sugar, so it tends to oversecrete insulin. Alcohol imbibed with sweet appetizers or sugary desserts can have an equally devastating effect on the body.

This exaggerated insulin response lowers blood sugar levels because it removes too much glucose from the blood stream. The end result is experienced as an appetite gone wild. In extreme cases, people may even black out. Since glucose is the sole food that nourishes the brain, we experience even the slightest deprivation of this essential sugar immediately. So when loads of insulin are released into the system and our bodies labor to remove sugar from our blood, our brains start emitting panic signals to the body's hunger-control center. It urges us to eat immediately in order to restore normal blood sugar levels.

A normal person who is given a solution of alcohol and sugar will develop reactive hypoglycemia between two and one half and four hours after drinking, and the resultant low blood sugar levels will heighten the intoxicating effects of the alcohol. This phenomenon is not observed when people are given alcohol with artificial sweeteners instead of sugar. The age-old practice of recommending large amounts of sugar-sweetened coffee to sober up is especially dangerous for some people in view of the fact that both sugar and caffeine contribute to a rapid and severe hypoglycemic reaction, including depression, increased appetite, sweating, shaking, and in severe cases, unconsciousness.

The presence of alcohol in our bodies interferes with the ability of the liver to break down its stored sugar into glucose. This makes it more difficult for us to recover from reactive hypoglycemia. The liver's inability to break down its glycogen to make glucose can be especially detrimental when the body has increased glucose requirements, as is the case during physical exercise or when attempting to elevate low blood sugar levels.

Alcohol will also inhibit *gluconeogenesis*, a fancy word meaning the manufacture of new blood sugar. As a result, blood sugar levels will remain low and drop even further unless food is eaten. A drop in blood sugar stimulates a craving for sweets, and once sweets are eaten, the presence of alcohol prods the pancreas into releasing insulin, thus driving the blood sugar still lower. This sets up a vicious cycle, forcing the person to overeat, especially on sweets, in an effort to elevate blood sugar, while at the same time the alcohol-sugar combination stimulates a heavy secretion of insulin to bring blood sugar levels down again.

Alcohol and exercise do not mix! During physical exercise the body's requirements for glucose are heightened. When alcohol is consumed during a period of high activity, it can produce hypoglycemia, even with people who are eating a balanced diet and are otherwise in good physical condition.

Like most people, when I'm at a party I feel more comfortable holding a glass. Maybe social scientists are right in claiming that one reason many people drink socially is to give them something to do with their hands. Or, perhaps a drink or two allows us all to loosen up a bit and let ourselves be silly and have more fun. At any rate, if you recognize that your after-party food binges are triggered by alcohol, try sipping unsugared fruit juices, mineral water, herbal teas, caffeine-free, sugar-free sodas, or plain water. In most parts of the country, where there is an awareness of some people being intolerant or sensitive to alcohol and others being health conscious, these drinks are often served.

A firm "I would prefer not to" (to quote Melville's *Bartleby the Scrivener*) will deter anyone from badgering you into accepting a cocktail against your will. So you don't have to let social pressure or wavering resolve thrust an alcoholic beverage into your hand. And, guess what, you might just discover that you enjoy parties even more.

In your more sober state you'll discover that the people boozing gregariously over drinks are not as fun-loving or interesting as they always seemed after you'd had a few drinks yourself. But the conversations you have with others who are sticking with the nonalcoholic drinks are going to start looking much more interesting to you. The fun you'll discover will be much more satisfying. As our culture moves increasingly in the direction of health consciousness, there's less emphasis on alcohol at social gatherings and more on people making contact and sharing stories about what really matters to them in their lives. Rather than being a deprivation, *not drinking* may just turn out to be a lot more pleasurable, and a lot more fun, than drinking.

Eight: Size of Meals and Frequency of Eating

When I was in high school I tried eating nothing during the day, drinking only diet beverages until I got home from school. I remember tearing down my driveway after the bus dropped me off, throwing my books into the air after I burst into the house, and sliding to the refrigerator like it was home base, where I gobbled indiscriminately and uncontrollably until I was overstuffed. Bloated and feeling guilty, I resolved to eat nothing until the next day, and then, I promised myself, I would only have a small snack after school. I was never able to keep my promise. I ate one huge meal a day for several years, believing I was controlling my weight, yet my weight continued to climb. When I later began studying the nutritional effects of food I learned that one meal a day acts as a weight-gain trigger.

It is not only what you eat, but when and how much you eat that will ensure a slim and healthy body. Research shows that people who consume the majority of their calories in one meal a day tend to weigh more and store more as fat than people who eat frequent small meals throughout the day. Skipping meals can lower your basal metabolic rate so that you burn fewer calories and store more as fat when you do eat.

There is an interesting study by Dr. Susan Roberts, chief of the energy metabolism laboratory at the Jean Mayer U.S. Department of Agriculture Human Nutrition Research Center in Boston. Dr. Roberts found that older women burn fewer fat calories than younger women after eating a large meal. But they burn the same number of calories after eating a small meal. Dr. Roberts concludes that as they age people apparently lose some of their ability to use fat as an energy source if the fat calories come from a large meal. Excess fat from such meals is deposited as fat reserves in the body. So eat several smaller meals during the day rather than one big one. This is a good idea for everyone, of course, but if you are over forty it's especially important.

If you need further proof, consider this study by the U.S. Department of Agriculture: Ten overweight women tried varying eating schedules as part of a weight loss regime. For three weeks they ate most of their daily calories by 11:30 in the morning; for another three weeks, they ate additional meals in the afternoon and evening. They also exercised throughout the day. Although the early-morning eaters lost slightly more weight, women who took in additional calories throughout the day and evening maintained more lean body mass. Lean body mass burns more calories, so in the long run this translates into greater fitness and ability to maintain your weight loss. This makes sense. By late afternoon, those who finished consuming their calories by 11:30 a.m. were forcing their hungry bodies to resort to protein catabolism to supply energy. What that means is that they were drawing from their own protein reserves, found in muscle tissue, to supply their energy needs. Not only does this cause us to feel hungry, which often gives way to binging, it reduces lean body mass and slows our metabolism so that we burn fewer calories, making it easier to gain weight.

There are so many benefits from eating more frequently that virtually any person interested in both health and weight management should be doing it. A major benefit is that it reduces the insulin and glucose responses after each meal. This may be because of what's known as the "Staub-Traugott effect," in which the closeness of one meal to the next partly determines our glycemic response at the second meal. In other words, the closer together the meals are, the better our glucose tolerance and the less insulin our bodies will release. Meals that are rich in fiber enhance the Staub-Traugott effect. The fiber in one meal improves carbohydrate tolerance, reducing the insulin reponse to the second meal, presumably by distributing the nutrient load between the two meals.

When there is too much time between meals, blood sugar will begin to drop. If our bodies don't get food at that time, glycogen reserves are called upon to release glucose. Then, as these reserves are exhausted, our blood sugar plummets, and we start experiencing hunger pangs and other undesirable symptoms, such as lack of concentration and mood shifts. When we do finally eat, we usually overeat.

Taking these factors fully into account, my Core Diet provides guidelines for eating at least three meals and two snacks a day so you will never feel hungry.

Nine: Coping with Natural Cycles

Accuse not Nature, she hath done her part; Do Thou but thine!
—Milton, *Paradise Lost*

If you are a woman trying to manage your weight, the chances are that you've already noticed how your menstrual cycle influences your eating habits. In fact, the monthly cycle is one of the most pernicious weight-gain triggers most women must deal with. To better understand this weight-gain trigger, you need to know something about how your menstrual cycle affects your nutritional needs. If you are a man with a wife, girlfriend, mother, daughter, sister, or best friend, then an understanding of how the menstrual cycle affects her eating will definitely make life easier for you. So don't skip this chapter just because you think it doesn't apply to you! You can be one of her greatest supporters if she is trying to diet or feeling unhappy about her weight.

It is about two weeks prior to your period, during ovulation, that we are most concerned with here. It is at this time that your estrogen production falls and progesterone is secreted in increasing quantities. Progesterone causes deposits of fat and glycogen to build up within the inner lining of your uterus. The purpose of this is to store nutrients for the egg, should it become fertilized. If the egg fails to be fertilized, the production of both estrogen and progesterone decline to low levels about two days before the end of your menstrual cycle, prompting the menstrual flow to begin once more.

During the first half of the menstrual cycle, and prior to ovulation, when your estrogen levels are high and your progesterone levels are low, your mood is enhanced and your energy is high. The second part of the menstrual cycle occurs after ovulation and is dominated by progesterone. During this phase, physiological changes occur that can have a powerful influence on how you eat. You have an increased appetite, you crave sweets, your body starts retaining more water, and your breasts enlarge. Depending on your size and metabolism, you will be able to eat 200 to 500 more calories per day than you normally would without gaining fat weight. This is because your metabolism is more active after ovulation, thus burning more calories. Water retention might cause a temporary weight-gain but this quickly normalizes as your period ends.

If we analyze the diets of women during their menstrual cycles, we find that their carbohydrate consumption increases by about 50 percent in the two weeks before their period. Women instinctively raise their caloric levels after ovulation by increasing their intake of carbohydrates. And yes, it is true, that our female hormones have something to do with our cravings for sweets. Fortunately or unfortunately, we women crave sweets much more than men do. It is one of the mysteries of life, but we can speculate that since our bodies are equipped for procreation, it is nature's way of ensuring that we will eat enough carbohydrate-rich foods to nourish a growing baby.

It is easy to understand why women would tend to eat more two weeks before menstruation since our bodies are metabolically more active at this time. At the opposite pole, estrogen inhibits appetite. Since we have increased quantities of estrogen prior to ovulation, which decreases after ovulation, we tend to eat less.

Changes in a woman's glucose tolerance also occur between ovulation and menstruation. Progesterone, secreted in increasing quantities after ovulation, alters the normal insulin response that regulates blood sugar, resulting in a greater tendency for hypoglycemia (low blood sugar). Those who have weight-control problems should not overlook this fact, for a low blood sugar reaction is almost certain to cause an intense craving for sweets.

Progesterone also slows down the movement of food through the gastrointestinal tract because it decreases muscular contractions that push food through the entire digestive system. This is one reason why most women feel so bloated during this part of the cycle.

Most dieting women believe they must stubbornly adhere to a certain daily caloric limit no matter how hungry or how ill they may feel, and they become guilt-ridden if one stray morsel exceeding this count should cross their lips. For this reason, it's important to keep in mind that once ovulation occurs, changes in your metabolic rate, glucose tolerance, and estrogen levels all necessitate caloric and nutrient changes.

If you ignore these changes and strenuously refrain from eating enough, or you resist your natural craving for essential carbohydrates, you are battling with your body's healthy needs. Because of your instinctual desire to obtain extra calories when you are metabolically more active, you may become so hungry that you overeat. In worst-case scenarios, I have seen the same cycle repeated every month, with women starting each cycle with strict dieting and ending with virtual orgies of overeating.

Although it is common to weigh slightly more during your pre-period week, and this varies greatly depending on your size and individual hormonal factors, do not panic. This temporary elevation in your weight does not reflect fat weight gain and will disappear once your period begins. This natural increase in weight stems from the normal increase in the uptake of sodium following ovulation. Scientists speculate that this may be nature's way of increasing your blood volume in anticipation of creating new life. Also, carbohydrates cause temporary water retention, contributing to false feelings of fatness. Just because your scale registers a little temporary water weight gain, don't be frightened into cutting back on calories when you need them the most. It is far preferable to raise caloric intake somewhat, ignore your scale, and resign yourself to feeling a bit puffy rather than set yourself up for a future eating binge because you fought your body's energy and nutrient needs. To cling to a suboptimal caloric level after ovulation not only starves the body, prohibiting it from operating at maximum efficiency, but also sets you up for health problems as well. When your diet is inadequate, menstruation can become irregular or cease altogether. There's also some evidence that under-eating during the menstrual cycle can contribute to the development of ovarian cysts.

The Core Diet will show you how to eat in a cyclically controlled manner so that you will not be fighting your body's normal and healthy needs. Many women following the Core Diet find that they reduce or even eliminate their premenstrual cravings and other uncomfortable symptoms they previously associated with their menstrual cycle. Attempting to restrict calories at a time when your body requires additional calories imposes stresses on your body, which contributes to PMS.

Warning! Do not use your natural preperiod changes as an excuse to overindulge. The weight gain you might then experience during this time would not be temporary. Discipline and common sense during the monthly cycle will definitely pay off, both in terms of keeping your food cravings manageable and in terms of rewarding you with a thinner figure.

Ten: Calories Too High

Most people are aware that overeating makes you fat, and that high-calorie food is a common weight-gain trigger. We certainly don't need to elaborate on this. Or do we? Do we take in more calories than we can burn because of certain weight-gain triggers that encourage us to do so, or are there nontrigger factors that cause us to take in more calories than we can burn? Although I know of no one whose difficulty regulating caloric intake is unrelated to weight-gain triggers, I can't say for certain that this is impossible. There may be people in this world who can eliminate every weight-gain trigger in their life and still have a problem regulating their weight. There could be actual physical damage to the appetite control centers in their brains. Or perhaps there are genetic anomalies that cause their obesity.

The Right Bite Program addresses this problem in a twofold manner: first by providing a trigger-free plan for those of you whose appetite is caused by weight-gain triggers, and second, by showing you how to calculate your caloric needs for maintaining or losing weight and providing guidelines for developing a calorie-controlled diet.

Eleven: Obesity

One of the most significant insights for many of my clients has been the realization that being overweight is itself a weight-gain trigger. While it's true that we have to succumb to perhaps many other weight-gain triggers to become overweight in the first place, once we've put on the pounds we have literally embodied our nemesis. We can't easily escape the weight-gain trigger that is most problematic for us because we have become it. That's the bad news; the good news is that when we address the issue this way and apply the Right Bite principles, we also become our own solution. Let's explore some examples:

When she was single, Sara watched her weight carefully, and her dress size always remained small. After she was married, however, she relaxed a bit and gained a few pounds every year. When she first got pregnant she was only ten pounds overweight, and during pregnancy she was careful about what she ate, though she also enjoyed eating anything she wanted. In the course of her pregnancy, she gained fifteen pounds. After the baby came, her weight stayed about the same, though she had returned to the same eating habits she'd practiced prior to her pregnancy. Despite the fact that she was eating more moderately, she could not get the weight off. Her own body was fighting her every effort to slim down.

Sara's situation is not unusual. Whether because of gains during pregnancy or indiscretion in our eating, we can't get around the fact that obesity itself becomes a weight-gain trigger. And it is a trigger for both men and women, by the way. Hunger itself is greater the heavier we are. Researchers at Johns Hopkins University maintain that people can have perfectly normal metabolisms when they start life, and can be thin for years. But once the pounds start creeping on, the resulting overweight metabolism makes getting back to their lower weight difficult. It is at this point that we discover the real power of the Right Bite Core Diet, which helps us reset our body's metabolism so that we can go back to our ideal weight.

If you are severely overweight or obese, don't just give in and join the currently popular strategy to "accept your body just as it is and don't worry about eating right and exercising." As you may already know, there is a glut of books on the market advocating this philosophy. Why have they become so popular? Undoubtedly because the problem of overeating or eating too many calorie-laden foods—primarily fast foods and convenience foods—has gotten so out of control in this country. The popularity of such philosophies is rooted in the very human tendency to accept problems as they are when we do not believe there are solutions. Certainly there are times in life when we do need to face the fact that we can't change things and so must learn to live with them as they are. For example, we can't do a whole lot to change our height, skin color, or eye color. If we suffer a terrible accident and lose a limb, we must come to terms with that, and if a loved one has died we can't change that, so must learn to live with how our lives are changed as a result. But everyone who wants to can do something about their weight. There are alternatives to accepting solutions such as the following, which so many books recommend:

✓ Accept your body as it is and forget about diets because diets don't work.

✓ You can't help being fat because you have the fat gene, so learn to love your body exactly as it is.

✓ You are fat for reasons presently beyond your control. These reasons and their solutions are yet to be discovered by scientists or psychologists.

It's easy to buy into any of these "give-up solutions" because it is true that no diets work that depend primarily on severely restricting calories or on a specific single food type, such as meat protein. Until we address weight-gain triggers, as only the Right Bite Core Diet does, the overweight person is going to be struggling with cravings that undermine even the toughest resolve.

Time and time again, I have consulted with people who complain that they simply can't accept themselves as obese, no matter how many books tell them it's okay. The fact remains that they are not comfortable with their fatness. If it's not physically uncomfortable being fat, it is a cold, hard fact that society does not accept us this way and will let us know every time we walk down the street, apply for a job, look at a magazine ad, turn on the TV, go to a mall, or squeeze into an airline seat. I don't know how many clients have told me that in the final analysis they believed that accepting their obesity was nothing but a big cop-out.

Maintaining your ideal weight is like anything in life that you want very badly. Most of us have to work for it. Believe me when I say that all the tools for success are at your fingertips. The obstacles that appear to be hindering your weight loss may presently feel insurmountable, but they will dwindle to molehills on the Right Bite Program as you control and eliminate the weight-gain triggers that have made you fat.

LEARNING FROM OUR DIETING HISTORIES

To better understand the relationships between obesity and weight-gain triggers, I'd like to share the experiences of a former client. As we journey through her history, I will note the name of her weight-gain triggers so that you can see the role they played in her obesity.

As a teenager, Ann had been slim and athletic. But after marriage and motherhood, she puffed up to as much as 195 pounds. Naturally, she became self-conscious about her figure. She remembered when she weighed 115 pounds, but even then she had felt dissatisfied when she saw pictures of models who were 5'10" and weighed 100 pounds. To Ann these models seemed to have everything in the world a woman could possibly want. So she started dieting, and this was where her weight problems began. (*Weight-gain triggers: Reducing below one's true set point, primitive brain, fattitudes.*)

At first Ann followed the latest fad diet her friends were following: reduce calories and drink high protein drinks. (*Weight-gain triggers: Calories too low, insufficient nutrients, stretch receptors, transient hypoglycemia, low SI foods, primitive brain.*) After only one week, her body, deprived of necessary calories and nutrients, rebelled, and Ann started binging, which was a new experience for her. (*Weight-gain triggers: Calories too low, insufficient nutrients, hypoglycemia, sugar, high glycemic foods, hyperinsulinism from spree foods.*) At this point, her muscle protein was already being catabolized, causing a shrinkage of her lean muscle mass, so that fewer calories were burned.

Ann entered college and was increasingly determined to lose weight despite the problems she was having. She learned about fasting, and fasted any time she went on an eating spree, returning the next day to her self-designed, low-calorie, high-protein diet. *(Weight-gain triggers: Primitive brain, fasting hypoglycemia, stretch receptors, specific dynamic action of food, calories too low, insufficient nutrients.)*

She was delighted to see her weight drop to her prespree levels, but the damaging unseen internal changes of fasting hypoglycemia had already crept in. Ann felt drained and hungry, so she began drinking diet colas with her first meal. *(Weight-gain triggers: Fasting hypoglycemia, reactive hypoglycemia, caffeine, meal size and frequency.)* Jittery, hyper, and ravenous, Ann would binge on sweets and salty junk food. *(Weight-gain triggers: Hyperinsulinism, high glycemic index foods, salt, reactive hypoglycemia, poststarvation hyperphagia, insufficient nutrients, seeing, smelling, thinking of food, lack of fiber.)* She could not understand why she never felt full though her insides were about to explode. *(Weight-gain triggers: Reactive hypoglycemia, hyperinsulinism, sugar, salt.)* Little did she know that the onslaught of sweets raised her blood sugar too high, and her body became hyperinsulinemic in a valiant effort to lower her blood sugar levels. The combination of high insulin and reactive hypoglycemia made Ann very hungry. All the internal changes that were initiated when Ann first began her diet were still stealthily progressing so that when she binged on sweets, many calories were deposited in fat cells.

Ann desperately tried to undo the damage of her latest spree by fasting again, but this time the scale did not return to its prebinge level. *(Weight-gain triggers: Primitive brain, calories too low, hypoglycemia, insufficient nutrients.)* Somehow Ann managed to go back on her diet without another binge the next day. However, she was bewildered. She was not losing weight very quickly, and when she did, she felt drained and sick.

Poor Ann was now fatigued all the time, yet managed to do well in college. Diet colas and strong coffee got her through finals. *(Weight-gain trigger: Caffeine.)* While these temporary spurts of energy from the caffeine helped her meet her academic challenges, she was nearly always hungry and tired. She started eating once a day, packing all her allotted calories into that single meal rather than spacing them out throughout the day. *(Weight-gain triggers: Meal size and frequency, thermic effect of food, calories too low, insufficient nutrients.)*

Ann decided she needed to exercise. She met someone who ran four miles in thirty minutes and thought that person had a terrific body. She tried running four miles herself but after only a few days of this she was exhausted, ravenous and sore. *(Weight-gain triggers: Overexercise, incorrect exercise.)* By the following week she decided to give up exercise until she felt better. *(Weight-gain triggers: Lack of exercise.)*

Time passed and Ann became increasingly lethargic and light-headed. She was also constipated. She wanted to speed up her weight loss and decided her constipation was preventing this. It never occurred to Ann that she was constipated because she was consuming inadequate fiber and also retaining water. Ann took a laxative and a diuretic the night before she weighed herself. *(Weight-gain triggers: Laxatives, diuretics.)* Although she felt absolutely horrible the next day, she was thrilled to see that she had lost three pounds. She decided that she would always use diuretics and laxatives the night before she weighed herself. What she didn't know was that the diuretics and laxatives were depleting her body's store of essential nutrients and electrolytes. Ann began to feel and look like a zombie. She and her friends chalked it up to the long hours she was studying.

Gradually, Ann got her weight down to 120 pounds, which she felt was fairly acceptable—at least for now. She maintained her weight only with great effort, sometimes fasting, sometimes going on high protein diets, always counting calories. In her senior year, she met Andrew and they were soon married. Ann worked part time at first, but she immediately became pregnant and quit her job. When she told her doctor about her dieting patterns, the doctor prescribed a standard nutritional diet with vitamin supplementation, which Ann followed carefully while she was carrying her baby. Her doctor became somewhat concerned when Ann quickly gained more than twenty-two pounds in her first trimester. The doctor monitored her weight carefully and in the week before Ann's daughter Sierra was born Ann weighed 180 pounds.

While nursing Sierra, Ann followed the diet her physician had given her, reducing it by a few hundred calories per day. It was only through careful discipline that she kept her weight below 165. As soon as she stopped nursing, Ann went back to her old ways, desperately wanting to be thin again . She set a goal to limit her intake to less than 1000 calories per day. She completed two consecutive 800-calorie days and began to feel optimistic that she could now be successful. *(Weight-gain trigger: Primitive brain, incorrect mind exercise, insufficient calories, insufficient nutrients, fasting hypoglycemia, stretch receptors.)*

After doing well on her diet for several weeks, the holidays rolled around. She and Andrew had not attended a social gathering for months, so he urged Ann to accept an invitation to a Thanksgiving party in their neighborhood. Though reluctant, she decided to go, mostly to appease Andrew. She purchased a loose blouse with a holiday print and wore it over black pants she'd worn during her pregnancy. Then she fasted the whole day of the party. *(Weight-gain trigger: Meal frequency, fasting hypoglycemia.)* She did not want to eat just before going because she would feel fat. *(Weight-gain trigger: Primitive brain.)* Plus, she wanted to be able to have something to eat and drink at the party.

As the hour of the party approached Ann felt increasingly nervous. Would people think she was fat and whisper behind her back? *(Weight-gain trigger: Stress.)* At the party she nibbled from a tray of raw vegetables, wishing she were not on a diet as she watched friends eating all the rich holiday foods. *(Weight-gain trigger: Seeing, smelling, thinking, hearing food.)* There were all kinds of warm drinks to enjoy around the fireplace, so Ann had an Irish coffee. *(Weight-gain trigger: Alcohol, sugar, caffeine.)* Boy, was she hungry now! She soon found herself stationed at the dessert table busily sampling one of everything. *(Weight-gain trigger: seeing, smelling, thinking hearing food, calories too low, marginal malnutrition, alcohol, caffeine, hypoglycemia, insulin.)* She was off and running! She moved away from the dessert table, gobbling down handfuls of chips—with clam dip made with sour cream. (Ann craved fat because of insufficient fat in her diet.)

Alarmed by her behavior, Andrew gently took his wife aside and asked what was happening. All she knew was that she felt disgusted with herself and told Andrew to take her home. At home, she craved foods high in sugar, salt, and fat—and consumed them ravenously. The next day, when she stepped on the bathroom scale, the dial spun around to 168 pounds!

Ann now thought that weighing 130 pounds didn't seem so bad at all. In fact, that was close to what she'd weighed when she'd met Andrew, and he had liked how she looked, even if she didn't. She rationalized that this was probably her true weight and decided to diet down to 130 instead of continuing to shoot for 115 pounds. She felt better thinking she just had 38 pounds to lose instead of 53.

When Andrew went out of town for a week-long training session for his company Ann decided she would "blitz" off some weight on a 500-calorie diet. *(Weight-gain trigger: Speed of weight loss, calories too low, insufficient nutrients, meal frequency.)* She reasoned that she should be able to maintain 500 calories for the week Andrew was gone, and when he returned she would resume a more normal diet. *(Weight-gain trigger: Fattitude, primitive brain.)*

The first two days went well. She lost five pounds. She felt encouraged. On the third day she was feeling weak, light-headed, and ravenous—and it frightened her that she was getting impatient with Sierra, who was crying more than usual. Ann broke her diet with a huge chef's salad with lots of dressing and crackers. *(Weight-gain trigger: Fat.)* She reasoned that it was better to break a diet with a salad and good food than with a pile of sweets, which was what she really wanted. The next day Ann climbed on the scale and the dial spun up to 178 pounds. She was devastated. She did not know that consuming large quantities of fat was actually worse than consuming large quantities of carbohydrates since our bodies store fat much more easily.

For over a year, Ann's eating habits fluctuated between periods of restrained eating (*Weight-gain trigger: Calories too low, hypoglycemia, insufficient nutrients*) and periods of overeating (*Weight-gain trigger: Hyperinsulinism, reactive hypoglycemia, poststarvation hyperphagia.*) At the end of the year Ann's weight had ballooned to 183 pounds. She now hated how she looked and felt like an utter failure. Moreover, she was certain her husband was starting to hate her as much as she hated herself. (*Weight-gain trigger: Primitive brain, fattitudes.*) To make herself feel better she made friends with people who were all overweight and who also felt and acted like her.

Andrew's concern grew as he noticed Ann's expanding weight and depression. He and Ann spoke often about this, and she considered going into counseling. She got a referral from a friend and attended her first counseling session. Her therapist asked her lots of questions and told her that it might take years to discover the root cause of her overeating, but meanwhile, to help her cope with her depression, he put Ann on an antidepressant and an appetite suppressant. (*Weight-gain trigger: Medication, appetite suppressants.*)

Ann continued her therapy sessions and from time to time was convinced that they were helping. She also continued her pattern of undereating and overeating. Nothing changed, except she was still gaining weight and now her therapist suggested that hidden conflicts with her husband might be causing her problems. Ann used to think that Andrew and she had a pretty neat relationship. Not now.

A year and a half after starting therapy, Ann weighed 157 pounds. She was taking antidepressants and appetite suppressants. She dragged herself around like the living dead, too lethargic to exercise. She spent hours watching TV, eating potato chips, dip, and other snack foods. She slept any time Sierra would allow it. (*Weight-gain trigger: Lack of exercise, high fat, medication.*) Andrew and she grew increasingly distant.

Ann felt totally defeated in every area of her life, so she decided to stop dieting and eat whenever and whatever she wished. She found that she still binged once a week, but was rather pleased to discover that she was eating less now that she had given herself permission to eat. She was alarmed, though, when her weight climbed to a distressing 186 pounds.

Ann decided to eat more low-fat snack foods and consume artificially sweetened soda and ice cream. (*Weight-gain trigger: Artificial sweeteners, diet foods.*) Her weight continued to increase, and she was hungry all the time.

She soon topped the 190-pound mark. A friend talked Ann into trying a popular diet program but she had trouble staying on it. Most menus were easy to follow, but after eating the diet drinks recommended she felt hungry and tended to overeat. *(Weight-gain trigger: Caffeine.)* The program did not recommend exercising, so she remained as sedentary as having a year-and-a-half-old child will allow. *(Weight-gain trigger: Lack of exercise.)* Worst of all, she didn't lose an ounce on the diet, while her friend lost over fifteen pounds.

Ann believed she had those fat genes people talked about. She resigned herself to always being fat. Ann's weight stabilized with this decision. She basically ate whenever and whatever she wanted and was pushing the 195-pound mark when she came to see me. The first thing she told me was that she accepted herself the way she was.

"Really I do," she insisted. "I am finally resigned to it and happy."

Resigned maybe, but happy? I didn't think so.

Ann's Escape from the Self-Perpetuating Cycle of Obesity

Ann's road to recovery began when she started reflecting on her past diet history and identifying the weight-gain triggers that had transformed her metabolism into that of a fat person's. With the Right Bite Core diet, she started losing weight right away, and continued to lose it steadily. She was amazed and pleased to discover that she had excellent energy and no longer suffered from the gnawing cravings that once caused her to binge.

One of Ann's most important insights had to do with fat itself as a weight-gain trigger. She learned that when any man has at least 24 percent body fat, and any women has more than 30 percent body fat, their body fat itself is the big weight-gain trigger that must be addressed. Unless we are able to recognize this fact, addressing one or two weight-gain triggers at a time will do very little good, and in fact, as we've seen, may only magnify the problem. When obesity itself becomes the trigger, lasting change can come only by addressing the whole person we are, with all our past history around food and eating. Ann changed her life and ultimately changed her metabolism, so that today she thinks, acts, and eats like the 115-pound person she really is. This process of education and transformation of her body began with the following realizations. Obesity itself becomes a self-perpetuating weight-gain trigger because:

✓ Basal metabolic rates have decreased following years of undereating (along with binging.) The body has slowed down to adapt to the chronic caloric and nutrient deprivation.

✓ Lean body mass has decreased, augmenting the decrease in the basal metabolic rate. Muscles burn calories, so the more you have, the more calories you burn.

✓ Lipoprotein lipase, a fat-depositing enzyme is present in higher levels in those who have imposed strict dietary restrictions. Whenever that person tries to eat normally, fat is deposited at an abnormally rapid rate.

✓ People who have become obese frequently do not exercise, or when they do they do so incorrectly or not long enough. They are not motivated to exercise because they find it extremely difficult to move the huge amount of weight they carry about, and because of embarrassment at being seen in public. Ever noticed how it is mostly lean people who attend health spas and that obese people look out of place there? The same overweight people may also labor under the misconception that diets without exercise are sufficient.

✓ Insulin resistance: Obese people are notoriously insulin-resistant. You may want to review what this means. First of all, recall what insulin normally does within the cells of your body. After a meal, it is released automatically. It then enhances the uptake of glucose, fatty acids, and amino acids, packing your cells with these. Insulin is intended to help your cells maintain normal balances of blood glucose and stimulate protein synthesis, glycogen synthesis in your liver and muscle, and fat synthesis.

Insulin resistance is a consequence of obesity. Obese persons require much more insulin to maintain normal blood sugar. As body fat increases and fat cells enlarge, they become sluggish in responding to insulin. As fat cells enlarge, they resist insulin, making it harder for excess glucose to enter. As a result, excess glucose remains in the blood longer than normal and rises still further. The excess glucose stimulates the frustrated pancreas into producing even more insulin—much more than is needed under normal circumstances to bring soaring blood glucose levels down to normal.

When the fat cells finally respond, a tidal wave of glucose floods into the fat cells and is stored as fat—too much fat because of the exaggerated level of insulin. To make matters even worse, these same swollen fat cells are also less sensitive to other hormones that promote fat breakdown.

Carbohydrate craving is accentuated when you are insulin resistant. Because adipose and muscle cells are unable to take up glucose easily, the obese person's cells continue to be hungry for glucose. Furthermore, because glucose is unable to enter cells, brain serotonin levels do not rise and the carbohydrate craving is intensified, causing the person to binge on sweets and other carbohydrates.

✓ Hyperinsulinism: People who are overweight tend to have higher insulin levels. Insulin is secreted in response to food but also in proportion to body fat. The more fat on your body, the more insulin you release. You will recall from reading about insulin earlier that its nickname is the "hunger hormone." So, just by having larger fat cells you will secret more insulin and feel hungrier, making it difficult to maintain a diet. Even if you maintain a diet, the higher insulin levels make fat loss more difficult for you than for someone with lower levels of fat because insulin prevents the breakdown of fat by inhibiting hormone sensitive lipase. Insulin also activates lipoprotein lipase, an enzyme that promotes the removal of fat from the bloodstream and its deposition in fat cells. To make matters worse, insulin levels are more elevated in overweight people, both in the fasting state and in the fed state. In other words, people who are fat are metabolically ready at all times to store whatever they eat.

✓ Fattitudes. Some people who are obese just do not have any desire to really lose weight. They may feel they want to be slender but they don't feel like making conscientious efforts to make the necessary changes to lose the weight or maintain a healthy weight once they do succeed in taking it off. They also have lots of excuses for why they are overweight, ranging from having to resolve old childhood conflicts to arguing that it is genetic— "Mom and my grandma were fat, too!" Losing and maintaining a healthy weight requires permanent changes in one's eating, exercise, and attitude. For some people this challenge outweighs the comfort or security of keeping things just the way they are.

Losing and maintaining weight is like anything in life that we might want very badly. Most of us have to fully open our eyes to what has to be done—and then do it. Believe me when I say that if you really want to find your perfect weight and maintain it, you will succeed with this program. In the pages ahead, you will find all the tools you will need to create the changes that you are seeking and will ultimately achieve exactly the body weight that you want.

Chapter Five

Heat-Seeking Missiles— Triggers That Seek Our Unique Hot Spots

As I see it, every day you do one of two things:
build health or produce disease in yourself.
—Adelle Davis, *Let's Eat Right to Keep Fit*

Weight-gain triggers can be as individualized as your fingerprints. You might never find a single other person in your life who reacts quite as you do to a particular food, food-related substance, or even a behavior that triggers your appetite. It's important to know this when you are trying to identify your own weight-gain triggers, since you might have to do a little detective work on your own to accurately pinpoint what your unique triggers are. I offer you this chapter in the interest of giving you a head start in this process. As you read this chapter, you might once again be reminded of how important it is to honor your own individual responses.

One: Nicotine

With certain smoke-sensitive people, nicotine acts as an appetite weight-gain trigger—even when it comes in the form of secondhand smoke. One of my clients, a college student, loved dancing and after she had completed her studies would go to a nightclub to dance. However, instead of returning home sleepy and ready for bed, she complained of feeling hyperactive and ravenous and would frequently binge. Sara didn't drink alcoholic beverages or drinks with sugar or caffeine. She just drank water. She also felt that the dancing was not strenuous enough to stimulate her wild post-dancing appetites.

In addition to the food binges, the day after dancing she always experienced what she described as a "gluey, fuzzy head." She claimed that as a teenager she used to go dancing frequently at a nightclub called Hullabaloo, where she never had any problems controlling her appetite and was content to return home and have a moderate-sized snack. She said no alcohol or cigarettes were allowed at that particular club. Because the only variable was that the nightclub she now frequented was filled with cigarette smoke, I believed that my client's problem was nicotine-related. I confirmed my belief when Sara attended a wedding reception in a smoke free hall and danced the night away without overeating afterward.

While reviewing the literature on the effects of cigarette smoke on our eating patterns, I was astonished to find a huge body of research showing that smokers had lower body weights than nonsmokers. Furthermore, when smokers quit, they tended to return to the weight they would have been had they not smoked. All that research almost made me want to run out and light up a cigarette. Almost—but not quite. Instead I dug deeper, hoping to find what happens to smoke-sensitive people, fat or thin, who may or may not be smokers. This is what I found:

1. Experiments were conducted with healthy individuals and with diabetics to determine if smoking affected blood sugar levels. It was found that in every case smoking a cigarette induced a rapid rise in blood sugar, followed by an unnatural drop. During oral glucose tolerance tests, smokers had higher blood glucose levels than did nonsmokers early in the test and lower values after two hours. Controlled trials were also run, in which it was shown that denicotinized cigarettes did not alter the smoker's blood sugar levels, whereas cigarettes with nicotine did destabilize blood sugar levels. The conclusion was that nicotine caused erratic fluctuations in blood sugar levels for all the people who participated in the test. It is believed that this happens because nicotine stimulates the release of epinephrine.

   If you are smoke-sensitive, and your blood sugar becomes abnormally elevated as a result of breathing cigarette smoke, you may notice that this reaction temporarily makes you feel more alert, animated, and not at all hungry. The reason for this is that a nicotine-induced rise in glucose signals your brain that you do not need to eat. Conversely, when the effect of the nicotine wears off and your blood sugar plummets, your body reacts with an intense craving for something to bring your blood sugar levels back to normal.

A rapid drop in blood sugar, with its accompanying appetite and withdrawal symptoms, is more than most smokers (particularly dieting smokers) care to tolerate. Rather than eating, they dull their appetite with another glucose-stimulating cigarette. So in addition to the addictive properties of nicotine, a fluctuating blood sugar level contributes to the pattern of chain-smoking.

It is no coincidence that many people feel hungrier after exposure to tobacco smoke, since the fumes, even when breathed by a nonsmoker, can raise havoc with blood sugar levels. After leaving a smoke-filled room where the lungs have steadily absorbed nicotine and other poisonous ingredients of tobacco, the innocent nonsmoker often experiences a drop in blood sugar. Without the smoker's recourse of another cigarette to temporarily quell a mounting appetite, the nonsmoker, often bewildered and ashamed, succumbs to a binge for which there seems to be no physical explanation.

2. According to another test by R. and J. Wurtman, nicotine increases appetite in another way. Like carbohydrates that we eat, nicotine increases brain serotonin secretion. Withdrawal from nicotine decreases it. Serotonin, you will recall, is a neurohormone in the brain that inhibits our carbohydrate cravings. Therefore, exposure to nicotine fosters satiety and "positive subjective responses," in short, feelings of happiness. Withdrawal promotes hunger and discomfort.

3. Cigarettes may also indirectly cause overeating by depleting the body of vitamin C. Serum levels of vitamin C are significantly lower in smokers than in nonsmokers, and this difference is not related to how much vitamin C they take in. This means that either less vitamin C is available for utilization by smokers, or smokers utilize vitamin C differently. Research has shown that each pack

of cigarettes can produce a deficiency of at least 500 mg of vitamin C.

Vitamin C plays a wide variety of roles in our bodies, including a crucial involvement with norepinephrine and serotonin—the latter being especially active in inhibiting carbohydrate hunger. It is not surprising that any deficiency in vitamin C, on which these neurotransmitters are so dependent, can produce signs of fatigue and hunger.

4. Tobacco smoke also causes fatigue because it depletes the body of oxygen. When you smoke, or are exposed to cigarette smoke, red blood cells that carry oxygen to the brain, as well as to the rest of the body, preferentially pick up carbon monoxide, a dangerous gas given off by cigarettes. This causes a shortage of oxygen in the blood stream, thereby depriving your brain and your body of that essential element.

The spongy tired feeling in your head after attending a smoky party, even when you have consumed no alcoholic beverages, is probably due to insufficient oxygen reaching your brain. You are essentially suffering from what I call a "cigarette or smoke hangover." In an attempt to throw off this heavy feeling, it is not uncommon to resort to appetite stimulants such as caffeine and sugar.

Studies of the effects of nicotine on habitual smokers show conflicting results, causing the speculation that many smokers develop a tolerance to tobacco through its chronic use. In addition, not every person's blood sugar will drop after being exposed to cigarette smoke. These variables in individual response may explain why some people overeat after being subjected to cigarette smoke, while others remain unaffected.

For those of you who are afraid to quit smoking because you have heard that you will gain weight, there is good news. As mentioned earlier you will gain weight up to the weight range you would be in if you did not smoke. Other research has shown that quitters who gained excessive weight and quitters who reported stable weight had significantly different health habits, both before and after they quit smoking. Those who did not gain weight were already trying to eat and exercise sensibly, whereas those who gained weight had poor eating and exercise habits.

Weight gain is not inevitable. By following the Right Bite Program, you will establish good eating and exercise habits, be able to quit smoking and control your weight. If you are already a smoke-sensitive non-smoker, then it is important that you avoid cigarette smoke.

There are many non-weight-related reasons to quit smoking, not the least of which is the cancer connection. But in addition, most people who wish to maintain a slim figure want to look attractive. Most people would agree that there is no faster way to ruin your good looks than to take out a cigarette and light up. Not only is a cigarette hanging off your lip unattractive, but there are also all the facial grimaces that go with nursing the smoke into your lungs and out again. I once thought a woman sitting across from me in a restaurant was in labor after watching her agonized facial expressions. She was not. She was merely smoking a cigarette.

Smokers wrinkle earlier and have more wrinkles than nonsmokers. This is believed to be due to chemicals in the smoke that prematurely age the skin, of which there are more than 4000, including forty-three carcinogens and more than 400 other toxins! Also, because cigarette smoke causes blood vessels to constrict, less blood reaches the skin, depriving it of an adequate supply of oxygen and nutrients. Anyone with eyes can see that the skin of nonsmokers looks more taut, soft, and wrinkle-free than the skin of smokers. And as smokers age this difference becomes ever more striking.

Two: Speed of Weight Loss

Some of the most popular food plans, the ones that always get dieters' serious attention, are the ones that promise fast weight loss. This includes fasting diets and high-protein diets. The rapid weight loss is largely due to loss of water in the tissues, and any pounds lost after the initial blitz tend to be from the muscles. Whenever you go off these kinds of diets, you will always not only regain the pounds you lost but gain additional ones—and with lightning speed. And as if this were not enough, the weight you'll gain will be all fat, so you will actually look worse than you did before you went on the diet.

All dieters want to get their weight off fast. Television ads lure innocent dieters into their programs with testimonials by beautiful people who claim to have lost ten or more pounds the first week. However, I have observed a weight loss principle that has always been true: *Fast weight loss results in faster weight gain.* I have never found a single exception to this principle in my practice. It is actually faster to lose weight slowly because you only have to do it once. People who lose weight fast lose the same ten pounds over and over and over again and never progress beyond a certain critical threshold in their weight.

Your body reacts to fast weight loss as a stress because of the radical changes in eating, exercise, and other behaviors associated with this practice. All the natural mechanisms that defend fat and promote its storage are activated and go into high gear. Your metabolism slows down, lipoprotein lipase levels and its activity increase, serotonin levels decrease (causing hunger), muscle mass shrinks, glycogen stores are reduced, and low blood sugar is experienced, also causing hunger. The end result is disastrous—overeating and a rapid weight gain plus additional pounds due to your more sluggish metabolism that has suddenly become more efficient than ever at storing fat.

The Core Diet is not a fad diet and weight loss will occur gradually but consistently, at a pace that will ensure that those pounds stay off permanently. You'll not just be losing weight you will also be learning to create a whole new relationship to food.

Three: The Thermic Effect of Food

Have you ever noticed that after you eat you sometimes feel hot? This is the result of what is called the thermic effect, associated with metabolizing the food we eat. The heat we feel after eating is how we experience the energy required to digest food, and absorb, transport, metabolize, and store nutrients. As all this is occurring, we are actually using some of the energy we receive from food to digest and process what we've just eaten. In fact, we use about 10 percent of whatever calories we eat just to process the food we consume. If we eat 2000 calories a day, the thermic effect burns up about 200 calories.

Some foods have greater thermic effects than others. Carbohydrates offer the greatest thermic effect, fat offers the least. While the thermic effects of the food you eat is not a weight-gain trigger in the sense of it stimulating your appetite, it is a factor that bears close scrutiny if you're to meet your weight goals. Take advantage of the fact that eating carbohydrates, particularly in the form of fresh fruits and vegetables, triggers the burning of more calories, not simply the storage of more fat.

The thermic effect is difficult to trace in other people, but I know best how it works for me, in my own life. For example, during the holidays I confess that I give myself permission to indulge a bit. And, yes, I confess, I periodically do so when there isn't anything to celebrate. It's fun and normal to indulge ourselves in this way from time to time, though if you are practicing weight management you learn to do it consciously, with full awareness of what you will do to get your weight back to normal in the days following.

Some years ago, motivated by scientific curiosity, I began weighing myself carefully before and after these holiday eating sprees. What I found surprised me. I never gained the amount of weight that I felt I should have, given what I'd eaten. I did observe, however, that when I overindulged on fatty foods, my weight went higher than when I ate mostly carbohydrates—and I'm not talking about grapefruit here. I'm talking about Aunt Mary's delicious holiday cookies. In the latter case—eating carbohydrates rather than fatty foods—my body was making use of the thermic effect of foods. This lesson has been a valuable one to pass on to my clients, for by choosing foods that have high thermic values, and avoiding fatty foods with low thermic values, they are able to enjoy special events and partake of some of the holiday foods without spiraling out of control.

The Core Diet makes the maximum use of the thermic effect by encouraging you to eat a healthy calorie level divided into three meals and at least two snacks a day. The result is a high level of satisfaction and sense of fullness, with all nutritional needs carefully balanced to avoid the pitfalls of other diets.

Four: Set Point Weight

Donna came to me at a hefty 160 pounds. For a woman of 5' 4", this was a lot of weight to carry. She had not been able to reduce her weight even though she was exercising moderately and eating what she considered to be a balanced diet. She neither overate nor binged, nor did she have any particular cravings. She described herself as "just a normal person who needed to lose about thirty pounds." She came to me wondering if she should just take her doctor's advice, which was to accept her present weight as normal for her, that is, her "set point weight."

After quizzing Donna about her diet and exercise plans, we came to the mutual conclusion that she had several weight-gain triggers that were affecting her ability to lose weight. In addition, the idea the doctor put in her mind, that she was already at her set point weight, programmed Donna to believe that her present weight was normal for her and nothing in the world was going to change that. Donna's physical exercise regimen included strenuously jumping around in front of her TV while she played her aerobic exercise tape. The trouble was that soon after exercising she became ravenous. I encouraged her to stop the aerobics for the time being and instead walk briskly for twenty minutes, three times a day. I discuss the reasons for doing this in Chapter 10.

In the first week of following our newly worked out plan, Donna lost an astonishing six pounds, which of course was largely water, but the improvement in her overall appearance was dramatic, and she was encouraged. Her face and eyes no longer looked puffy, and her pants at her waistline were not quite so snug. Donna continued to drop weight steadily, and eventually reached 122 pounds, which was eight pounds less than she had ever been in her life. She has held her weight at 122 pounds but says that if it falls below that she feels fatigued and tends to eat more. From this we concluded that Donna's true "set point" weight was 122 pounds, not 160. The Right Bite program that Donna and I worked out for her eliminated several weight-gain triggers, but the biggest revelation for her was the one about her set point weight. Through the program, she discovered her true set point and was astonished to find that it was far lower than she had ever weighed in her adult life.

Our set point is the point above which we tend to lose weight, and below which we tend to gain weight. Most research seems to indicate that our set points are determined by genetic and environmental factors. The body sends out signals to establish, regulate, and maintain our set points, defending a particular set point weight whenever it is challenged. Experiments have shown that when people are made to overeat so that they gain weight, they spontaneously lose any weight they've gained when they return to normal patterns. Many overweight people erroneously believe they are at their set point weight when they are actually far from it. They come to this conclusion about their set point because they have not been able to reduce without rapidly regaining those lost pounds. The erroneous belief that they are at their set point actually becomes a weight-gain trigger for those people. Working with such clients over a period of months, we soon find that it is not their set point but their diets that are making it difficult for them to find their true set point and maintain that particular weight. However, until they gain this new insight, they find themselves harnessed to the false set point number and so remain overweight.

Keep in mind that your true set point is determined by your body's inherent set of checks and balances, which seek a specific weight. For most people, it is not these internal regulators that encourage them to overeat, but dietary habits such as suboptimal calories, inadequate nutrients, and caffeine and other destabilizing agents. Also, when you are at a certain weight for a year or more, your body temporarily adapts to that weight by developing all the systems needed to sustain it. Accordingly, your body tenaciously defends this weight, and any drastic decrease in calories will set defense mechanisms into action to keep things as they are.

If you go on a quick weight-loss diet based on low caloric intake, you will never achieve your true set point weight. In a study at Harvard Medical School, Jeffrey Flier, M.D., found that thirty-three obese patients who had lost 18 percent of their weight on quick weight-loss diets had enzyme levels that were nearly the same as those they'd had prior to their weight loss. You may remember from our previous discussions that the enzyme lipoprotein lipase increases the rate of fat deposition. What this all comes down to is that the person who loses weight by drastically restricting calories alone actually boosts this enzyme's activity when she follows low-caloric diets. Bottom line? You guessed it; when she starts eating more normally, these enzyme systems pack away the fat. In addition, all the systems that were in place for handling a larger body are still present following the quick-weight-loss program, now triggering the body to eat more to make up the loss.

With weight reduction achieved on a nutritionally and calorically adequate diet, you will ultimately reach your own, unique biologically true set point weight. Below this point, your body will rebel by overeating or by manifesting abnormal psychological and physical symptoms, such as depression, headaches, and lethargy. You might think you are doing yourself a favor but you're not. Reducing your weight below your true set point is always going to act as a weight-gain trigger.

The Right Bite Program will allow you to achieve your slimmest healthy weight—your set point. Your set point on the Core Diet will not be a fat weight. Weight loss will occur steadily on this nutritionally sound and adequate caloric diet. Once you are at your true set point weight, however, trying to reduce further will act as a weight-gain trigger.

Five: The Fat Gene

I had a thirty-year-old pen pal from Lithuania. Jura was eventually able to come to the United States to visit for a year. After she had been here for several months I asked her what she thought of America—what had made the greatest impression on her. Her response took me by complete surprise, as I expected her to heap praises on our lovely country. Instead she said, "Everyone here is *fat*. Even other Lithuanians who have lived in America for a while are fat. You never see fat people in Lithuania. Now I hear about this fat gene that makes everyone fat. What! All my friends come to America and 'catch' this gene and get fat now?"

Although you can't *catch* the fat gene, scientists have pinpointed some rare genetic flaws that make some people fat. These defects do their damage by *slightly* slowing the body's use of calories. There may be anywhere from eight to thirty genes that can contribute to obesity. While it is probable that no single gene causes obesity, people who inherit several such genes are likely to have a tendency toward having weight problems. Even so, researchers have found little or no evidence that these fat genes exist in any great numbers in obese humans or that they contribute significantly to being overweight.

Perhaps more myth than reality, the fact remains that *the very idea* of possessing a fat gene can be a weight-gain trigger. However, as often as not, the trigger can be traced to learned behavior rather than genetics.

If one of your parents is overweight, you have a 40 percent chance of being overweight. If both your parents are overweight, your chances are 80 percent.

I used to blindly accept the idea that fat genes could affect our weight until I hired Melanie, a nineteen-year-old to assist me one summer. She was 5'8" and 180 pounds and very large boned. Upon learning that I was a nutritionist she said that everyone was overweight in her family and that she had been fat for as long as she remembered. As Melanie went about her day, I couldn't help noticing the way she ate. She would frequently arrive at my door with candy bars and malts. She ate sugary cereals for breakfast and pizza for lunch. During her spare time she would lie on the couch and read bridal magazines since she was getting married in a year.

One day I heard Melanie sigh out loud and say how she wished she could be slimmer for her wedding. I casually remarked that she should try eating right and exercising for the summer and see what happens. Although she thought it was hopeless, she began to follow the Core Diet and started taking walks in her spare time. By the end of the summer she was down to 154 pounds. So much for fat genes!

Several years ago I was invited to the housewarming of a family whose various members were all quite obese. I had watched the children grow up, wondering if they would become overweight like their parents. By the time three of the children were ten they were all overweight. The fourth child, Ramona, remained fairly thin up to her early teens, and I thought she was going to escape her family's destiny of fatness. When I went to the housewarming, Ramona had recently turned seventeen, and I was saddened to see that she too had become obese.

After seeing Ramona I decided to do a little sleuthing. I wondered what kinds of foods a family whose members are all obese would keep on hand in the kitchen. I slipped unnoticed into the kitchen and began opening cupboards and the refrigerator and freezer. Everywhere I looked I found high-fat foods or huge quantities of sweets, ranging from ice-cream to pastries and cookies. Glass jars lined the counter, filled with an assortment of candy. Chocolate milk and sugar-rich sodas filled the refrigerator shelves. I thought that perhaps all this food was for the housewarming, but the hostess never served these foods to the guests. The closest thing to vegetables that I found were frozen French fries. The experience was quite sobering. Ramona had never even had a chance. She was surrounded by foods that supported obesity.

Today I am convinced that a genetic inheritance is not destiny and should not be used to rationalize being overweight. In fact, many skinny people have been found to have the defective fat genes and most fat people do not have them. This mere biological susceptibility to being overweight can be overcome by healthy diet, exercise, and a good attitude. There is an unfortunate tendency for people to believe that genetic factors absolve them of personal responsibility. Be assured that if you have a genetic tendency toward being overweight you are not doomed to a lifetime of obesity. You merely have to be a little more vigilant than someone who does not have this tendency.

Fat genes exert themselves in two ways: physically and psychologically. First of all, if you are one of the rare people who actually possesses one or more fat genes, your body will have a slightly greater tendency to gain weight than a person without those genes. But don't get carried away with the impression that you are powerless in the face of it. You're not. Your *belief* that fat genes are in control of your life, even more than your actual genetic makeup, is the trigger you need to address if you really want to be thin. The truth? With or without these genes, you don't have to be fat.

My visit to the party given by my overweight friends provided a valuable lesson in these issues. My conversations with a number of the members of that family convinced me that the prevailing attitude among them was that since their fatness was due to their genes, there was nothing to do but accept it. As one person said, "You can't fight biology! So you might as well go with it." As near as I could tell, these people not only weren't fighting biology, they were immersing themselves in a virtual sea of fatty and sugary foods. And there were frequent comments in the family about the "family genes," and how, if you're going to be fat anyway you might as well enjoy yourself.

The combination of having fat genes, or just laboring under the myth that you do, plus eating any way you choose and not exercising, all comes together to create about as powerful a weight-gain trigger as I can imagine. But I have to say that I have never met an obese person— fat gene or not—who was unable to lose weight with my program.

Six: Additives

Food additives should not elicit feelings of fear and anxiety when they are listed on a package, but rather feelings of caution. Additives consist of antimicrobial agents (to keep food from molding or getting bugs), antioxidants (to prevent food from going stale), nutrients, food coloring, artificial flavors, and flavor enhancers. These are added to some foods in order to extend their shelf life, make them safer, more visually appealing, more palatable, or to "improve" them in some other way. It is the flavor enhancers that concern me the most, because these seem to be triggering taste bud stimulators for some people.

There are over 2000 flavor enhancers—the largest single group of food additives. The downside of flavor enhancers is that they stimulate our taste buds and our appetites, making food much more appealing than it would be if left alone. This contributes to what I refer to as "pleasure eating"— eating to satisfy a sensory need and not true hunger. You may remember a potato chip ad that challenged, "Try to eat just one!" That's a perfect example of how flavor enhancers can affect us. How many times have you felt quite full but kept eating just because the food tasted so good? It is probable that you were a victim of flavoring agents and enhancers.

One of the best-known and most popular flavor enhancers is MSG, commonly associated with Asian foods but also used in hundreds of "convenience" foods. I have observed that certain people suffering from weight problems react to monosodium glutamate (MSG) by overeating. Research has demonstrated that mice that were fed MSG became obese. Following a glucose load, there was an increase in glucose deposited in the fat tissue of the mice given MSG. By four months of age, fat stores were increased by 45 percent above normal levels. That would be like a 120-pound woman gaining fifty-six pounds in four months. Perhaps the increased glucose deposition caused the mice to eat more because of lower blood glucose values. What is baffling is that many diet products contain MSG. This is a wise move by the manufacturer, since it makes the food more palatable—and the more their food is consumed the more money they make. If manufacturers really want to help dieters, however, they would leave out the flavor enhancers and make their diet products a little less enticing.

Several years ago, a client of mine had been very successfully losing weight on the Right Bite Program and had identified several weight-gain triggers that had caused her to lose control and overeat in the past. She was doing so well that she decided to add some treat foods to her diet. She found a potato chip that was oven baked instead of fried in oil, as most potato chips are. The caloric value was about half that of the fried chips, so she decided to buy some.

For the first couple times she ate the chips, she was okay. But then she called me one afternoon to tell me that two nights before her appetite had spun out of control and she could not seem to satisfy her food cravings. She was horrified and fearful that the program had ceased to work for her. It was then that I asked her if she'd added anything to her program lately. Yes, she had added the baked potato chips, but she had only been eating the recommended amount to keep her calories in check.

I asked her to find the bag of chips and read me the ingredients. She did. There, at the end of the list of what the chips contained, written in fine print, were two innocent looking words: "monosodium glutamate." MSG! I told her what was happening and suggested that she get rid of the remainder of these chips, find a substitute that had no MSG, and that was low in salt, and test to see what would happen. She did this and reported back the following week that she was back on track with her program.

The Core Diet is free of MSG and avoids most prepackaged and processed food. It also encourages enjoying foods that are whole and as close to their natural state as possible. Your taste buds, your internal mechanisms, and your newly slimming figure will be delighted!

Seven: Diet Products

Grocery stores and health food stores are filled with low-fat and low- or no-sugar foods. Here is a partial list of these:

1. Low-fat cheeses
2. Low-fat or no-fat chips
3. No fat cereals
4. Low sugar or fruit juice sweetened jams and jellies
5. Low-fat or sugar-free cookies
6. Low-fat or sugar-free ice cream and yogurt
7. Sugar-free chocolates and other candy
8. Low-fat or no-fat mayonnaise and other spreads

Many of these foods can lull us into a false sense of security and can even sabotage our efforts to lose weight. For example, researchers have found that some people who favored foods containing sugar substitutes, such as no-calorie sodas, made up for the loss of sugar calories by eating an average of 11 percent more fat. Other people who read "low-fat" or "low-sugar" on a label think it gives them a license to eat as much as they want of that product without consequences. Consequently, they may consume more calories in sugary and fat stuff than they might have with regular food that didn't make such claims.

The fact of the matter is that many of the foods that are marketed to dieters have about the same number of calories as their regular counterparts. Just check the labels and you'll quickly discover that "no-fat, low-fat, low-sugar," or "no-sugar" does not mean no or low calories. Next time you are in the supermarket, notice that foods you have seen on the shelves for years and years suddenly have labels blazing claims such as "low-fat" or "no sugar added." Often these are in bright yellow, pink, or red lettering—yet the ingredients and calories are exactly as they were when you were a child.

Your fat cells love overeating of any kind, regardless of what the label on the package says. Once your meal total exceeds 600–700 calories, the excess calories, even from nonfat foods, will be stored in your fat cells, especially when you overeat before bed. There is little your body can do to burn off the calories during sleep.

Secondly, because most of these items are snack foods, many of us like to eat them instead of healthier whole foods such as fruits, vegetables, and grain products.

Lastly, since many "low-cal" foods are also "low-fiber" foods, in addition to being calorically dense, nutrient sparse, and delicious, it's easy to eat too much. A handful of unfilling low-fat pretzels is equivalent in calories to a bowl of more satisfying and nutritious oatmeal. One low-fat cookie can range from 80 to 150 calories—the equivalent of a glass of skim milk or an apple. Have you ever tried to eat just one cookie? One half cup (4 oz.) of sugar-free, fat-free frozen yogurt or ice cream runs anywhere from 90 to 120 calories, the equivalent of two cups of strawberries. And would you be satisfied by just four little ounces of frozen yogurt?

Food companies have more recently come out with substances that replace fat. One of the most popular new snacks on the market is a fat-free potato chip that really tastes fried. Also, there are butter flavor sprays that have no calories. When used wisely, many of these products can help you control your weight. When used unwisely, they can be powerful weight-gain triggers. For example, wise use of a low-fat diet product would be eating a baked potato with no-fat sour cream and butter flavoring rather than with real butter and real sour cream. You will avoid hundreds of calories and still feel satisfied. Unwise use of a diet product would be eating low-fat cookies without taking into account that while they might be low in fat they are still high in sugar. Also, there is a tendency to eat more of a low-calorie food just because of the erroneous perception that it isn't going to be fattening. I can't tell you how many clients I've had who binged on low-calorie cakes and cookies that they kept on hand just in case they had a craving for sweets. One woman ate fifteen low-calorie cupcakes from her freezer before even waiting for them to fully defrost. Total intake added up to more than 1000 calories.

The Core Diet does not eliminate all diet products, but educates you on how to incorporate them into your food plan so that they aid, not retard, your ability to control your weight.

Eight: Medication

One of my clients had surgery three years ago, and a month or two afterwards she came in for an appointment with me, distressed that in spite of her surgery she was gaining weight. "I am the only person I know who *gains* weight after surgery," she said, "Everyone else I know *loses* weight!"

I asked her if she was still on any kind of medication. She was: a steroid drug and a pain medication. After consulting my medical references, we quickly determined that both medications had increased appetite and weight gain as potential side effects. I suggested that my client ask her doctor if she could cut back, discontinue, or find alternatives to these drugs. As it turned out, she was able to completely discontinue them over the next three weeks, after which her appetite and her weight quickly returned to normal.

The above case is not an isolated one. Few of my clients have surgery but many do take medications of one kind or another, whether over-the-counter or prescribed. For that reason, I always ask them about any medications they are taking during our initial interview. I am convinced from these interviews that this decade should be called the Decade of Medication. It seems that we are becoming increasingly reliant on medication to ensure that body parts that formerly worked very nicely by themselves continue to work effortlessly. We drink caffeinated beverages during the day to give us pep rather than going to bed earlier when we are tired. We drink alcohol or take sleeping pills or tranquilizers to unwind or fall asleep, rather than exercising or giving up the coffee, sugary foods, and cigarettes that contribute to our tension. Rather than eat a high-fiber diet, we resort to laxatives to ensure that we have a daily bowel movement. Rather than watching our intake of difficult to digest foods, we devour greasy spare ribs and carry a bottle of antacids in our purse. We consume too much salt, often contributing to high blood pressure and edema. Not to worry— we have diuretics and blood pressure pills for that.

All this pill-popping is bound to affect us adversely since there is no such thing as a medication without side effects. None of them are 100 percent safe. Most medications have consequences other than those for which they are intended. If you are having difficulty controlling your eating and your weight and you are currently taking any kind of medication, over-the-counter or by prescription from a doctor, it is important to explore the ways that some medications can act as weight-gain triggers, and what you can do about it.

Medications can cause malnutrition by interfering with food intake. Others influence appetite, alter our sense of taste or smell, cause irritation in our mouths or intestinal tracts, increase or decrease saliva, or induce nausea or vomiting. Some drugs increase food intake and lead to undesirable weight gain. Also, the food we eat can enhance, delay, or reduce the absorption of certain drugs. Conversely, drugs can enhance, delay or reduce the absorption of nutrients. The worst offenders for causing weight gain are psychiatric drugs, antihistamines, antihypertensives, and steroids.

PSYCHIATRIC DRUGS

I cannot give you brand names of all drugs that can cause problems in this category. But here are the generic names of drugs commonly prescribed for depression and other emotional difficulties that are known to affect weight gain: amitriptyline, bupropion (9–13 percent weight gain to be expected); phenelzine sulfate, paroxetine, clomipramine, and alprazolam (2–27 percent weight gain possible). Luckily, a weight-gain response to one drug doesn't mean you will react the same way to any of the others, so talk to your doctor if you are on one of these drugs and you notice a weight gain. Be particularly clear with your physician if these drugs are being recommended and you also have concerns about your weight. As I tell my clients, I'd hate for you to be taking a strong antidepressant because you are feeling depressed about your body weight, only to discover that one of the side effects of that drug was that you would gain even more weight.

ANTIHISTAMINES

Newer antihistamines seem to be particularly prone to causing weight gain. They are popular because they don't make you feel drowsy. Unfortunately they can affect the part of your brain that controls appetite. Two such drugs are *astemizole* and *loratadine*. Older antihistamines are probably your best bet but they are more likely to cause drowsiness.

ANTIHYPERTENSIVES

Blood pressure drugs can often cause us to gain weight because of how they affect our kidneys. Any change in kidney function can lead to water retention, frequently resulting in edema. Some antihypertensive drugs cause weight gain without inducing water retention, though the mechanism is not clearly understood. *Guanadrel* has been reported to cause weight gain in almost half of everyone who takes it. Because drug reactions are very individual, don't be discouraged. Talk to your doctor about switching to an alternative if you are gaining weight or unable to lose it. Other drugs that you might try include methyldopa, guanethidine, betaxolol, and pindolol.

STEROIDS

I am not referring to anabolic steroids that give you a bodybuilder's physique but corticosteroids that are used to treat asthma, arthritis, and allergies. They cause weight gain in a number of ways:

✓ By causing your body to retain water

✓ By increasing your appetite.

✓ By causing your body fat to be redistributed to less flattering parts of your body, such as your face or hips.

Some of the drugs that fall into the above category are: prednisone, beclometh diprop, and flunisolide.

Steroid drugs such as leuprolide acetate, nafarelin acetate, and danazol, are used to treat endometriosis. These drugs can cause weight gain because of water retention or increased appetite.

Tolmetin sodium, a nonsteroidal drug used to treat arthritis, can also cause weight gain.

OTHER DRUGS

On the previous pages, I discussed four categories of medications that cause weight gain because of their direct and immediate effect on one's appetite or water balance. The following is a list of medications that act as weight-gain triggers by another route—*through their effects on the quality of your nutritional status.* (I've also included alcohol since many people use it like a medication, to calm down, dull their worries or anxieties, or to simply feel a little better than they presently do.) In most cases the impact of these medications on our bodies may not at first be noticeable but over time they can be devastating. This process is a little like soil erosion—you don't notice it until you can't grow crops there any more. The gradual depletion of certain nutrients is subtle but it becomes increasingly significant over time until your health and your energy levels decline and your appetite flies out of control.

✓ **ALCOHOL:** Causes deficiencies of the B vitamins, vitamin D, calcium, potassium, magnesium, and zinc.

✓ **ANALGESICS:** (Many drugs contain salicylates, aspirin being the purest form of it.) These drugs can cause deficiencies of thiamine, vitamin C, and vitamin K. Long-term use of aspirin lowers the amount of folate in the blood and causes iron and potassium losses through occult blood loss—which simply means low levels of concealed blood loss caused by the salicylates themselves.

✓ **ANTACIDS**: They can increase the excretion of calcium and phosphorus and may accelerate the destruction of thiamine. Depending on the type of antacid, magnesium, iron, and vitamin A absorption may also be compromised.

✓ **ANTIBIOTICS**: Antibiotics interfere with your absorption of amino acids, folate, fat-soluble vitamins, vitamin B12, calcium, copper, iron, magnesium, potassium, phosphate, and zinc. These drugs increase your excretion of niacin, potassium, riboflavin, and vitamin C. They destroy vitamin K-producing bacteria and thus reduce vitamin K production.

✓ **CAFFEINE**: (Found in coffee, some teas, and some soft drinks, also contained in many drugs, such as some analgesics, cold medicines, diet pills, and drugs to prevent drowsiness.) Caffeine inhibits the absorption of iron and accelerates calcium excretion.

✓ **SEDATIVES (BARBITURATES)**: These drugs increase the rate at which folate, thiamine, and vitamins D, B12, and C are used by the body.

✓ **CHOLESTEROL-LOWERING MEDICATIONS**: These may cause the decreased absorption of vitamins A, D, E, K, plus folate and iron.

✓ **ANTI-INFLAMMATORY MEDICATIONS—STEROIDS AND CORTICOSTEROIDS**: These drugs cause an increased excretion of protein, potassium, calcium, magnesium, zinc, vitamin C, and vitamin B6. They cause an increase of sodium in the system and water retention.

✓ **DIURETICS**: These drugs cause you to excrete potassium, calcium, sodium, magnesium, chloride, thiamine, and zinc.

✓ **LAXATIVES**: (effects vary with type) Laxatives reduce your ability to absorb glucose, fat, carotene, vitamin D, calcium phosphate, and potassium, plus they increase the excretion of all unabsorbed nutrients.

✓ **ORAL CONTRACEPTIVES**: They reduce your absorption of folate and lower your blood concentrations of vitamins B2, B6, B12, C, and folate.

Because of the tens of thousands of drugs available, it is impossible in a book of this kind to list all medications, their biochemical pathways, and their nutritional consequences. But be aware that all drugs have both positive and negative side effects, all of which can have an impact on your health as well as your weight. Take any drug only when medically necessary. This holds true whether the substance is prescribed by a doctor or purchased over the counter, and whether it falls into the category of mainstream medicine or "natural," as in herbs or tinctures.

What can you do if you are taking one or more medications and are trying to lose weight? Start by checking with your doctor to make sure that the medications you are taking are really necessary. Then inform yourself about how the medication works in your body and what effects it might have on your nutritional status. Ask your physician, druggist, or health consultant about the nutritional impact the drugs you are taking. Or do your own research on the Internet.

When a medication is dispensed to you, ask the pharmacist for the brochure that accompanies the medication. Brochures such as this, prepared by the company that makes the drug, listing the known side effects, are required by law. More recently, pharmacists are required to discuss any newly prescribed medication with you and answer any questions you might have. You may also wish to check out the *Physicians' Desk Reference* (PDR), which gives complete information on every drug prescribed today.

If you know that a drug causes you to excrete a certain amount of a vitamin or mineral, you can at least partially counteract this, in most cases, by taking a vitamin supplement to make up the deficit. Always make certain you are eating a diet that is nutritionally dense, with adequate calories, and that tastes good to you. By following the Core Diet that I describe in Chapter 8, you will be optimally fortified if you are taking most medications.

Nine: Diet Pills

I first learned about diet pills during my freshman year at college. In my dorm was a girl who was about fifty pounds overweight when she arrived. But as the weeks passed I also noticed that she became thinner and thinner. Her behavior also became increasingly strange. Whenever I would get up in the middle of the night to use the rest room down the hall, I always noticed this girl wandering about in what seemed like a daze or trance. By the end of the quarter, she was really thin but she looked hollow-eyed and would make yipping sounds like a dog with a tick in its ear.

Since I still had a few pounds to lose myself, I decided to ask her how she managed to lose so much weight. She told me she had used diet pills and took out little white pills that had an X marked on them. I asked her if I could sample one as I thought I would get more of these if I liked them. She handed me one of her little white pills and as a precaution, I only took one half of it. Well, I certainly did not feel hungry and had more energy than I ever had in my life.

Full of energy that Friday evening, I went dancing at nine o'clock at a discotheque (as they were called then) and friends told me that I was dancing so hard they thought I would bore a hole in the floor. When I returned home in the early hours of the morning, I was unable to sleep. In fact, I could neither sleep nor eat for three days. When the pill wore off I was scarcely able to get out of bed the next week, and boy was I hungry! I ate everything I could get my hands on.

I would never take diet pills again. I later learned that what I had taken was an amphetamine, which was illegal. I remember thinking that I could never run for a political office now because someone might find out I'd "used drugs," and nobody would ever vote for me. As for the young lady— she flunked out of school her first quarter and I never saw her again.

Although diet pills are considered a medication, I am discussing them under a separate heading because of their popularity. There are many weight-loss drugs on the market and more being developed every day. With the proliferation of diet pills, one would think we would be a nation of thin people. But we are not—we are a nation of fat people, with obesity reaching epidemic proportions.

Why are weight-loss drugs ineffective?

First of all, the short-term (weeks or months) treatment of obesity with drugs of this kind is generally ineffective since most people will soon regain whatever weight they lose once the drug is discontinued. This is because the underlying problems that caused the original weight problem have not been corrected. People predictably resume unhealthy diets, exercise incorrectly or not at all, and engage in behaviors that per-petuate their overweight condition. In addition, the effectiveness of weight loss drugs tends to plateau after six months.

In experiments in which rats were administered amphetamines, rats displayed transient appetite inhibition and weight loss. A week later, however, after their weight returned to normal, the rats overate and gained weight. Within three weeks they were eating 7 percent more than normal, became 3 percent overweight, and had a 5 percent increase in body fat. Their increased appetite lasted for two months after they'd stopped taking the drugs.

Taking weight-loss drugs is somewhat like taking sleeping pills. Rather than discovering and correcting the underlying problems that are keeping the person awake, such as too much caffeine or stress, the person continues consuming caffeine or engaging in stressful activities before going to bed. Predictably, if you don't take away the cause you are going to have to continue living with the effect. Diet pills are no exception.

Appetite-suppressing medications are ineffective for a second reason. Most people who take such drugs eat lopsided diets while they're on them, instead of simply eating smaller portions of a balanced, nutritional diet. The combination of taking these medications while eating a lopsided diet will lead to internal processes like those we explored in Chapters 2 and 3. These are:

1. Blood sugar levels are disrupted, causing predictable cravings, binging, and other physical and psychological symptoms.

2. Serotonin levels are decreased causing carbohydrate cravings.

3. Muscle protein is broken down creating a propensity to become overweight.

4. Metabolic rate is decreased, which slows down the burning of calories.

5. Lipoprotein lipase, an enzyme that facilitates fat deposition, is increased.

6. Malnutrition or marginal malnutrition develops, resulting in physical abnormalities and distorted thinking.

Some appetite-suppressing medications cause a false sense of energy, causing you to unknowingly stress yourself.

To be both successful and safe, any drug for weight loss must have the following qualities:

✓ It must be able to decrease body fat by decreasing hunger.

✓ It must continue to be effective over the long term.

✓ It must NOT produce a drug tolerance or rebound effect.

✓ It should prevent any decrease in basal metabolic rate.

✓ It should be able to help people reduce their intake of dietary fat, which is now regarded as a major cause of weight gain and regain.

✓ It should have no dangerous side effects.

So far, there is no drug that meets all these criteria.

In a recently published study, an expert panel[1] reviewed twenty studies of antiobesity drugs and concluded that none of them should be used

---

1. "Long term weight loss: the effect of pharmacologic agents" *American Journal of Clinical Nutrition*, 1994.

routinely for any obese patients, and they should not be used at all for anyone who just wanted to lose a few pounds. The panel also concluded that even when the drugs are used appropriately, they must be used in combination with a healthy diet and exercise program.

Diet pills are unnecessary if you are following the Right Bite Program because the diet itself will remove or control weight-gain triggers that formerly caused you to overeat or gain weight. Eating nutritiously, exercising, and working to maintain a healthy attitude is the result of a conscious effort and is an active ongoing process. Over time, taking a pill is a passive and ineffective process for most people.

In the long run, the ultimate solution for managing your weight is to control and eliminate the weight-gain triggers that are causing your increased appetite and weight gain. I realize it is much easier to ask what pill you can take to lose weight than to ask what you can do to improve your health and lose weight. But taking a pill will only make you weak and dependent on medications. To succeed in the long term, you need to become an active participant, to look at the weight-gain triggers that are throwing off the normal and healthy inner mechanisms that can keep you healthy and slim.

The Right Bite Core Diet works. You don't need pills or magic formulas. All you need is you and the Right Bite Program.

Ten: Aging

Aging is a fact of life, one that very few of us want to face until we absolutely must. For most people, aging inevitably means more wrinkles, less energy, and becoming overweight. But do we really have to get fat? Unfortunately, metabolic changes that encourage us to be overweight begin when we are still quite young—in our thirties. One of these changes is that our lean muscle mass begins to decrease, slowing our metabolisms but not our forks. Once we hit our mid-thirties, we can lose as much as one-third of a pound of muscle a year. This steady, but gradual decline in our lean body mass causes a reduction in our calorie-burning capacity because pound for pound our bodies simply have less metabolically active tissue. You need fewer calories to function, and any excess calories are easily stored as fat. What to do? Exercise will prevent the age-related decline in lean body mass. See Chapter 10 for more on this.

As we age, most of us tend to become more sedentary. Once the kids are out of the house, our active lives become less intense. We are now able to sit through a meal, watch an entire television program, or take a nap for the first time in twenty years. This slowing down to smell the roses will put a few inches on your waistline unless you make it a habit to exercise.

For women, aging is more complicated. A woman's estrogen and progesterone production begins declining between the ages of thirty-five and fifty. After menopause women lose about 66 percent or more of their estrogen production and 50–60 percent of their androgen or testosterone production. As estrogen declines, you will see some changes in your body fat. Your pear-shape fat pattern with fat around your hips and buttocks suddenly becomes more apple-shaped as fat moves toward your middle. Also, the enzyme lipoprotein lipase begins to increase in upper-body fat and starts to decrease in the lower-body fat tissue, thus contributing to increased upper-body fat.

It is the changing ratios of the ovarian hormones, estrogen and testosterone, combined with less physical activity, more food than we need, and a lowered metabolism, that causes weight gain in women as they become older.

Tampering with your hormones, as we do with certain popular diets, or with erratic yo-yo, lose-and-gain diets, can not only affect your future shape and weight but also your future physical and psychological health. Our hormones are very sensitive fellows. Not only do they change naturally as we age, but there is something that we do that also alters them in deleterious ways. Our hormones are affected *adversely* by unhealthy dieting, which lowers our hormonal levels and can throw their delicate balance out of whack.

What should we women do to stay healthy and not become over-weight as we age? First of all, by choosing the Right Bite Program and enjoying the Core Diet, you will be eating and exercising in a manner that will maximize your weight loss and maintain lean body mass, thus increasing your basal metabolic rate. Secondly, I recommend discussing with your gynecologist the correct hormonal regimens and strategies to keep you healthy and feeling and looking your best—and yes, preserving your beloved pear shape into old age. By being informed, you and your gynecologist can develop a plan that is best for you.

What about men? The male "change of life" is referred to as "andropause." However, men are lucky when it comes to testosterone. For most men, testosterone production diminishes very little. So, weight gain for men is mostly due to the natural slowing of metabolism and reduction of muscle mass that comes with aging. But high on the list of why men become heavier are a more sedentary life-style and an overactive fork.

Contrary to popular opinion, aging does not have to be as powerful a weight-gain trigger as it has been in most countries. The Right Bite Program will help you stay slim and healthy for a very long and happy life.

Chapter Six

Needles in a Haystack— Triggers Rare but Prickly

Folks differs, dearie. They differs a lot.
Some can stand things that others can't. There's never
no way of knowin' how much they can stand.
—Ann Petry

I once heard it said that all people are alike: We're all made of flesh, bones, and dinners. Only the dinners are different. Well, I suspect there are a few more factors than that involved, but the pundit certainly makes his point. When we are identifying weight-gain triggers in our own lives, these different dinners can determine our success or failure. Each of us is different. And each of us responds in a particular way to her or his own unique triggers.

It is important while reading this chapter to realize that most of these uncommon triggers occur at the extreme end of the dieting spectrum— they are *rare*, but because I do have clients who have trouble with these triggers, I want to make sure that you are aware of them. Knowledge of *all* the triggers is important because it just takes ONE to sabotage your weight-loss efforts.

One: Overexercise

It is not often that I meet people who exercise too much, but it does happen. And when it does, I am reminded once again that too much exercise too soon after starting the Core Diet can sabotage one's best efforts.

The best example of overexercising that I've ever encountered was with a young lady named Julie, an insurance agent who wanted to lose thirty-plus pounds she had gained since starting a new job. She had recently joined a fitness center in her efforts to lose weight but came to me because she was troubled by periods of overeating and also was not able to maintain her exercise program as she'd planned to do.

Before going on with Julie's story, I want you to know that this is an extreme case. While you may not fully identify with it in your own life, I tell it because it illustrates the process by which this trigger works. For some people, even moderate physical exercise can be excessive, impeding their early efforts to succeed with the Core Diet. For example, for someone who is massively obese, brisk walking would be overdoing.

According to Julie, she went to the fitness center daily. One day she saw a young woman named Laurel who seemed to always be there no matter what the time of day. Julie admired Laurel's figure and reasoned that all she had to do to look just like her was duplicate this woman's workout. The shapely woman was very flattered by Julie's interest and gladly wrote out and explained her workout. Julie returned to the center the next day, invigorated and excited that she had finally found the exercise program that would give her the dream figure she had always wanted. The workout consisted of stretching for thirty minutes, working out with weights for three hours, jogging two miles, and an hour-long aerobics class at the end. Julie now understood why her friend was always at the fitness center—she had little time for anything else!

Because Julie was a novice when it came to exercise, this workout took her six hours to complete. By the time she got to the aerobics class she could hardly move. During the aerobics class, her friend, who was energetically doing jumping jacks at her side, kept telling Julie she had to exercise more intensely. Julie said by then she was so tired her feet stayed in place while her arms barely fluttered from her sides. She barely managed to drag herself home and in to bed. She was so sore and exhausted she did not return to the fitness center for an entire week. During the week she felt starved and overate almost every day. She tried the exercise program one more time and again dragged herself home weak, sore, hungry, and discouraged.

Not to be deterred, Julie devised a new workout for herself—less time-consuming and less arduous. She decided to jog five miles a day.

Although she maintained this program for two weeks, ultimately she became physically exhausted and again very hungry. She frequently succumbed to eating sprees and did not understand why because she had always read that exercise reduces one's appetite.

Julie went on to describe her pattern of overexercising and then ending each program with what she thought was a "baffling eating spree." How was Julie's exercise program acting as a trigger?

Muscles burn a combination of fat and glucose. To keep fat burning you need a little glucose. Those who are fit rely less on stored glucose and more on stored fat for energy, thus conserving their precious glucose reserves. Fit people have developed more muscles and fat-burning enzymes through healthy eating and correct exercise.

If you are not fit, however, your body is going to use more blood glucose for energy and will resist dipping into the fat reserves. When you are less than fit, your body's ability to use fats for energy is diminished, particularly if you have been sedentary and/or have been following a radical diet or series of diets. Muscles have to be conditioned to burn fat, and if you are not exercising regularly they simply are not going to be very good at that. Instead, they'll bypass the fat and burn your precious glucose. Because those who are overweight or out of shape, as Julie was, use up their limited supplies of glucose more quickly than people who are fit, their blood sugar tends to be low; thus, they more often feel hungry than people who are fit. Those who are fit often experience a decrease in hunger.

So what's the solution for the person who is overweight and unfit? Chapter 10 discusses how to exercise in a way that won't act as an appetite and weight-gain trigger. You will learn how to exercise to increase your lean body mass and enhance your fat-burning capabilities while conserving your body's use of glucose so that you will experience a decrease in your appetite. What's more, the healthy Core Diet, combined with the exercise program described in Chapter 10, will help your body increase the synthesis of fat-burning enzymes.

Until your muscles are sufficiently built up and your system is producing the fat-burning enzymes, exercise is not going to take off the weight. In fact, the main result you will get is that your muscles will resist the burning of fat while burning off glucose, which your brain needs to function well. You will experience this sugar shortage as hunger, headaches, and/or slight disorientation caused by diminished brain function.

Fat-burning enzymes are very fragile and easily destroyed. Lack of exercise, very-low-calorie diets, and radical diets such as the high-protein diets, all damage these enzymes. Under such conditions, you will lose muscle mass and your ability to burn calories, so you'll get fat more easily.

Moderate, prolonged exercise in conjunction with a healthy diet stimulates the synthesis of fat-burning enzymes, while intense exercise, especially on an inadequate diet, inhibits this synthesis.

Now, regardless of your physical condition, glycogen reserves are not inexhaustible, and if exercise continues long enough at a high enough intensity, your muscle and liver glycogen stores will run out almost completely. Glycogen depletion usually occurs in less than two hours of vigorous exercise. Once stores have become depleted, you will experience: low blood sugar and a craving for sweets, binging, or psychological symptoms that characterize eating disorders.

Dieters who exercise for prolonged periods or too intensely are at a disadvantage. Unless you are on a carefully designed diet, you will be taking in fewer calories and fewer nutrients than the exercise can support. So the chances are pretty good that your glycogen stores will already be partially or even completely depleted. Exercise performed under these partial fasting conditions rapidly creates low blood sugar with its craving for sweets.

Our glycogen reserves amount to an average of 1800–2000 calories and these reserves are affected by what we eat. If you eat a high-fat diet for three days and then exercise until exhaustion, you would only be able to exercise for approximately fifty-seven minutes. If you were to eat a mixed diet of carbohydrates and fats for three days and then exercise until exhaustion, you'd be able to do so for approximately 114 minutes. However, if you went on a high carbohydrate diet, you would be able to exercise the longest—167 minutes until exhaustion. What does all this tell us? It tells us that muscle tissue requires lots of carbohydrates.

For many people, exercising on the first day of a low-calorie or low carbohydrate diet is the easiest. This is because your body has sufficient glycogen reserves from the sweets and other carbohydrates you've recently eaten. As the days go by, however, and your glycogen stores are used up and not replenished, you will, like Julie, find physical exercise increasingly difficult, while feeling increasingly hungry afterwards.

If you are eating a suboptimal diet and overexercising, you may actually begin to notice that your muscles are atrophying. You will start losing muscle mass rather than body fat, just the opposite of what you think should happen. This seemingly paradoxical process occurs because you have used up your immediate glycogen stores and your body has turned to breaking down its own protein (muscle tissue) in order to get the glucose it needs. Your muscle mass and basal metabolic rate decrease as the result of losing this lean body tissue, so the only thing exercise will achieve for you under these circumstances is a wasted, flaccid appearance. Even on an adequate diet, overexercise can stress your muscles so that they are not able to repair themselves, the end result being the same cycle of losing muscle tissue and reducing your ability to burn calories.

Some dieters are in the practice of consuming a dose of a sugary food to give them energy just prior to exercise. This behavior is unwise. If you consume sugar within three hours of exercise the sugar will stimulate excessive insulin, causing your blood glucose to drain away so that the likelihood of your experiencing hypoglycemia while you are exercising becomes more likely. Besides that, a sugary drink taken before exercise can reduce your performance by as much as 25 percent.

Since it is counterproductive to overexercise whether you undereat or not, you should learn how to recognize when you are beginning to overtrain. The following are the ten most common symptoms of an overexercised state:

1. Lack of interest in exercise
2. Chronic physical and mental fatigue
3. Overeating or binge eating and/or loss of appetite
4. Persistent joint and/or muscle soreness
5. Insomnia
6. Illness and/or injury
7. Deterioration of motor coordination
8. Increase in resting pulse rate
9. Increase in blood pressure
10. Irritability

Two: Anaerobic Exercise

Because Jill was sixty-five pounds overweight she had joined a health club, determined to exercise her weight away. Her instructors showed her how to use all the equipment and she diligently went in every day to lift weights, do situps, leg presses and extensions . . . and much more. Her workout lasted an hour and fifteen minutes. When she returned home, she was exhausted and hungry. That's when she overate.

Because Jill was having difficulty losing weight and controlling her appetite she came to me, referred by one of her trainers. I explained the Right Bite Program to her and she was quite excited about getting started. I told her that she would have to add aerobic exercise to her routines, that weight lifting was anaerobic, and while it was good to have the strength training she was getting from these exercises, the aerobic exercises would have even greater benefits for her. As she became aerobically fit she would be better able to manage both her appetite and her weight.

Jill changed her workout to twenty minutes of brisk walking every other day with fifteen minutes of weight lifting twice a week. She also started the Basic Core Diet. A year later she had attained her weight goal of 130 pounds. She is now getting her aerobic exercise by jogging forty-five minutes, five days a week, and getting anaerobic exercise by lifting weights for another fifteen minutes, three days a week. She loves her workouts and feels totally satisfied with her dietary program.

As you start the Right Bite Program, it's important to know the difference between aerobic and anaerobic exercise. When you exercise, the amount of glucose you are able to burn as fuel depends on the availability of oxygen, which depends on the intensity of the exercise. During *moderate* exercise, your lungs and circulatory system have no difficulty providing sufficient oxygen for the muscles to extract all available energy from both glucose and fat. The exercise is said to be "aerobic." During aerobic exercise, fatty acids supply much of the energy and glycogen reserves are conserved more efficiently. Examples of aerobic exercise are power walking, jogging, cross-country skiing, and bicycling. Aerobic exercises are best for losing fat weight.

In contrast to aerobic exercise, "anaerobic" means "taking place in the absence of oxygen." In anaerobic exercise, muscle exertion is so great that the heart and lungs are not able to supply oxygen fast enough to support aerobic metabolism. Therefore your muscles must instead draw mostly on your body's limited supply of glucose. Fat cannot be used to meet the increased energy needs. Only glucose calories are burned for energy, thus depleting your glycogen rapidly. Because anaerobic exercises only burn glucose, they deplete your glycogen reserves faster than aerobic exercise. If, for example, you are only doing weight training—which is anaerobic—you will experience low blood sugar and hunger quickly. Other examples of anaerobic exercises are sprinting and racquetball.

Anaerobic exercise is detrimental to weight control unless you use it correctly. What is important to remember is that aerobic exercise primarily burns fat, and anaerobic exercise burns glucose, which results in depleting your glycogen reserves more quickly so that you will experience hunger sooner as your blood sugar drops.

According to fitness expert Covert Bailey, an anaerobic exercise such as weight lifting is excellent to add to your aerobics program as you become increasingly conditioned. The reason for this is that it builds muscle, thus increasing your lean body mass—which burns calories. Besides, the increased physical strength you gain from weight lifting makes it easier for you to perform in other sports. People who concentrate solely on anaerobic exercise will not achieve maximum fitness and will not be successful at losing weight, since it is the aerobic effect that burns fat.

As the *intensity* of exercise increases—weight training being the most intense—less and less of the energy you burn is contributed by fat. In aerobic exercise, fatty acids (from the fat stored in your thighs, buttocks and belly) provide much of the energy needed to sustain the exercise, thereby conserving your limited glycogen stores. When you spare your glycogen stores, your blood sugar will not drop and you will not experience the symptoms of low blood sugar, including hunger. Generally, the longer the duration of exercise—walking five miles instead of two, for example—the greater is the percentage of energy contributed by fat. The key word here is moderation. When you think of aerobic exercise (walking, running, stair-stepping, etc.), think, "It burns my fat and saves my glucose."

Three: Artificial Sweeteners

I first became aware of the connection between artificial sweeteners and overeating when I began counseling. I had several clients who overate or broke their diets soon after chewing eight or ten pieces of artificially sweetened gum. At first I thought that they were using the gum in place of food, as is a common practice among dieters. The gum temporarily satisfied their hunger and reduced their appetites. After experimenting with different suspected triggers, and varying their calorie intake, however, we were not able to head off their overeating episodes. Then we removed the sugarless gum from their diets and hit the jackpot. The artificial sweeteners turned out to be the villain, and with the discontinuation of the gum their overeating ceased.

What we learned is that for some people artificially sweetened foods may stimulate the desire for an intensely sweet taste. I cannot help but wonder about the fact that since the advent of artificial "low-cal" or "no-cal" sweeteners, Americans' consumption of sugar, fructose, corn syrup, and other calorie-rich sweeteners has risen to about fifty pounds per person per year!

My experience has been that for some people, but not all, a sweet taste can increase the motivation to eat. Some of my clients have reported being hungrier and responding with an increased appetite after ingesting artificial sweeteners. Other clients find that artificial sweeteners help them control their appetites by satisfying their need for something sweet without adding calories.

Some people who eat foods containing sugar substitutes tend to feel that since they are taking in fewer calories in sugar, they can eat more with no adverse consequences. They don't actually think this out or make a conscious decision about it. Just knowing that they are eating a calorically reduced food seems to give them permission to eat more of the fattening foods that they prefer.

My advice is that if you are using artificial sweeteners, or are eating artificially sweetened foods, take heed! They *might* be the culprits responsible for triggering your appetite. If you have any suspicions that this might be true, cut out the foods with artificial sweeteners and see what happens. If your cravings cease, you've identified the problem.

Artificial sweeteners are not all bad, because some people find them an aid in losing or maintaining their ideal weight. A study published in the *American Journal of Clinical Nutrition* suggests that most people who used artificial sweeteners lost significantly more weight overall and regained significantly less weight during maintenance and follow-up than those who did not use the sweeteners.

The Core Diet prohibits the use of artificial sweeteners for the first three months. After three months you can try artificial sweeteners to see how they work for you. If you discover that they act as triggers, then you will know to avoid them.

Four: Allergies and Food Intolerances

Rhonda craved bread with desperate urgency. Every time she ate even a half a slice she ended up consuming the whole loaf. She became so terrified of bread that she forbade her mother to buy any. However, since other members of the family had no problem with it, her mother continued to buy it but hid it away so that it wouldn't tempt Rhonda between meals. However, Rhonda kept finding the bread and would devour the whole loaf before she even realized what she was doing. Because Rhonda's behavior was so bizarre I sent her to an allergist to determine if she had an extreme food intolerance or a severe wheat allergy.

Here I need to distinguish between "food intolerances" and food "allergies." The former are adverse reactions to foods that do not involve the immune system. Signs of food intolerances may include the same symptoms as those experienced in an allergic reaction, but they do not involve the immune system. A true food allergy is an adverse reaction to certain foods that occurs when our immune system, whose job it is to locate and destroy microorganisms that might harm us, falsely identifies a food protein as an enemy. The result is that our immune systems produce antibodies, histamines, and other defensive agents to destroy the "offender." In the case of severe allergies, this can produce symptoms such as rash, difficulty breathing, or even anaphylactic shock, which in extreme cases can be deadly. There's the possibility that compulsive eating may be the result of an allergy.[1] The same food allergy may cause different reactions for different people, even as to what part of the body is affected.

How do you determine if you are allergic or intolerant to certain foods or substances? Turn your attention first to the foods you eat most often and in greatest quantities, the foods you binge on, and the food you crave or love . . . and the foods you hate. If you are allergic to a food it may make you hungry, thirsty, or physically uncomfortable, and affect your mental state.

It is impossible to remove from the Core Diet every food that has allergic potential. If we did that, we would end up with a diet that would be about as appealing as eating sawdust, and impossible for most people to follow. Always keep in mind that if the food isn't palatable, or if preparing it is too complicated, the chances are that it's not going to work, regardless of how "healthy" it might be.

Also, there are particularly rare cases in which people are allergic to so many foods that they must follow complex rotation diets in which the same food cannot be eaten again until at least four days have passed. Not everyone is affected by food allergies and food sensitivities, but they definitely exist, and may be exacerbating your eating problems. If you suspect that you suffer from allergies after following the Core Diet, and are unable to determine which foods you are sensitive to, I urge you to consult an allergist. You may be allergic to not only a particular food but also a nonfood substance that is acting as an appetite trigger.

Five: Laxatives

Even though laxatives are a medication, I am highlighting them as a specific trigger because of their widespread use as a "diet aid." Having worked with dieters for over twenty years, I know that in their desperation to lose weight, many people are routinely using laxatives for this purpose, not knowing that they may actually be causing food cravings as well as disrupted metabolisms. The following is a good example:

Jenna was sent to me for a consultation after a particularly embarrassing incident at school. She was trying to lose weight and had bought a bottle of mineral oil, which is a common laxative. She had drunk the whole bottle before bed after consuming her usual amount of food. She awoke the next morning, expecting to be cleansed of all the calories she consumed the day before. Instead, she was disappointed because nothing happened at all. Feeling bloated, Jenna got dressed and went to school.

---

1. For more on this, see *It's Not Your Fault You're Fat*, by Marshall Mandell and Fran G. Mandell, 1983; New York: Harper Trade.

Jenna's day progressed normally and she forgot she had even taken the laxative. When the lunch bell rang Jenna stood up and heard giggles and gasps. People were pointing at her. Her very perceptive teacher quickly escorted Jenna out into the hall and to the ladies' room. Jenna was horrified at what she saw when she looked in the mirror. All the mineral oil had leaked out and had made the back of her white skirt almost completely transparent. It was like looking through a window. After telling her teacher what she'd done, Jenna was sent to the nurse's office, where her parents were contacted.

I will never forget another patient, Shirley, who wished to lose about forty-five pounds. She confessed to me that she was always constipated and had to use laxatives. When I asked her if she ate foods that contained fiber, she looked indignant and annoyed with me for asking such an obvious question.

"Of course I eat fiber! Everybody knows you need fiber in your diet in order to have healthy bowel movements. Even though I have fiber in my diet, I am still constipated," was her reply.

"Well, then," I said, "why don't you tell me what foods and how much of them you eat that contain fiber."

"Why, I eat a tablespoon of bran mixed with juice every day!" she said seriously.

Out of compassion, I had to bite my tongue until it hurt so that I would not smile after hearing this. I didn't know where she had gotten such misinformation but I had to tell her that her bran and juice were giving her about the same amount of fiber as a single teaspoon of bran flake breakfast cereal—in short, almost no fiber at all.

However, most people who are trying to lose weight don't take laxatives to relieve constipation. At the extreme end of the dieting spectrum are those who take laxatives because they have been told it will speed weight loss by getting rid of food more quickly. Also, some take laxatives because doing so makes them feel thinner. The empty, concave feeling that dieters feel in their stomachs and abdomens after taking laxatives is appealing, and eventually they come to think of this feeling as "normal." The sensation of food in their stomach and intestines makes such people feel as though their stomachs are protruding, even when they are not.

Unless a doctor prescribes or recommends laxatives for you because you have hemorrhoids, are bedridden, or have some other medical condition, laxatives are usually not necessary. And while we are on the subject, some people take laxatives because they believe that everyone should have a certain number of bowel movements per day. There is a wide variation of what's "normal," however, so one should never take laxatives only for this reason. Always check with your doctor if you are troubled by persistent constipation or any other bowel changes. In normal healthy people, bowel movements are promoted by a diet that has adequate fiber, fluid, and physical exercise.

Taking laxatives can have serious nutritional consequences, with a number of triggering effects on your appetite. Here is a list of them:

1. Laxatives reduce your nutritional status by decreasing nutrient absorption. Food passes so quickly through your intestines that your body cannot make use of the nutrients. When dieting, most people are already compromising their nutritional needs. Taking a laxative in addition to dieting can bring you dangerously close to severe malnutrition, ultimately triggering cravings and binges.

2. Laxatives disturb your body's fluid, salt, and mineral balance. The effects can be dramatic, throwing off the electrolyte balance, which you will experience as dizziness, dehydration, rapid heartbeat, and weakness. Many dieters then resort to weight gain triggering stimulants to pep them up.

3. Depending on which laxatives you are taking, they may cause nausea and abdominal cramps, which can act as triggers by causing you to restrict food intake when you need to be replenishing lost nutrients.

Unless you have a physical condition that warrants the use of a laxative, most people just need adequate fiber in their diets. The Core Diet ensures that you get enough fiber in your diet so that you will never have to worry about being constipated or malnourished.

Six: Diuretics

In recent years there's been a great deal of talk about "water retention," and how that makes us feel and look fat. As a result, it has become popular among dieters to take diuretics so that they don't retain as much water. Unfortunately, while taking diuretics might make you weigh less and feel thinner, this practice does nothing in terms of reducing the fat on your body. As a so-called "diet aid," they should definitely be looked upon as an *abused medication*. As a weight-gain trigger, they will inevitably make you feel hungry.

Sheila came to me about a problem she was having with bloating. Whenever her period started, she told me, her weight went up several pounds. To counteract this, she had begun using diuretics about a year before. She had begun this practice when her period and a special event at work coincided. She had to give a presentation to a large group and wanted to look her best. But she knew that she would be bloated because of her problem with water retention. Given the circumstances her doctor gave her a prescription for diuretics.

Sheila took a pill before going to bed the night before the event. When she got up she was happy to learn that she was not bloated, and she was still at her normal weight. The only trouble was that she felt lethargic, light-headed, and hungrier than usual.

The night of the event she was still feeling a little dizzy and lethargic. But her clothes fit her perfectly and she was happy about the way she looked. As the evening progressed, however, she became thirsty and hungry, and continued to drink one beverage after another, and ate far more than usual. By the time she was to do her presentation, her clothes were feeling tight and uncomfortable. Nevertheless, her presentation went well enough, and she was relieved that the event was over.

For three or four months after that, she continued to take diuretics during her period to help with water retention. But she was shocked to discover that her appetite was getting more and more out of control, and she was gaining weight at an alarming rate.

It did not take long to identify Sheila's weight gain trigger when she came in to see me. She discontinued the diuretics, went on the Right Bite Program, and soon noticed not only that her weight was dropping and her hunger was gone but also that she had almost no noticeable bloating associated with her period.

Sheila's experiences are not all that unusual, unfortunately. Many women use diuretics to reduce water retention. Some don't even know what they are taking, however, because diuretics may be found in diet pills or in medication for PMS. On occasion, some doctors prescribe them for women who complain of bloating during their periods.

Diuretics work by inhibiting your body's absorption of sodium and chloride, the result being that you urinate more. Physicians sometimes prescribe them to reduce high blood pressure, but these medicines also have many side effects that can have serious consequences for the dieter:

1. Diuretics promote malnutrition. The increased flow of urine causes water-soluble nutrients and some minerals to be excreted quickly, preventing their full assimilation and thus promoting malnutrition. (Water-soluble nutrients are those that your body does not store but which you must consume daily in frequent small doses.) We have already discussed how different deficiencies affect a person emotionally and physically. If you are undereating or restricting your diet in any way, diuretics will compound and intensify the risks of malnutrition.

2. Diuretics can intensify your appetite because of their effect on carbohydrate metabolism. Some diuretics produce hypoglycemia, or low blood sugar, with its accompanying craving for sweets.

3. Diuretics produce other undesirable symptoms such as: dryness of mouth, thirst, weakness and lethargy, drowsiness, restlessness, muscle pains, muscular fatigue, hypotension, and even depression. Such symptoms can make you crave caffeine in an effort to boost your sagging energy and spirits, again undermining your nutritional status even more and exacerbating any eating problem you may have. Don't use diuretics unless your doctor prescribes or recommends them for you.

Seven: Vomiting

Most of us look upon intentional vomiting with extreme repugnance. In spite of this, I include it in this discussion of triggers because it is all too often employed as a form of weight management—and not just by bulimics! As many as 14 percent of all women, and 4 percent of all men have used vomiting for this purpose. Judging by the women I have seen in my practice over the years, I am convinced that the real figures are much higher than that because people are anything but comfortable with talking about this all too common practice among chronic dieters.

I want to make it clear that I am not just talking about the condition we know as bulimia, whereby people routinely use vomiting to rid themselves of unwanted calories. Many nonbulimics have confessed to me that they have at least tried, or occasionally use, vomiting as a means of weight control. Vomiting is a powerful trigger with devastating effects.

Vomiting causes uncontrolled eating, binging, or weight problems because it rids the body of needed calories and nutrients. We have already seen how depleting our bodies of calories and nutrients results in malnutrition, low glycogen reserves, low blood sugar, and low serotonin levels. All of these are potent triggers that can cause hunger and binging. By depleting your body of needed calories in the form of carbohydrates, vomiting will also cause your body to cannibalize its own tissues in order to get glucose, resulting in muscle atrophy. I know I'm repeating myself, but here's yet another reminder that as you lose lean body mass, your metabolism will slow, making it easier for you to gain weight when you eat.

Your body reacts to vomiting as it does to undereating or any other radical behavior: it accelerates lipoprotein lipase activity and synthesis and hangs on tenaciously to your fat stores.

Vomiting upsets your electrolyte balance, which can cause dizziness, dehydration, depression, and even death by a heart attack. People have also been known to suffocate on their own vomit.

The only way to stop overeating is to stop vomiting. Vomiting creates overeating and weight gain. Vomiting sets up a vicious cycle of binging and purging. The only way to terminate this type of binge is to stop vomiting.

Bulimics, some dieters, and bulimic-anorexics vomit in an effort to "get rid of calories" that they believe will make them fat and because vomiting makes them feel slim. Purging in this manner gives them a false sense of slimness. I must stress that in addition to causing the problems I've already noted above, vomiting can trigger internal changes that will eventually result in obesity, the very condition that the dieter is trying to prevent by vomiting. In all my years of counseling, I know of no one who remained slender using chronic vomiting to control their weight.

Eight: Marijuana

When I was in college I was invited to an off-campus party. During the evening, someone brought out a little plastic bag filled with something that looked like green tea or maybe Italian seasoning. But it wasn't either one. The same person produced a little white square of paper, sprinkled some of the herb into it and twisted it into a crude looking cigarette. At this point, everyone gathered around in a circle, taking turns puffing the cigarette, inhaling deeply and holding their breath. When it came to my turn I took a puff, but I swear I didn't inhale. There was no way I was going to take that foul smelling smoke—or any foul smelling smoke—into my lungs. Instead, I puffed up my cheeks like a blowfish and then exhaled as I handed the joint to the next person. I nodded my head and smiled, as the others smiled and made remarks such as "Cool, man!" or "Hey, this is great stuff!"

As time passed, the people who had smoked the marijuana became increasingly silly or mellow. The mellow ones went off in the corner, as one person said, "to veg out!" One couple started necking. As for me, I didn't feel much different than I ever did. I sat there wondering why everyone was making such a big deal of it. Since I wasn't enjoying myself, I decided to go back to my dorm room. About halfway there it hit me, a hunger greater than any I'd ever experienced. I had to find something to eat—RIGHT NOW!

I ran to my room, grabbed my coin purse and bolted for the vending machines. I poured coins into the slots, tore open the wrappers of the goodies the machine gave up, and wolfed them down as fast as I could. Everything tasted delicious, extraordinarily delicious. But then my coins ran out, and I was still famished. I checked out the garbage cans as I made my way back to the room, on the outside chance that someone had left something delectable there. Nothing.

Back at my room, I began searching every nook and cranny for food. A few slices of bread were left, along with a can of tuna. I thought about it, then dismissed the idea. The tuna would make the room stink. My roommate even had a small, sealed package of tofu—yuk! I was really getting frantic when I remembered her fresh boxes of raisin bran . . .

The Center for National Health Statistics estimates that 5 percent of the U.S. population over the age of twelve currently smokes marijuana. However, the accuracy of this figure is suspect and probably conservative because there are undoubtedly many smokers who won't admit their indulgence.

A major side effect of marijuana is its stimulation of your appetite. For patients with wasting diseases such as AIDS this effect is a benefit. However, for the majority of "tokers" marijuana induces the "munchies," which you surely don't want if you are concerned about your weight.

Nine and Ten: Anorexia and Bulimia

Because the focus of this book is weight control and not severe eating disorders, I will discuss these two triggers in detail in Appendix B for those who are scientifically interested, for those who feel these triggers may apply to themselves, or for those who may have a loved one or friend suffering from these afflictions. Suffice it to say that, both anorexia and bulimia are the cumulative results of triggers and become triggers in and of themselves. *If* one survives untreated anorexia, the victim inevitably becomes a bulimic, ranging in weight from normal at first to obese as the disease progresses.

Going Forward

Now that you have become familiar with a wide range of potential triggers, you probably have a good idea which ones may be affecting you. In the next chapter I will be taking you a step further, walking you through the process of identifying your own unique set of triggers, or combinations of triggers, which you will eliminate in the weeks ahead.

Chapter Seven

Five Steps to Freedom— Taking Control of Your Weight-Gain Triggers

I am never afraid of what I know.
—Anna Sewell

As a result of her hectic schedule as a surgical nurse in a large hospital, Becky subsisted on bird-sized helpings of packaged foods and caffeinated drinks, including both coffee and colas. In spite of eating a meager 700 calories during the day, she was a whopping 80–100 pounds overweight, and she was miserable. A typical day consisted of a piece of toast (white bread) and coffee for breakfast, a sandwich consisting of two pieces of bread (white) and one slice of low fat bologna at lunch, a small bagel for a snack, and a chicken breast and salad with low-calorie dressing for dinner. The problem was that even though she ate these birdlike meals, she found herself binging at least twice a week, and she didn't know why. She was astonished when I told her that she must eat more to weigh less and that she was a victim of the trigger I call "insufficient calories."

Along with eating more, Becky also eliminated caffeine from her diet. Consuming 1400 calories per day, she lost seven pounds the first week. Not a bad beginning!

"I know that three of my weight-gain triggers are insufficient calories, insufficient nutrients, and caffeine. But how can I be sure I don't have others?" Becky asked me after her first week on the program.

She was asking the same question that is probably on most readers' minds at this moment—how to accurately identify my unique set of weight-gain triggers?

Identifying your weight-gain triggers sounds more difficult than it really is. In fact, I want to assure you that it is easier to do than to explain. There are five skills that we apply to identify our triggers:

1. **Common sense:** Being observant and giving thought to our eating behavior

2. **Oops, I forgot!:** How to handle errors and misjudgments

3. **Testing the rules:** Honestly testing the guidelines for maximum benefits in a methodical and controlled manner

4. **Expanding the diet:** Adding new foods and assessing our reaction to them

5. **Analyze to isolate:** Using our own analytical abilities to identify and isolate triggers

I encourage you to keep a journal in order to better understand and isolate all your weight-gain triggers.

Common Sense

A teacher of mine once told me that common sense was an oxymoron because the faculty we are talking about when we use this term isn't common at all. Given that this is the case, I always start by telling my clients exactly what I mean when I use this term. For me, common sense is:

✓ Paying attention and observing what's happening around us and to us, then acting as wisely as we can at that moment

✓ An acceptance that certain weight-gain triggers will be applicable to most of us most of the time, particularly for those of us with weight issues. For example, we know that eating three pieces of chocolate fudge is not only going to put flab on our hips, it is going to send our entire system out of control.

✓ Observing that if we are losing weight on our new diet then chances are that this has something to do with our new way of eating and exercising

✓ An ability to compare our old habits to any new ones we are developing and note what we are doing differently now

Common sense can be helped along by writing notes to yourself about your old eating behaviors, how you have altered them, and how those alterations have benefited you. These changes will point you toward various weight-gain triggers that you have eliminated from your diet. For example, if in the old diet you never ate breakfast and you used to binge at lunch, and now you do eat breakfast and you don't binge at lunch, then the weight-gain trigger we refer to as "meal frequency" is applicable to you. Similarly, if you never drink beverages containing caffeine, and never have, common sense should tell you that these triggers would not be applicable to you unless you started using them and had an adverse reaction.

Adopt common sense as your watchdog. Life is full of surprises, many of which are beyond our control, and common sense can serve you well at such times. For example, what if you were thirsty and the only beverage available was a diet soda with caffeine? You might go ahead and drink that, knowing that the caffeine was going to trigger unusual hunger afterward. Knowing the source of this hunger would help you make better choices about what you eat to satisfy that hunger.

Common sense is particularly important when we encounter a brand-new weight-gain trigger, that is, at those times when we eat or drink something that is new to us that sends us into a tailspin.

First and foremost, exercise your best common sense in this or any other diet. Most people who have tried the Core Diet follow the program so carefully for the first three months (Phase I) that they never experience anything unusual. They easily control their weight or lose weight for the first time in their lives! They are not having any problems: no overeating, binging, reactions, sudden weight gains, or extreme weight fluctuations—nothing unusual at all. Everything is working so well that when it comes to expanding their diet in the next phase of the program they don't want to change a thing. They may even jump to the conclusion that since this first phase of the Core Diet is getting such good results, maybe all the weight-gain triggers apply to them. What if in isolating their specific weight-gain triggers they make a mistake, and the diet ceases to work for them?

Between your common sense and the guidelines in the pages ahead, you can successfully isolate your specific triggers and expand your diet accordingly. It's important to trust this process since expanding your diet, in the second phase of the plan, gives greater variety to what you can safely eat, ensuring your continued success.

Oops, I Forgot!

It is human nature that the care we initially invest in any new endeavor gradually diminishes over time. Remember how careful and focused you were when you first learned to drive a car? That same pattern of behavior applies to any new diet. I have observed that overwhelming success during the initial weeks can sometimes result in getting overconfident as the pounds melt away and the program becomes more of a daily habit. One day we simply "slip." We invite a friend out to lunch on her birthday, and she orders a piece of chocolate cake. You take one bite just to be sociable and decide it tastes so good you order a whole piece for yourself.

By mid-afternoon you're starving, and over the next few days you have returned to your old eating habits and are gaining weight again. The usual explanation is, "I knew better than to eat that huge piece of chocolate cake, but I didn't think it would hurt anything." Like flying on automatic pilot, we forget about occasional turbulence and fail to keep our seatbelt buckled. The *oops!-I-forgot* syndrome gets us into all sorts of trouble.

I remember one client who was an avid coffee drinker before he went on the core diet. When his friend offered him a cappuccino from his new espresso machine, temptation got the upper hand. "Oh, why not? One time can't do any harm." For the rest of the day he battled the demons of ravenous hunger.

Another *oops-I-forgot* situation occurs when we get particularly busy. Up to that point, we were being very careful about spacing meals and snacks appropriately so that not too much time elapsed between them. Then we skip a meal because we feel we can't stop what we're doing to eat. When we finally do sit down to eat we overeat or binge.

If you do get into an *oops-I-forgot* situation, don't give yourself a bad time about it or jump to the conclusion that you can't follow this eating plan. Instead, remind yourself that even these times are valuable learning experiences. Go back to the Core Diet rules, identify any triggers that set you off, and note the situations that you particularly have to watch.

We all slip from time to time. I am embarrassed to say that when I started working on this book, I became forgetful. At 6:30 p.m. I would stick my meal in the microwave, think of something I needed to write and race back to my computer. Before I knew it I was deep into my work and had forgotten all about eating. Like Beethoven, who was so preoccupied with composing that he often paid his bill at restaurants and ran back to his studio before he had eaten, I would emerge from my office hours later, starving and wondering why. It was not until I opened the microwave to warm my bedtime snack that I would find the now cold dinner sitting there uneaten. By then I was so famished that I had to exercise every ounce of common sense I still possessed to not head for the cookie jar.

Handling the *oops-I-forgot* situations that will inevitably arise in our lives is a challenge, no doubt about it. Your awareness of these *oops* episodes and what causes them is your first step toward knowing both what you must avoid and what you can do to get back on track when you, in effect, "fall off the wagon."

Testing the Rules

There is a right and a wrong way to test the rules. The right way is to alter the rules according to the guidelines that I have described in the Right Bite Program. These guidelines are designed to help you more accurately isolate or confirm which foods or beverages are your weight-gain triggers. The wrong way is to alter rules according to your own whims, which can lead to confusion and disastrous consequences.

For example, some dieters find it difficult to believe that they can lose weight by eating as much food as is actually required on the Core Diet. So they deliberately reduce their intake of food. They remember the dangers of *insufficient calories*, which we explored in Chapter 2 but do not believe it applies to them. They are in a hurry for faster weight-loss results and think that slashing calories while avoiding other weight-gain triggers will allow them to reach their weight-loss goal more quickly. But I must warn you, as I did in Chapter 2, that on the Core Diet, insufficient calories will always be a weight-gain trigger—sooner or later. Each time you test this rule you will find it to be true. So *relax* and enjoy eating, feeling full, and losing weight.

Maybe you deliberately alter or test a rule either on your own or according to instructions in the Core Diet Program and are completely surprised when you start overeating or gaining weight. You think that this reaction is a *coincidence*, so you test the rule again, with the same results. Even then, you may not be convinced and you continue testing the process until the cause-effect link is firmly established in your mind.

My rule of thumb is this: If you change a rule once and have an adverse reaction, it might just be a coincidence. If you alter that same rule a second time with the same results, you can rest assured that it is not a coincidence but due to a weight-gain trigger.

Be aware that some weight-gain triggers work cumulatively. You might successfully skip a meal one day, but this does not mean you can skip a meal every day without dire consequences. Many people who purposefully decrease their calories to a dangerous level, for example, successfully maintain this level for a few days. When they eventually overeat, binge, or just feel downright rotten, they attribute their adverse symptoms to something else—for example, to a difficult emotional experience rather than to insufficient calories. So be aware when you alter a rule that involves a period of time, such as the hours between meals. The unpleasant repercussions may not show up immediately, and when they do it is all too easy to attribute an eventual consequence to an unrealistic cause. The deliberate and guided alteration of the Right Bite rules in order to determine direct cause and effect relationships will enable you to define your own unique set of triggers.

Expand the Diet

For the first three months it is critical to follow the Right Bite Program and instructions exactly. After three months, you will be expanding the diet by following my guidelines, in order to individualize it and make it a way of eating you can happily live with for the rest of your life. While honoring the fundamental principles of the diet, you will begin adding one food at a time in order to find out if any of them are trigger foods for you. But let me warn you never to try several new foods or beverages at the same time. Doing so makes it difficult, if not impossible, to pinpoint the culprit food in the event of a reaction. By carefully controlling the timing of the food additions, you should have no difficulty determining when a food or behavior acts as a weight-gain trigger.

Analyze to Isolate

You may believe that you are following the Right Bite Program perfectly—not being careless or forgetful and not altering the rules. In spite of your best efforts you find, to your horror, that you have slipped. Somehow a weight-gain trigger made a sneak attack, and you are not at all certain what that trigger was. You're faced with a real dilemma. How do you discover what went wrong? Maybe, just maybe, it was even a weight-gain trigger that was not explained in this book! How are you ever going to figure out what the problem is? There are several steps you must take to analyze and isolate what it was that happened:

1. Before drawing any conclusions, gather as much information as you can surrounding the incident. Consult your journal to help you recall details. Go back in your recent food history to the time when you were eating successfully. Review your menus, your physical exercise, and the mind exercises you were doing. Take a new look at what was going on in your life at that time—your health status and any other factors you feel may have been affecting your eating and your weight. Now move forward in time

to the point where you started having trouble. What were you doing when the slip occurred that was different from the times when you were trouble-free?

Look at all the food factors, flavor enhancers, nonfood factors, such as activities, and even emotional issues, such as a recent fight with your boyfriend and good or bad news of any kind. Perhaps you were on vacation at the time trouble occurred, and you were eating unfamiliar foods.

Make a list of all the different variables you have discovered that occurred just prior to and during your slip. Learn all you can about them. Reread sections in this book. Expanded knowledge will give you the answers and solutions you seek.

2. Review the chapters on weight-gain triggers and the Right Bite Program and its guidelines.

3. Put together the information you have gathered in steps 1 and 2 and develop your own theories about what trigger or triggers caused your problem. Make sure you are following the Right Bite Program exactly as you did in the first three months. Do not test each variable by duplicating the situation you feel may have caused the problem or ingesting the culprit food or beverage. It would be counterproductive to needlessly risk increasing your appetite. Furthermore, it would be unnecessarily traumatic or even dangerous to duplicate certain situations such as running into your ex with his new girlfriend when you look your worst. That would send anyone running for cover—and a comforting pastry! If you breathed bug repellant accidentally sprayed in your face and followed this with orgiastic eating you can be certain the bug spray was the cause. Instead of duplicating the problem that triggered your appetite, trust whatever theories or conclusions you come to about the cause and act accordingly so that you can get back on track.

Sometimes reactions involve multiple variables that are important to examine. For example, when one of my patients first began expanding her diet, she found that if she ate ice cream after a Core Diet main meal, she could enjoy a small bowl of it without stimulating her appetite or increasing her weight. But if she ate the ice cream too long after eating her regular meal, her appetite zoomed out of control.

Reactions may or may not occur just because of a minor alteration in a circumstance or food. One client always overate when her in-laws made unannounced visits to her home at times when the house was a mess. However, if the visits were planned ahead so that she could get the house in order, my client felt relaxed and did not feel the compulsion to overeat. Another client, who loved chocolate, only had trouble maintaining her diet when she saw the chocolate bunnies that come out at Easter. She was grateful that Easter only came once a year. And in case you might be wondering, she was not similarly moved by chocolate Santas.

Sometimes the triggering cause and effect are so immediate that we can draw conclusions about them on the spot and resolve never to make that mistake again. One woman I know forgot to take her birth control pills for a couple of days. Her doctor told her to double up on the dose until she caught up to the proper day. For two days this poor woman took the pills and was absolutely famished, eating ravenously and gaining several pounds. Her appetite ceased when she got back on her normal schedule of pills.

Sudden weight gain can be health-related. Many years back, my college roommate gained seven pounds rather quickly, and continued to gain. Her doctor ran some tests, found she was hypothyroid, and soon corrected the condition.

Any time you have a change in appetite or weight or experience any worrisome symptoms check with your doctor. Many health conditions can cause changes in appetite and weight. Have your doctor evaluate them and take measures to correct them.

4. Follow the guidelines in this book for controlling or eliminating the weight-gain triggers you feel are responsible for your trouble area.

5. If you have unearthed a trigger not discussed in this book, which is possible with the rapid development of new foods, processing methods, and additives, you may need to formulate your own instructions for controlling or eliminating that weight-gain trigger. This is easy to do. For example, if you find that, after sprinkling a new substance on your potato, you experience an increased appetite or a weight gain the following day, then you can assume that this new substance is a trigger for you.

To illustrate this analytical process, I will take you through two true examples.

EXAMPLE #1

I once had a client named Annette who complained, "I feel weird today. I've been feeling more hungry than ever and don't know why."

I started by asking her to review with me all of her food data for the two weeks prior to feeling "weird" as well as during the week that she had begun to feel "weird." The first week seemed very routine, but during the next two Annette had consumed the bulk of her calories prior to 5:00 p.m. and ate little or nothing the rest of the evening. There was nothing wrong with the quality and quantity of the diet, however. The caloric totals were approximately the same daily.

I then asked Annette to define what she meant by "weird." She replied that she felt strange, uneasy, tired. Not depressed, but my spirits do not feel the same." In addition, she woke up at night and couldn't get back to sleep.

While most areas of her life were going well, she had a huge amount of school work to do. She had stopped exercising to make more time for her studies and was not getting to bed until midnight or later. As for the stress she was feeling, she was at a loss about what to do to relieve it.

Annette was eating dinner before 5:00 p.m. in order to devote all of her attention until midnight to her school studies. That meant she was going nearly seven hours without food or sufficient calories to meet the needs of her increased study schedule, which was both stressful and intellectually demanding. And don't forget, both increased stress and increased intellectual activity burn calories.

You may remember, from the chapter on insufficient calories, that insomnia is often a symptom of insufficient calories. Even if you manage to fall asleep, the quality of the sleep is poor, and you will feel tired and "weird" the next day.

Lack of sleep, the additional stress of exam week, and insufficient calories had teamed up to become a major burden for her. I reminded her that the brain is a glucose hog under these circumstances.

"Your brain at rest uses two-thirds of your available blood glucose," I told Annette. "During exams, it will use considerably more. No wonder you are feeling weird!"

In spite of being glucose-deprived, Annette was able to complete her own analysis of what had gone wrong. "I've broken at least three of your guidelines," she reflected. "First, I'm getting insufficient calories. Second, I'm not making any adjustments in my diet to take care of the stress. Third, I've dropped the one thing that could have helped me reduce some of the stress, that is, my physical activity program."

"There is one more," I reminded her. "You have set up a situation where you have very poor spacing and frequency between meals and snacks."

During the week ahead, Annette increased her caloric level to better meet the demands of this stressful period in her life. She distributed her caloric intake more evenly throughout the day, even including a bed-time snack.

Annette began going for a ten-minute walk just after eating her evening meal and before she settled down to her studies. She found she had more energy than before and was able to concentrate better, so these few minutes of exercise more than made up for the time away from her studies.

Since stress is such a powerful weight-gain trigger, it is sometimes necessary to counsel clients on how to handle it. I described to Annette a way to plot out each semester on her calendar so that she could see in black and white what she had to accomplish. By doing that for the fol-lowing semester, she was able to schedule everything that would be required of her in the weeks ahead.

Annette's peculiar feelings ceased as she adjusted her diet and exer-cise program. The following semester was a breeze for her. She contin-ued to lose weight, increased her energy, and did great with all her studies.

EXAMPLE #2

One day a client named Emily phoned me and said, "I nearly had a binge. I just bought a bag of cookies, ate one, and threw the rest out the window. I called you when I realized that I was about to lose control. I don't know why I bought these cookies and what tempted me to start eating them. What happened?"

Emily was in her late thirties and recently divorced. She was the co-owner, with her best friend, of a craft shop in Bangor. She had been doing very well on her program and had already lost fourteen pounds, so she was bewildered by her sudden impulse to eat a cookie.

Together we reviewed Emily's diet history and did not see anything abnormal. The quality and quantity of the diet seemed sufficient, and the spacing of her meals was correct.

I then asked her if she had experienced any recent change in her rou-tine. She had spent the weekend with her partner at her parents' home in Bar Harbor. During this weekend she stuck to her diet, exercised reg-ularly, and slept well. Then Emily chanced to mention that after every meal her friend and her family ate desserts. Over the weekend Emily had done pretty well, managing to excuse herself gracefully from the dessert rituals, preferring to stick to the Core Diet. In addition, during the ride back to Bangor that evening of her near-binge, a chocolate cake was sitting in the front seat between her and her friend. She said that she could smell it the entire trip.

"How did you feel, being around desserts so much?" I asked.

"I felt really full and content after each meal . . . that is why I was so surprised to see how hungry I later became. After the desserts were served I found myself watching others eat them and wishing I could eat them too. On the way back home I was mostly busy concentrating on my driving and chatting with my partner, but at all times I was aware of the smell of chocolate."

It seemed very obvious to me that Emily was a victim of seeing, smelling, and thinking about food, and in this case a very enticing, rich chocolate cake. When I mentioned this to her, she was surprised. She had not known that seeing the desserts and smelling them could be triggers for her. She had never prepared herself to be around desserts all weekend, much less sharing the ride back home with a chocolate cake. Since she came from a family that never served desserts with meals, it was easy to see how she could have overlooked the need to do the proper mental exercises (Chapter 11) to ward off the desire for tempting treats.

After this experience she vowed that before she spent another weekend with her partner, she would make sure any chocolate cake or cookies were stored safely in the trunk of the car where she wouldn't smell them. She would also formulate her own "gross-out" images to counteract the temptations of any desserts that might be paraded in front of her. By the end of this session with her, Emily had created all the insurance she needed to ward off sneak attacks from the dessert corps.

You may think that all this strategizing is unnecessary in the normal course of things. But may I submit that you never know when a Girl Scout is going to show up at your front door selling your favorite chocolate mint cookies, or when Auntie Marge might drop by with homemade chocolate eclairs.

Proclaim Your Freedom from Triggers

I am positive that by applying the principles in this chapter you will be able to identify your own unique set of triggers. You'll be able to lose weight and keep it off by controlling or eliminating them forever.

Chapter Eight

Be a Happy Loser Today— the Trigger-Free Right Bite Diet

*To tend, unfailingly, unflinchingly towards a goal,
is the secret of success.*
—Anna Pavlova

Lee was a busy executive, running her newly formed company while doing her best to be a good mom to her infant twins at home. Unable to lose the extra sixty pounds she'd put on during her pregnancy she came to me complaining, "I am at the end of my rope!" Fatigued and frustrated, the whole world seemed pretty gloomy to her.

"I just can't find a diet that I can work with," she told me. "They are all so inflexible. The menus are either too restrictive or they require that I buy special foods. How am I supposed to drink a liquid diet when I take a client out to lunch? It's awful. Besides all that, I feel like a refugee. I'm starving all the time. I'm OK for a while, and then I start craving a particular food and pretty soon I'm binging and totally out of control again. I hate cooking, but even if I loved cooking I don't have time to assemble fancy menus for my family or myself. I know that in order to lose weight and maintain it I must make permanent changes in my eating and exercise habits, but I can't find a single program that appeals to me or that I have been able to stay with permanently. What I really need is a food plan that I can adapt to my lifestyle.

I introduced Lee to the Core Diet, and it was love at first bite. One year later, she had lost sixty-three pounds, had abundant energy, and was thoroughly delighted with herself. She has no abnormal cravings, never feels even the least tendency to binge, and is more than satisfied after every meal or snack.

Like so many other clients over the years, Lee's success came about not just by rigidly following a single set of food *dos* and *don'ts* but by employing a multistrategy approach. This approach consisted of three parts: the Right Bite food plan, described in this chapter and the next, physical exercise, described in Chapter 11, and Mind Exercises, described in Chapter 12.

Before you get started, I want to provide you with a picture of what lies ahead. In that way you'll get jump-started so that you can enthusiastically anticipate the different phases of the program. Let's start with the Core Diet that I've divided into two sections, Phase I and Phase II.

In the present chapter, we will be exploring Phase I.

Phase I is the most rigorous part of the diet, which you will follow for three months, immediately getting down to the business of transforming your metabolism from that of a fat person to that of a thin person. This scientifically sound program is based on a desperately needed synthesis of the most comprehensive nutritional information available about weight management, and it makes a quantum leap ahead of any quick-fix weight-loss diet ever invented. Nowhere does it fall back on tricks for artificially manipulating your natural physical processes or on single-strategy schemes that are effective only in the short term, if at all. The Right Bite Program will set you firmly on a path that will convert your biochemistry from the fat-storing to the fat-burning metabolism it was meant to be. By fully honoring your biological roots, and what your body was designed to do best, you can achieve a lifetime of slim, vigorous health enjoying delicious foods and never feel that you are starving yourself.

With the program I am going to describe, you will achieve five important goals:

1. You'll completely control and/or eliminate your appetite and weight-gain triggers, releasing you from cravings and hunger pangs that entice you to breach your diet.

2. You'll undo the damage of any previous diets, repairing and healing damaged tissue and regaining your natural ability to burn away your fat stores.

3. You'll correct malnutrition and straighten out your body's diet-impaired biochemistry, terminating weight-gain and erasing food cravings that caused you to yield to food temptations in the past.

4. You'll speed up your metabolism so that you will be burning more calories each day.

5. You will increase your lean body mass, replacing fat with muscle, not only increasing your energy and stamina but adding beautiful toning and fat-burning capacity.

The science of nutrition teaches us that there is a strong correlation between permanent weight loss and good fitness and health. You won't have permanent weight loss with a diet that is based on unsound food plans that obtain their results by damaging and manipulating your body's natural processes. If you have ever experienced fad diets aimed at quick weight loss you will have learned this lesson firsthand: You may quickly drop some weight but at the expense of feeling dreadful and deprived. As soon as you stop the diet you immediately gain back the weight you lost, plus a few pounds. That is not going to happen on the Right Bite Program because you will be controlling and eliminating weight-gain triggers that undermined your past weight-control attempts. This comprehensive strategy will enable you to manage your weight and know that you are also doing something good for your body.

One of the first things you'll notice in the three-month period of Phase I is that you will lose both weight and inches. You will feel far better, physically and emotionally, than you have in years. This is because the diet respects and conforms to the physiological processes that have been the foundation for human health for thousands of years. Success is built into the Core Diet because you are required to eat when you feel hungry, stop when you feel full, and eat three meals and at least two snacks every day. If anything, you may be concerned that you are too full, since some people erroneously associate feeling full with gaining weight or not losing it.

The Core Diet shows you how to translate your body's signals, enabling you to distinguish true hunger and satiety—something many chronic dieters have forgotten how to do. If you count yourself in these ranks, don't despair; you'll soon become skillful and confident with the choices that will make you an expert weight manager. You will be acquiring knowledge that dispels nutritional myths, misconceptions, negative emotions, and unnatural eating behaviors. All of these camouflage true hunger and become devastating weight-gain triggers. For example, I'm sure you already know the consequences of the typical dieter's pattern of skipping breakfast, then getting a caffeine charge by drinking sugar-laden black coffee or a caffeinnated cola drink. Between the sugar and caffeine you won't be able to get a reliable reading on your physical and mental status. Instead you'll be inundated with conflicting and confusing messages, torpedoing your best resolve. Phase I of the Core Diet will take you back to the basics, putting you in touch with your body's own wisdom, freeing you of triggering foods, substances, and actions, and keeping you right on track for achieving your weight goals.

In the Core Diet Phase I, I've chosen foods that are nutritionally dense, that are satisfying, and that eliminate weight-gain triggers. You will discover that these food choices are wide and varied, with satisfying flavors that will keep your taste buds happy. I refer to the foods in this phase of the program as "Standard pleasure foods." These are foods that are vital to building optimal health for managing your weight and that really appease your hunger yet cause you to lose weight immediately. The part you'll like most of all is that it is impossible to overeat standard pleasure foods because they are designed to satisfy genuine hunger, not just your capricious appetite.

You might be thinking that if there are Phase I Foods, there must be other phases of foods as well. And you are right. You'll soon graduate to the different phases as you expand your program. Future food selections offer an even greater variety of delectable choices, while simultaneously controlling your weight-gain triggers and melting way the pounds.

Basic Core Diet: Phase I

In Phase I of the Core Diet, you will accomplish two things:

1. You will master the Basic Core Diet along with the essential physical exercise and mind reeducation exercises discussed in Chapters 11 and 12;

2. You will begin to recognize your highly individualized personal weight-gain triggers and learn how to avoid their destructive influences.

How Long It Takes to Complete Phase I

One of the things that people love about the Right Bite program is that you can proceed at your own pace. I've developed signposts to watch for, however, that indicate when you have completed one level and are ready to move on to the next. For instance, you will know that you have completed Phase I of the Core Diet and are ready to begin Phase II when:

1. You have become comfortable with the Phase I Core Diet, along with its related exercise program and mind exercises, and these have become effortless and routine for you.

2. Your eating is under control.

3. Your weight is under control.

4. You are experiencing no side effects. If you were on an extreme diet just prior to going on this one, you may find that you are experiencing side effects that are caused by the previous diet. I have observed that the people most susceptible to side effects during Phase I are those who previously were following very unbalanced, low-caloric diets and/or high-protein diets. Also, most dieters who have consumed large amounts of caffeine, sugar, and alcohol, or those who have used nicotine, usually experience withdrawal side effects. Following are some common side effects that can last anywhere from one to seven days.

Headaches

These often occur after removing caffeine, nicotine, and sugar from your diet.

Temporary Weight Gain

A small number of people gain between one and seven pounds in the first week. If this happens to you, keep your cool. This gain is temporary! There are a number of reasons for this:

✓ **Water-weight gain:** If you have been following a high-protein diet, a very low-calorie diet, or have been taking diuretics you will probably experience a temporary water-weight gain after embarking on the Core Diet. Recognize that if you were formerly engaging in any of these diet practices, your previous weights were based on the fact that you were dehydrated. Since 70 percent of the human body consists of water, eating a high-protein diet or undereating negatively affects one's water balance, resulting in dehydration. After a healthy water balance is restored, the scale will register your body's new cellular rehydration. Visualize your formerly thirsty cells as shriveled raisins and then as grapes after sufficient water has been restored.

✓ **Glycogen depletion:** As we've discussed in previous chapters, glycogen is a form of glucose stored in your liver and muscles. It has its own cellular weight. Rigorous dieters quickly reduce their stored glycogen. Once a normal eating pattern is resumed the body automatically begins storing this important energy source again, and you see the numbers on your scale go up when you weigh yourself.

✓ **Actual weight of food digesting in stomach and intestines:** Again, many dieters weigh themselves after they have been undereating for a prolonged period so that there is little if any food in their stomachs, or fecal matter in their intestines. Once regular eating resumes, our bodies will be continually processing food in various states of digestion and, quite naturally, this will show up on the scale. Also, the Core Diet is high in fiber content, and fiber holds considerable amounts of water as well. You will note this if you weigh yourself before and after a bowel movement. Scientifically curious dieters often report losing two or three pounds after a bowel movement.

✓ **Preperiod:** If a woman weighs herself fourteen days before her period is due, she will likely note a weight gain. This is due to the fact that her body naturally retains more water during this time.

✓ **Increased lean body mass:** Lean body mass means muscle—and don't forget that muscle is one of your greatest allies for burning fat. Keep in mind, though, that muscle is heavier than fat, so as muscle replaces fat on your body you may see it reflected either in higher numbers on your scale or in no appreciable weight loss. But don't let this fool you. With muscle gradually replacing fat, you will look thinner, feel better, and have more energy, even if your weight temporarily increases.

✓ **Rebound water-weight gain from radical dieting:** If you have been dieting prior to starting the Core Diet, your water-deprived body may start grabbing and storing all the water it can. It goes into survival mode for awhile, sort of like a camel that's found a watering hole after wandering on the desert for thirty days. So it's possible that your body will overhydrate for several days, retaining water because it believes it must do so in order to protect itself from the next journey across the arid desert.

Milk Sensitivity—Lactose Intolerance

Research has demonstrated that the severity and prevalence of lactose intolerance are grossly exaggerated by the media. In a similar vein, congenital lactase deficiency is extremely rare. In case you were wondering, lactase is an enzyme, produced by your body, which must be present to properly digest milk and milk products. I have found that the most common form of lactose intolerance experienced by clients is something known as "secondary lactase deficiency." This is a temporary and transient condition resulting from diseases or conditions, such as radical dieting, that damage the intestinal mucosa where lactase (the enzyme that breaks down lactose) is present. Once the physical conditions are resolved, lactose digestion improves.

Many dieters eliminate milk products for personal reasons so that when they first begin consuming them again they are lactose intolerant—that is, unable to digest the milk sugar lactose because they lack the enzyme (lactase) for doing that. Some people experience gas, bloating, and cramping or diarrhea during this period of early adjustment.

If you are not sure if you are lactose intolerant and are experiencing unusual gas, bloating, or cramping, check with your doctor to rule out any medical conditions that may be causing it. Or you may wish to remove all milk products from your diet for a day or two. If your symptoms lessen or disappear altogether, you can be pretty confident that milk and milk products are the culprits, and you would then want to temporarily remove them from your diet.

Usually an actual lactase deficiency shows up somewhere between two and twenty years of age. Even if you were lactose intolerant, it would be extremely rare for you to be unable to occasionally consume milk products. While you need to experiment so that you will know your own threshold for milk products, most lactose intolerant people find they can tolerate the equivalent of about one cup of milk or milk products a day. Also, cottage cheeses and yogurts are tolerated better than milk.

There are several ways to remedy lactose intolerance. The easiest is to take milk off your diet for several days, then gradually increase the intake of lactose-containing foods. This continued exposure to lactose seems to enhance the efficiency of colonic bacteria to metabolize lactose and increase your body's production of the lactase enzyme. Completely eliminating lactose-containing products will worsen lactose intolerance. If you have difficulty digesting milk and milk products and want to be able to enjoy these foods, you can get a liquid lactase preparation to add to your milk, or you can take an oral enzyme replacement tablet at the beginning of a meal that includes milk products. You can also buy lactose-free milk products.

Constipation

Some people, especially those who have been on high-protein or other severe diets, do not have bowel movements for several days when they begin the Core Diet, despite the large amounts of fiber in this diet. This is because your intestinal flora and enzymes make adjustments every time there is a structural change in your diet, or whenever you take medications. If your intestines are not used to processing lots of carbohydrates, as would be true if you'd been on a high-protein diet, the enzymes that otherwise would be used to disassemble them are temporarily deficient. Once carbohydrate foods are reintroduced via the Core Diet, your body will start calling forth the enzyme workers to do their job. Sooner or later a bowel movement will occur—and be prepared—it will be "the mother of all bowel movements." After that, all systems will return to normal.

Excess Bowel Movements or Urination

Some dieters experience loose bowel movements and more frequent urination as they start the Core Diet. This is more likely to be true if you have been on a radical diet prior to starting this program. In about a week, your body will magically produce new enzymes and bacteria, and your system will soon be in shape to handle the nutritious and abundant foods you are now eating. Your digestive system will settle into a regular and comfortable rhythm.

Depression

A few dieters have reported that they experienced some depression during the first week. In every case that I've examined, this has been the result of coming off sugar, caffeine, alcohol, and/or highly processed foods, and then adapting to new nutritious eating. Any changes in mood generally level out and vanish entirely in the second week.

Fatigue

Some dieters at first feel a type of fatigue similar to that one experiences after major surgery. They may go through a period of being chronically tired, sleeping longer than usual, and resisting getting up in the morning. The reason for this is that when you have been undereating or using caffeine and other stimulating drugs for a prolonged period, your body responds to this stress by releasing stress hormones. Stress hormones are "hyper" hormones. Stress, which, thank heavens, is ordinarily a temporary state, creates no major harm, so it is okay to be hyper once in a while. But imagine your formerly diet-abused body religiously pumping out stress hormones day and night for months, if not years. Your body never gets a chance to rest. Your true fatigue level has been completely camouflaged, and your body has not been able to repair itself properly. Suddenly, on the Core Diet you begin to eat adequate calories of the most nutritious foods possible, and you are not taking detrimental stimulants. What does your body do? It gives a big sigh of relief and decides to convalesce—it rests and repairs. Thankfully, as your body normalizes through the Core Diet, the fatigue you initially experienced is replaced by a new level of energy.

The Basic Core Diet—Phase I

The Basic Core Diet consists of eight food categories. These are:

Category I—Dairy
Category II—Protein
Category III—Fruits C
Category IV—Fruits A
Category V—Vegetables C
Category VI—Vegetables A
Category VII—Grains and Starches
Category VIII—Oils

There is an abundant variety of food preferences and tastes represented in these eight groups, and from them you will be able to choose meals that are both satisfying and nutritious. At the beginning of each chart, I have provided you with a note for the *minimum number of servings* you will need to select from that chart each day. Notice that I say "minimum number of servings." Sometimes the total recommended servings per day might seem like a lot of food to you. These food lists have been carefully calculated and tested and used with great success by my clients, and me, for over twenty years. To get immediate and permanent results, be sure to follow the food plan and instructions exactly. It is important to choose at least the minimum quantities per day, except under special circumstances:

✓ You are too full: Please refer to Guideline #2 under Instructions, and also refer to Modifications to the Core Diet, at the end of the chapter.

✓ You are still hungry: Please refer to Guideline #2 and #9 under Instructions. In addition, refer to Basic Core Optional Fruits and Vegetables list and Modifications to the Core Diet section at the end of this chapter.

It's important to accurately follow the measurements and quantities I give you in these charts. Get a food scale and measure your helpings at first. Within a week you'll be able to estimate the size of your helpings by sight rather than measuring them out. After that, you'll only need to measure new foods for which you haven't yet established a mental picture of portion sizes.

Now, let's examine each of these categories in detail.

Foods for Phase I—Basic Core Diet

CATEGORY I: DAIRY PRODUCTS

Minimum Servings Per Day: 2
Nutritional Values: 12 g carbohydrate, 8 g protein, trace fat, 80–90 calories.

Low-fat cottage cheese (1% fat or less) . .1/2 cup
Nonfat milk (skim) . . . . .1 cup
1/2 % milk . . . . .1 cup
1% milk . . . . .1 cup
Low-fat buttermilk . . . . .1 cup
Evaporated nonfat milk . . . . .1/2 cup
Nonfat instant dry milk . . . . .1/3 cup dry
Low-fat yogurt with no sugar added . . . .1 cup

CATEGORY II: PROTEIN

Minimum Servings Per Day: 2

Nutritional Values:	Protein (g)	Fat (g)	Calories
Low-fat cottage cheese: 1/2 cup . . .	14	2	80-90
Bluefish: 2 oz.	14	3	90
Bass: 2 oz	14	2.5	83
Catfish 3 oz.	16	1	90
Clams: 4 oz. raw	14	1	84
Clams, canned/drained: 2 oz	14	1	84
Clams, steamed: 14	16	1	93
Cod: 3 oz poached	18	1	90
Crabmeat: 3 oz	18	1	90
Flounder: 3 oz	20	1	100
Grouper: 3 oz	21	1	100
Haddock: 3 oz	22	1	100
Halibut: 3 oz	22	1.5	120
Lobster: 5/8 cup steamed . . .	19	1	90
Lobster: 4 oz steamed	23	1	110
Octopus: 4 oz raw	17	1	93
Oysters, Pacific raw: 1/2 cup	12	3	100
Eastern raw 1/2 cup	9	2	85
Oysters Pacific: 4 oz broiled	11	2	92
Eastern: 4 oz broiled	9	2	82
Perch: 3 oz	20	1	103
Pollack: 3 oz baked or broiled	20	1	96
Salmon: 1/4 cup canned	13–14	3–5	70–110

Nutritional Values: **Protein (g)**   **Fat (g)**   **Calories**

Note: If choosing salmon, eliminate one oil serving for that day.

2 oz. Fresh (after cooking)

	Protein (g)	Fat (g)	Calories
Atlantic	12	7	115
Chinook	15	7.5	130
Chum	15	3	80
Coho	14	5	100
Pink	15	3	80
Sockeye	15	6	120
Scallops: 4 oz raw (before cooking)	15	1	96

Shrimp:

	Protein (g)	Fat (g)	Calories
Cooked, boiled, 6	18	1	85
Canned, drained 1/2 cup	15	1	76
Snapper: 3 oz	22	1	108
Surimi: 4 oz	17	1	112
Tuna, water packed: 3 oz	22	1	100
Chicken: light meat: 2 oz	16	2	100
dark meat: 2 oz	15	5	116
Chicken, Swanson, canned in water: 3 oz can	16	1	80
Turkey, light meat: 2 oz	17	2	90
dark meat 2 oz	16	4	106
Egg Beaters®: 1/2 cup	15	4	106
Egg whites: 4	16	0	70
Soybeans: 1/3 cup	10	0	100
Tofu: 1/2 cup	10	0	94

Legumes: (kidney beans, pinto beans, etc.) Although also considered a source of protein, because of their starch content, these foods will be listed elsewhere.

CATEGORY III: FRUITS "C"

Fruits in this group are recommended because they are a delicious source of Vitamin C. Vitamin C from fruits helps in collagen synthesis, which helps to strengthen joints and connective tissue and fortifies blood vessel walls, heals damaged cells, and creates the matrix for bone growth. It is an antioxidant, helps our bodies resist infection, and assists in the absorption of iron.

Minimum Servings Per Day: 2
(Each serving contains 15 to 20 grams of carbohydrates)

Nutritional Values	Calories
Grapefruit: 1	80
Honeydew: 1 cup cubes	60

Nutritional Values	Calories
Kiwi fruit: 2	.80
Mango: 2/3 cup	.70
Orange: 1 1/2 or 1 cup sections	.90
Papaya: 2/3 cup	.90
Pineapple (fresh) 1 cup	.75
Raspberries: 1 cup fresh	.60
Strawberries: 1 cup fresh	.60
Tangerines: 2	.80
Watermelon 1 1/2 cups	.80

CATEGORY IV: FRUITS "A"

Fruits in this group provide Vitamin A. This vitamin helps us maintain healthy skin and mucous membranes, as well as the outer layers of cells around many of our internal organs. It is also important in maintaining healthy teeth and bones, and in maintaining good immunity and reproductive functions. You will note that some fruits and vegetables are placed in both "A" and "C" categories because they are excellent sources of both of these nutrients.

Minimum Servings Per Day: 1
(Each serving provides 15 to 20 grams of carbohydrate.)

Nutritional Values	Calories
Apricots: 4 fresh	.70
Cherries: water packed, fresh,	
frozen, sour: 1 cup	88
Cantaloupe: 1/2 melon	.93
Mango: 2/3 cup	.70
Papaya: 2/3 cup	.90
Peaches: 2 or 1 cup fresh	.70
Tangerines: 2	.70
Watermelon: 1 1/2 cups	.80

CATEGORY V: VEGETABLES "C"

These vegetables are excellent sources of vitamin C.
Minimum Servings Per Day: 2
(Each serving contains about 10 grams of carbohydrates)

Nutritional Values	Calories
Asparagus: 1 cup	.45
Broccoli: 1 cup fresh or frozen	.45
Brussels sprouts: 1 cup fresh or frozen . .	50

Nutritional Values	Calories
Bok choy: 1 cup cooked	.20
Cabbage: 1 cup red raw	.20
1 cup cooked	.32
Cauliflower: 1 cup cooked or raw	.30
Kale: 1 cup cooked or raw	.40
Kohlrabi, raw: 1 cup	.38
cooked: 1 cup	.48
Mustard Greens: 1 cup cooked or raw	.22
Parsley: 1 cup raw	.22
Pepper, green: 1 cooked or raw	.20
Pepper, red: 1/2 cup	.20
Snow peas: 1 cup	.60
Tomato: 1	.26
1 cup	.38
Turnip greens: cooked, fresh, 1 cup	.30
frozen: 1 cup	.50

CATEGORY VI: VEGETABLES "A"

These vegetables are excellent sources of vitamin A.
Minimum Servings Per Day: 1
(Each serving contains about 10 grams of carbohydrates.)

Nutritional Values	Calories
Asparagus: 1 cup fresh or frozen	.45
Snap green beans: 1 cup	.40
Beet greens: 1/2 cup cooked	.20
Broccoli: 1 cup fresh or frozen	.45
Bok choy: 1 cup cooked	.20
Carrots: 1 large carrot	.31
1/2 cup cooked	.35
Chard: 1 cup cooked	.35
Collards: 1 cup cooked, fresh	.35
frozen	.31
Dandelion greens: 1 cup cooked	.35
1 cup raw	.25
Escarole (endive): 4 cups	.32
Kale: 1 cup cooked, fresh or frozen	.20
Romaine: 4 cups (seems like a lot, but remember, just a few leaves take up a lot of space when cut for a salad)	.32
Mustard greens: 1 cup cooked, fresh or frozen	.20
Pepper: red 1/2 cup	.30

Nutritional Values	Calories
Pumpkin: 1/2 cup	.40
Spinach: 3 cups raw	.36
1 cup cooked	.45
Winter squash: 1/2 cup	.48
Tomato: 1	.26
Turnip greens: 1/2 cup cooked, fresh	.30
1/2 cup cooked, frozen	.50

CATEGORY VI: GRAINS AND STARCHES
Minimum Servings Per Day: 6
(Each serving contains about 20 grams of carbohydrate.)

Nutritional Values	Calories
Barley: 1/2 cup cooked	.100
Buckwheat groats, 1/2 cup cooked	.90
Corn: 1/2 cup	.90
Corn grits: 3T. dry	.105
Cracked wheat cereal: 1/4 cup dry	.90
Multigrain oatmeal: 1/3 cup dry	.90
Old-fashioned Quaker oats: 1/3 cup dry	.100
Shredded wheat and bran: 2/3 cup	.90
Brown rice: 1/2 cup cooked	.108
Bulghar wheat: 3/4 cup cooked	.113
Oat bran: 1/3 cup dry	.100
Whole-wheat spaghetti: 1/2 cup (cooked)	.90
Whole-wheat elbow macaroni: 1/2 cup (cooked)	.90
Whole-wheat shells: 1/2 cup (cooked)	.90
Whole-wheat spinach spaghetti: 1/2 cup (cooked)	.90
Whole-wheat spinach egg noodles: 1/2 cup (cooked)	.90
Whole-wheat spirals: 1/2 cup (cooked)	.90
Millet: 4 oz cooked	.135
Wheatena: 1/4 cup dry	.120
Red River Cereal: 1/4 cup dry	.120
Sweet potato—medium-sized, baked in skin: 5" x 2"	.118
Wheatgerm: 1/4 cup	.110
Bulgur wheat with soy grits: 1/4 cup dry	.110
Potato: 5 oz	.100
7-grain cereal (usually found in health food stores): 1 serving	.130
4-grain cereal (usually found in health food stores): 1 serving	.130

Nutritional Values	Calories

Wheat bran: 1/4 cup—may be sprinkled freely on any
of the above but not counted as grain serving 30

Note: It is important to find a good source for whole grain foods, including pastas. My favorite source is Hodgson Mills.

Legumes: 1/2 cup (must be chosen once a day) 100

Great Northern beans, kidney beans, navy beans, lima beans, black-eyed peas, garbanzo beans, black beans, lentils, split peas, pinto beans

To fulfill your legume requirement, I heartily recommend my lentil soup as a core component of your daily diet. (See Chapter 10 for menus and recipes.)

CATEGORY VIII: OILS

Minimum Servings Per Day: choose 3–9

Nutritional Values: Each teaspoon of oil contains 40 calories.

Flax seed oil: ....1 teaspoon
Canola oil: ....1 teaspoon
Olive oil: ....1 teaspoon

Basic Core Diet Condiments and Seasonings Allowed

Flavor makes the experience of eating enjoyable. However, many commercially processed foods are heavily seasoned, often with flavor enhancers that act as weight-gain triggers. As a result, it can be difficult, if not impossible, to tell when you are truly hungry or full. When our taste buds are overstimulated by special seasonings, we have a tendency to eat even when we are no longer actually hungry. For this reason, I have selected condiments that enhance the natural flavors and wholesome tastes of the Basic Core Diet selections. These condiments satisfy our desire for tastes without triggering a hard to control appetite. Your taste buds are in for a wonderful surprise.

SALT SUBSTITUTES:
> ✓ Vinegar—be sure to try out specialty vinegars such as balsamic, herbed vinegars, and rice vinegar. But always check the labels to avoid excess salt.
> ✓ Herbs and spices that do not contain sugar or artificial sweeteners, MSG, or large amounts of salt—for example, Mrs. Dash®, onion powder, garlic powder, cinnamon, basil, thyme.
> ✓ Calorie-free spray-on butter flavor
> ✓ Lemons or limes
> ✓ Salsa—use as a condiment in moderation, not as a sauce!

✓ Spaghetti sauce that is sugar free, such as Classico®
Tomato and Basil: 1/4 cup. Also see Hal's Spaghetti Sauce
in the Recipe Section.

✓ Potassium chloride salt substitute

Basic Core Diet Beverages

✓ Water
✓ Naturally flavored, sugar-free sparkling waters
✓ Decaffeinated tea and coffee
✓ Herb tea
✓ Skim milk

Basic Core Optional Fruits List

When you have met all your Core Diet requirements and if you are still hungry, you may go back to the Core Diet food categories in Phase I, and select two more items from Dairy and two more from the Protein. There are no restrictions on your selections from the Fruits, Vegetables, and Starch category. Also, instead of, or in addition to supplementing your diet with foods from the Core food categories, you may supplement from the following Optional Fruits and Vegetables List. You may not count these fruits as your main fruits because they are not as nutrient dense as the others.

Nutritional Values   **Calories**
(Each serving contains 15 to 20 grams carbohydrates.)

Apple: 2 3/4" diameter 81
    1 cup 63
Banana: 1 (11 calories per inch) 80
Blackberries: 1 cup, fresh 86
Blueberries: 1 cup, fresh, ...85
Cranberries: 1/2 cup 30
Water-packed fruit or fruit pack
    in natural fruit juice: 1 serving . .Refer to label
Green Grapes: 20 grapes 70
Nectarine: 1 70
Pear: 1 fresh: 2 1/2" diameter 98
Plums: 2 fresh 72

Basic Core Optional Vegetables List

The following are vegetables that you may include with your meals but that are not to be counted as your main vegetable. Just as with the Optional Fruits List, the vegetables on this list are not as nutrient dense as the ones on the main vegetable list.

Nutritional Values   **Calories**
(Each serving contains approximately 5 grams of carbohydrate.)

Alfalfa sprouts: 1 cup 10
Artichokes: 1 60
Bamboo shoots: 1 cup 25
Yellow or wax beans: 1 cup 44
Bean sprouts: raw, 1 cup 31
Bean sprouts:boiled: 1 cup 26
Beets, fresh, sliced or diced: 1/2 cup 37
       canned, sliced or diced: 1/2 cup 26
Celery: 1 stalk 6
Cucumber: 7 slices 4
Eggplant: 1 cup cooked 45
Lettuce—all varieties: unlimited 10
Mushrooms, raw, sliced: 1/2 cup 9
       cooked: 1/2 cup 21
Okra: 8 pods 27
       1/2 cup 34
Onions: 1/2 cup raw or cooked 45
Radishes: 10 8
Turnips: 1/2 cup, cooked 14
Spaghetti squash: 1/2 cup 22
Watercress: 1/2 cup 2
Yellow squash: 1/2 cup 25
Zucchini: 1/2 cup 20

Vitamin Supplements

One multiple/vitamin mineral supplement a day: In addition to taking a high-quality multivitamin-mineral supplement, I recommend also taking 500 mg of vitamin C, 400 IU of vitamin E, and three 500–600 mg tablets of calcium if you are female.

Foods to Avoid During Phase I of the Basic Core Diet

Phase II Foods: See Chapter 9 for a complete definition and list. These consist of Medium-Pleasure Foods and High-Pleasure Foods.

Deviation Foods and Substances: (I will address these in greater detail in the next chapter.) Most of the foods and substances on the following list are considered deviation foods and substances:

- ✓ Eliminate the following sugars unless they occur naturally in the food you're eating: honey, syrup, corn syrup, molasses, raw sugar, cane sugar, brown sugar, confectioner's sugar, sucrose, lactose, fructose, dextrose, dextrins, corn syrup solids, nutritive sweeteners, maple syrup, heavy syrup, invert syrup, caramels, malt, maltose, sorghum, sorghum syrup, refined sugar. Also if package says "sugar cured," "cured," or "mild cured," it means that the product contains added sugar.
- ✓ Foods high in fat
- ✓ Refined, bleached, or unbleached white flour
- ✓ Coffee, tea, colas, Mountain Dew®, Dr. Pepper®, and any other beverage containing caffeine
- ✓ Alcohol
- ✓ Monosodium glutamate
- ✓ Cocoa powder or chocolate
- ✓ Sugar-free chocolate
- ✓ Salt (See Guideline #6 under "Instructions.")
- ✓ Nicotine
- ✓ Illegal drugs
- ✓ Medications not approved by your physician

Obviously it is *impossible* to list all foods not allowed because of the enormous quantity of edibles already on the market and because new food products are being developed every day. The following elaborates on the previous list.

PROTEIN TO AVOID
- ✓ Cheese spreads
- ✓ Cheeses except those listed as "allowed"
- ✓ Cottage cheese containing sweetened fruit
- ✓ Most cold cuts or lunch meats (See details in Phase II Food List.)
- ✓ Pickled or spiced meats such as pastrami, corned beef, sauerbraten
- ✓ Bacon
- ✓ Sausage, kielbasa, frankfurters

- ✓ Turkey roll, chicken roll
- ✓ Fried chicken
- ✓ Ready-made salads such as egg, chicken, tuna
- ✓ Fish cakes, deviled crabs, breaded fish
- ✓ Breaded veal
- ✓ Glazed baked ham, canned ham
- ✓ Meat with flour-thickened gravy
- ✓ Presweetened or flavored yogurt
- ✓ Chocolate milk
- ✓ Dry roasted or canned nuts that contain sugar (Note: Although nuts are high in protein, we steer away from them in the Basic Core Diet because of their high fat content.)
- ✓ Most canned soups: Read labels. There are some health food varieties that are acceptable. Others contain many of the items on the above list.

FRUITS NOT ALLOWED
- ✓ Any canned or frozen fruit that contains sugar
- ✓ Applesauce that contains sugar
- ✓ Jams, jellies, preserves, except sugar-free varieties (See Chapter 9.)
- ✓ Maraschino cherries
- ✓ Fruit drinks containing sugar
- ✓ Canned pie filling that contains sugar

VEGETABLES NOT ALLOWED
- ✓ Baked beans
- ✓ Canned vegetables in sauce, or containing MSG or sugar
- ✓ Vegetables frozen in sauce, or containing MSG or sugar
- ✓ Pickles
- ✓ Candied yams

CARBOHYDRATES NOT ALLOWED
- ✓ White, bleached, or unbleached bread products
- ✓ Breaded foods
- ✓ Crackers containing taboo ingredients such as sugar, MSG, or high salt content.
- ✓ Cake
- ✓ Candy
- ✓ Cookies
- ✓ Cereals except those listed under "Grains and Starches Allowed"
- ✓ Sweetened desserts

✓ White refined bleached flour
✓ Gelatin deserts
✓ Jams or jellies containing sugar
✓ Ice cream
✓ Noodles made from white bleached flour
✓ Pancakes made from bleached four
✓ Pastries, cupcakes, donuts
✓ Rice pudding
✓ Tapioca pudding
✓ Peanut butter containing sugar and/or hydrogenated fat

BEVERAGES NOT ALLOWED
✓ Alcohol
✓ Beverages containing caffeine
✓ Sugared sodas
✓ Lemonade
✓ Punch
✓ Postum®
✓ Ovaltine®
✓ Chocolate milk
✓ Hot chocolate
✓ Kool-Aid®-type drinks
✓ Fruit-juice-type drinks sweetened with sugar

FATS NOT ALLOWED
✓ Butter whipped with honey
✓ Imitation dairy products
✓ Mayonnaise, unless specified
✓ Prepared salad dressings that are sweet: Thousand Island, French, honey mustard, etc.

DRUGS AND MEDICATIONS NOT ALLOWED
Check with your doctor and take only physician-approved medications or drugs. NO NICOTINE!

EXCEPTIONS TO FOOD NOT ALLOWED
1. Sugar in bread: Sugar is added to bread in order to make the yeast rise. If you see sugar on a bread label, and it is not listed as a main ingredient, the bread is acceptable. However if you pick up a bread called "Honey Bran Bread" or cinnamon loaf, and sugar or honey is listed within the top five ingredients, it means the bread is high in sugar, and it is not acceptable. You will know that extra sugar has been added

beyond the rising needs of yeast. In Phase II you may add whole grain bread to your program.

2. The sugars occurring naturally in fruits, milk, and other carbohydrates are acceptable. If a product contains 1 gram or less of sugar per serving, you may use that product if other ingredients are acceptable.

The Instructions

1. FOLLOW YOUR PHASE I—BASIC CORE DIET, DAILY FOR THREE MONTHS

Admittedly, this will probably be a "boot camp" experience for you. The diet has been carefully researched and tested to make certain that all potential weight-gain triggers are eliminated and controlled—even the ones that may not apply to you. Although the diet requires more attention than simplistic and ineffective single-strategy diets, the payoff is extraordinary for anyone wishing to achieve permanent weight-loss and complete weight-management. You'll enjoy insights about yourself and your relationship to the food you eat, greater knowledge of your own body, an increase in your energy and sense of well-being, and a renewed sense of your own power to have the body and the life that you dream of.

Phase I of the program helps to restore to their natural powers the metabolic processes that may have been harmed by prior diets, including the more detrimental damage of high protein diets. Because of the importance of this phase of the program—truly the healing phase—it's particularly important that you stay focused and stick close to all the recommendations. After achieving biological harmony over the three months duration of Phase I, you will be ready to expand your diet through the upcoming phases described in the next chapter.

2. EAT WHEN HUNGRY; STOP WHEN FULL!

Eat whenever you experience hunger. Do not wait for your next scheduled meal or snack. I do not recommend a specific, total caloric intake but rather a range to work within. Larger, taller people, or those who are more physically active, or people whose metabolisms are balanced and healthy, will require more food than a person who is short, has a sluggish metabolism, or is physically inactive. If you are not confident that you recognize true hunger, consider the following.

Hunger

True hunger reflects a genuine need for sustenance, even though you may still feel your last meal or snack in your stomach. Hunger can also cause an empty feeling in your stomach, even if you don't have a strong urge to eat. When you are genuinely hungry, you may feel lethargic or fatigued several hours after eating, even though you have not engaged in any draining activity or experienced a more conscious desire for food. Unexplained headaches or irritability are frequent symptoms of hunger. Initial hunger pangs will not feel intense if you have been closely following the Right Bite Program.

Insomnia is often hunger-based. There are at least four nutritional causes for insomnia: too few calories in your diet, insufficient oil in your diet, caffeine, and, in a small percentage of cases, the food additive *aspartame*. Unexplained depression or sagging spirits can be caused by hunger. Feelings of being light-headed, faint, cold, or shaky, or an inability to concentrate may be hunger-based. Hunger may be a craving for food, especially for sweets or greasy salty carbohydrates. When you tell yourself, "I am not hungry, I just feel like nibbling" you may be experiencing hunger.

Hunger is sometimes rather difficult to determine for people who have been chronic dieters. They have stoically ignored or resisted hunger for such long periods of time that they are almost unable to recognize it. Many people believe that hunger occurs only when they experience an empty feeling in their stomach, complete with rumblings and groanings of their digestive machinery. This is just one manifestation of hunger, and if you wait until your stomach has indeed become hollow or concave, you're sure to make it overly convex with later bouts of out-of-control overeating.

In some rare cases, there are people who truly can't tell for sure when they are hungry, who simply cannot trust their own judgment about what is true hunger. If you feel you fall into this category after being on the Core Diet for two weeks, please see Appendix A for guidance.

WARNING! If you *abnormally* or ferociously crave any specific food listed on the Basic Core Diet or find that a particular food makes you hungrier, causes sudden weight gain, or produces any other undesirable symptom, you may be dealing with a food addiction or experiencing a food intolerance. Immediately remove any such food items from your diet. The only sure way of controlling or eliminating an allergic or addictive food is through avoiding that food completely.

Consume and *enjoy* all of the allowed foods listed on your program until you are comfortably *full or satisfied*. At first, many of you will not be able to fulfill all the diet requirements because you feel satiated. This is because your metabolism has slowed down from past radical and very low-calorie dieting. As your metabolism speeds up, you will burn more calories and feel increased hunger. IMPORTANT! It *is acceptable* that you don't eat the total *quantity* of each Core category requirement, but you must eat portions from each of the required food categories. In other words, just eat smaller helpings of each required food. Do not eliminate a food category because you feel full, just eat less of it.

Many long-term dieters have forgotten what it means to be "full" or "satisfied." I define these feeling as follows.

Full or Satisfied

You are full or satisfied when your physiological desire for food has ceased. Your stomach no longer gurgles or feels concave. A meal or snack has relieved the peculiar lethargic feeling that is a signal of food deprivation.

It is important for you to learn to distinguish between diet-related fatigue and the normal fatigue associated with working a full day in the salt mines, of getting up at the crack of dawn, or of concentrating hours at school and studying late into the night. There is no one who can feel more fatigued than a mom who has had young children careening around her all day. Also, you will need to know the difference between the fatigue from poor dieting and the fatigue that can engulf you once your body is no longer under the self-imposed stress of poor dieting.

It is not unusual to feel tired when you first begin to eat nutritiously and have given up false stimulants like coffee and nicotine. Your body desperately needs a period of time to convalesce and repair. When you no longer crave sweets, when you are no longer light-headed, when you feel alert and are able to concentrate without caffeine—these are indications that you may be "full" or "satisfied." One thing is for sure— being full does not mean overstuffing yourself with as much food as you can shove down your gullet.

3. EAT A *MINIMUM* OF THREE MEALS AND TWO SNACKS A DAY

I strongly encourage you to enjoy more than three meals and two snacks a day, if you desire. Just for the record, here's how I distinguish between meals and snacks.

Meal: A meal is any gathering of four or more foods from the different categories I've listed in the previous pages of this chapter. For example, a breakfast of oatmeal and milk is unacceptable. However, a breakfast of oatmeal, milk, an orange, and a teaspoon of canola oil sprinkled on top is acceptable.

Snack: A snack is defined as any protein or protein/carbohydrate source combined with a carbohydrate. For example, a glass of milk is unacceptable for a snack. A glass of milk with a half cup of strawberries is acceptable. This combination of protein and carbohydrates help us maintain stable blood sugar levels.

4. Plan Ahead

If you have a job or go to school, you will need to take the time each day to pack a lunch with snacks or be familiar with restaurants in the area where you will be spending your time. I have never been to a restaurant that was not able to provide food cooked to the customer's specifications. Most restaurants serve baked potatoes, grilled fish, and steamed vegetables. When I eat at a Chinese restaurant, I always request no MSG, and ask that my vegetables be prepared steamed or without thickened sauces.

If you are going on an extended outing, or are attending a party, plan ahead. Never assume that your proper food or beverages in the correct amounts will be available at your destination. Check and double-check. Don't disrupt your diet because of poor planning, lack of foresight, laziness, or carelessness. Chapter 13 provides detailed guidance for eating out and discusses other trouble spots for dieters that may arise.

5. Read All Labels

Read all labels to make sure you are not consuming any contraband item that a food processor has sneaked into your food. Don't take anything for granted. If in doubt, don't eat it.

6. Use Salt Moderately

Be moderate in your sodium intake but not fanatical about avoiding it. Sodium occurs naturally in foods and in some of the products listed in this book. When you want a more salty taste use a no-salt alternative.

7. Eat a Variety of Foods

You will be much happier with the Core Diet and feel more satisfied if you explore a wide range of the foods in the categories I list. It might seem easier to focus on the same foods every day, but in time you will get bored and even feel deprived. Because variety ensures that you are getting an adequate balance of nutrients, and satisfies deep inner desires associated with food, choosing from a wide range of foods and tastes will help keep you happily on track.

8. Use Optional Choices Correctly

You may include Basic Core Optional Vegetables or Fruits with your meals, but don't count them as your A or C vegetable or fruit. Eat the required A and C groups, as prescribed as well, because Optional Fruits and Vegetables are not as nutritionally dense as those in the required groups.

9. What to Eat If You're Still Hungry

If you complete the Basic Core Diet requirements and are still hungry, you may choose additional helpings from the Phase I—Basic Core

Diet or from your Basic Core Optional Fruits or Vegetables List. But do not choose more than two extra servings from the protein and dairy food groups. Make sure that any of your additional helpings come only from starches, fruits, and vegetables.

10. Weigh or Measure Your Food

Initially, weigh or measure your food to insure that you are getting the exact requirements and are not undereating or overeating. After you measure portions for a short time you will be able to estimate portion size without weighing or measuring.

11. Plan for Social Events

Attending social events can pose some particular challenges while you are on the Core Diet. Please refer to Chapter 13 for how to effectively deal with these issues. A general guideline is to make sure you have a small snack before you leave home so that you won't be tempted by bacon-wrapped water chestnuts, liver pate, or chocolate-covered macadamia nuts.

12. Have a Physical

Before starting any diet, it's always a good idea to have a complete physical examination to rule out any physical problems that need attention, particularly hormonal imbalances and thyroid malfunctions. Check with your doctor to make sure any medication you might be taking is necessary. If weight gain is a side effect of your medication, ask your doctor if there is an alternate drug that can accomplish the same thing.

13. Abstain from All Alcohol Consumption

Even small amounts of alcohol will undermine your best efforts on this diet.

14. No Caffeine!

15. No Smoking!

Using any kind of tobacco product, or smoking marijuana, will disrupt your best efforts on the Core Diet. In addition, you must limit your exposure to second-hand tobacco smoke as much as possible.

16. Incorporate Regular Physical Exercise in Your Program

Follow my guidelines, outlined in Chapter 11. Always obtain permission from your doctor before embarking on any exercise program.

17. TAKE YOUR VITAMINS

Take them with breakfast or lunch and never on an empty stomach.

18. DEVELOP YOUR MIND EXERCISE PROGRAM

Develop your mind exercise program according to the guidelines I set forth in Chapter 12. You'll be learning all about these in that chapter, but for now it's enough to know that you will perform these daily, repeating them whenever the opportunity arises. And those opportunities are many: before falling asleep at night; while you are exercising, showering, driving, waiting in line, or on hold on the telephone. You will be surprised at the amount of idle time your brain can take advantage of. Use this time productively.

19. BE AWARE

Use your knowledge of weight-gain triggers that cause uncontrolled eating or weight gain, such as knowing when you need to move away from people who are smoking or remembering to have a snack or meal before attending a party. Your heightened awareness will be a powerful tool for helping you to achieve your ideal weight and manage your weight thereafter.

20. KEEP TRACK OF YOUR PERIOD

For menstruating women not on the pill: Mark your calendar for the first day of your next menstrual cycle. Then count two weeks back from the anticipated onset of your next menstrual period. This will be the estimated time of your monthly ovulation. The days from this point to the estimated beginning of your next period are your preperiod days. It is normal to feel hungrier and to crave carbohydrates during this preperiod portion of your cycle. If you experience preperiod hunger, do not fearfully ignore it. Raise your caloric intake a modest amount in the form of carbohydrates. Your appetite will decrease once your period begins. But be careful! Do not use your preperiod as an excuse to overeat.

I have occasionally had clients who experienced a preperiod hunger that is not appeased by food, no matter how much they eat. If you are one of these rare individuals and this hunger plagues you, establish an upper limit on how many extra calories you are going to consume. I recommend an additional 200 to 500 calories per day. I can assure you that on a day when you are experiencing this type of curious hunger, you will still feel just as hungry on 5000 as on 500 extra calories. I have observed that this abnormal hunger usually never lasts more than one to two days so hang in there!

21. Listen to Your Body

Listen to your *body* and its own internal *wisdom*. Do not listen to the ignorant brainwashed segment of your brain that may be feeding you doubts, misconceptions, negativisms, and unhealthy emotional responses. You will find that these two opposing forces are sometimes at war—your higher wisdom, with its more educated brain cells, and your childlike, gullible brain. Never let the unenlightened part of your brain win this battle. There will be numerous times throughout your day when it will test you. It will even brazenly tempt you with the thoughts of triggering foods or substances. You must allow your greater wisdom to win this battle. These are the times when your mind exercises are most helpful—when you are under siege, not just when you are idle. Never ignore the healthy demands of your body. Keep your antennae tuned to your body and the informed part of your brain.

22. Guidelines for Stress

Over the years it has become clear to me that one of the most common ways people cope with stress is by overeating. For that reason, developing tools for dealing with stress is a crucial component of the Right Bite program:

- ✓ Follow the Core Diet guidelines because the best protection from stress is a nutritious, adequate caloric diet, coupled with an exercise regimen.

- ✓ Try to identify your stresses and when possible avoid them, eliminate them, or make adjustments in your lifestyle to minimize them.

- ✓ Don't try to "do it all." Ask for help when possible.

- ✓ Set aside time each day for yourself, whether it be for a nap, reading, a walk in the park, or a few moments of quiet meditation. It is important to distance yourself from your normal routine from time to time throughout the day. In this way, you stay in touch with the greater wisdom of your body and mind.

- ✓ Have someone in your life you can trust to talk about your concerns and anxieties. This might be a special friend, a spouse, a parent, a brother or sister, or even a counselor. Just expressing your feelings helps to put stressful situations into perspective. Often a wise second party who has your best interests at heart can offer you valuable insights and solutions that can lighten your stressful concerns.

✓ Get organized! A common cause of stress comes from the dread that you cannot get everything done. Grab a calendar and organize your schedule, marking in important deadlines as well as the dates you will begin to work toward those deadlines. Believe it or not, when you see your schedule in black and white it helps you to realize that you can accomplish your goals.

✓ Be selective. Develop a scale of 1 to 10 for prioritizing what is important. Maybe now is the time to bow out of that neighborhood garage sale or to throw away the invitation to Jane's twelfth plastic ware party. Unless you are indispensable at these festivities it might not be essential for you to stand in grim attendance at every graduation, funeral, wedding, birthday, housewarming, anniversary, clambake, confirmation, bar mitzvah, circumcision, or holiday celebration.

✓ Try to develop a more relaxed outlook on how you perceive stress. Adopt fresh attitudes to prevent stress buildup from overwhelming and debilitating you. I realize that for certain stress agonies, such as the death of a loved one, there are no escapes, but for everyday trivial stresses, you can determine to change your perspective. For example, when my children were small, it was easy to become nearly frantic every time one of these treasured babes broke a dish or spilled goo on my furniture, barfed on my bosom, drew on the white wall with a banana, or gleefully mistook the carpet for a potty chair. I knew I had become skillful at handling high stress levels when I watched serenely as a rubber ball hurled by my two-year old sent grandmother's hand-painted china teapot to its final destination on the ceramic tile floor! Had I not learned to cope with unimportant stresses, I would have been under medication by now or locked up in an institution. Temporarily, my dishes all became plastic. I've painted my walls with washable paint, and I've learned that in the greater scheme of things material objects have to take second place to peace of mind and love for our children.

✓ If you can calm yourself enough to eat intelligently during periods of stress, do so. But eat only what your stomach can easily handle. Then try to eat small, frequent snacks to meet your energy and nutritional needs.

✓ Be sure to drink ample fluids to flush excess sodium from your body.

✓ Because all nutrients are compromised during the stress don't forget to take your vitamins.

✓ When the stressful situation has passed, replenish your depleted nutrient stores by conscientiously continuing to follow the Core Diet.

✓ As stress diminishes and if you are physically able, you must make an effort to regain lean body mass that was lost during the stressful episode. Physical exercise and healthful eating are extremely important at this time. If you are not physically compromised during a stress, it is a good idea to exercise moderately because exercise helps to relieve tension.

23. DEVELOP WAYS TO COUNTERACT TEMPTATION

Develop ways to counteract the temptation to eat that is stimulated by the sight, smell, or thought of food. Useful strategies include both mental imagery and defensive behaviors that will prevent your pancreas from secreting insulin, the hunger hormone. Here are some helpful guidelines:

✓ When possible, try not to hang out where food is being displayed and eaten. If you are at a party or social function, avoid standing close to tables loaded with goodies: move elsewhere, go powder your nose, dance, start a conversation with someone. Use the power of your imagination to keep your mind off the food.

✓ Think of the food in the same way you think of furniture or children's plastic replicas of hamburgers—objects that occupy space and are not to be eaten. Such copies of delicious desserts and entrees are extremely realistic, but because we know they are not real, they do not stimulate appetites. Pretend that all tempting morsels, particularly those that are your weakness, are nothing but inedible plastic or clay.

✓ Our appetites respond strongly to the tantalizing scents of food. Sometimes, if we are to not be swayed by tempting smells, we have to dissociate those tantalizing smells from the food they represent and the pleasures of eating them. Yes, I know this sounds like a ridiculous concept, but it can be put into practice. Let me give you an example. My daughter once brought home some delicious-smelling food-scented crayons. Brown was chocolate; black was licorice; red gave out the odor of maraschino cherries; white smelled like creme soda. However, being no fool, I knew they were wax crayons and was not tempted to eat them. And in spite of the tantalizing scents, my body did not respond to them as food. The same principle can be applied to foods that you must refrain from eating. Allow yourself to believe that the scents enticing you are the result of totally inedible compounds mixed up in a chemist's lab. Haven't you ever smelled a bar of chocolate scented soap? How many of you would be tempted to lose control and sink your teeth into it?

✓ The hostesses of most social functions now provide foods that are acceptable to people who are dieting or who do not eat sugary or oily foods. For example, carrot and celery sticks are pretty commonplace. Place items such as these on your plate and nibble on them throughout the evening. Sip on a glass of water with a slice of lemon.

✓ Use outrageous mental imagery to suppress your appetite. I am not trying to entertain you by being gross, but this strategy really works. It is sometimes necessary to conjure up repulsive images in order to stay in control. If you have a tremendous weakness for beer, you might want to imagine the beer you see as glasses of urine. If you can't resist anything made with peanut butter, imagine the peanut butter as earthworm spread. If you find chocolate irresistible, try thinking of it as ground up flies, cockroaches, or mouse droppings formed into cake or candy shapes.

I am sure you can think of your own mental "gross outs" that will take even the heartiest appetite away and save you at moments when you are on the verge of tearing off all your clothes and flinging yourself headlong onto a white chocolate cake. If you have children, they can be wonderfully helpful at assisting you in finding disgusting ways to view the foods that tempt you the most. And don't worry that these images will prevent you from enjoying chocolate again later. I have yet to see anyone lose that ability!

✓ If you are in charge of the kitchen at home and food temptations abound because of nondieting family members, place their mouth-watering goodies in opaque wrappers, climb on a stool and put them on shelves too high for you to reach without effort. Or enclose them in canisters that do not allow you to see or smell them. I keep my son's favorite cookies in an oatmeal container.

24. CRAVING GREASY FOODS

If you are craving greasy foods you may not be getting enough essential oil in your diet. Take care that you do not cut back on or completely eliminate oil from your diet.

25. MEAL PLANNING

Meal Planning Guidelines:

- ✓ Eat a minimum of three meals a day.

- ✓ Eat a minimum of two snacks a day.

- ✓ Never wait more than three hours between meals or snacks. Spacing of meals and snacks is very important.

- ✓ Make sure that the sizes of your meals and snacks are adequate so that in general you are comfortably able to wait a few hours in between. You don't want to eat breakfast at 7:00 a.m. and find yourself ready for lunch at 8:00. If you find that you are hell-bent on consuming your breakfast, snacks, lunch, and supper all in a couple hours, this should alert you to the fact that you are still not consuming enough at each meal.

- ✓ Never eat solely a carbohydrate for a snack. Include a protein source. Protein is antagonistic to insulin. In other words, it will help keep your insulin levels down, while stabilizing your blood sugar levels.

- ✓ Never eat solely a protein for a snack. Include a carbohydrate source. This will help maintain your blood sugar levels and prevent the protein from being converted to glucose.

- ✓ Eat legumes *at least once a day*. They are filling, high in fiber, carbohydrates, and protein, and are low on the glycemic index. They are foods that help you stabilize your blood sugar and lose weight.

- ✓ Vary your menu. Keep your food selections interesting and satisfying by making new selections every day.

✓ If you crave sweets, eat a carbohydrate from your Basic Core Foods along with a small serving of protein: oatmeal and milk, watermelon or strawberries with cottage cheese, and so on.

✓ Take the time to plan your menus until you are automatically familiar and comfortable with your program and can accurately prepare meals.

26. Do Not Vomit If You Binge, Overeat, or Feel Overfull

This will only cause you to binge again. While I hate to keep mentioning this, if you are one of the 14 percent of dieters who routinely use this method for controlling your weight, STOP!

27. Eat Slowly

It takes twenty minutes for your stomach to tell your brain that you are full.

28. Drink at Least Eight Cups of Fluid a Day

You will also get water from the foods you'll be eating on the Core Diet. Remember that thirst can manifest as hunger, and being adequately hydrated helps to prevent overeating. However, be sure you do not overuse fluids to make yourself feel full when you are truly hungry.

29. Keep a Journal

My favorite journals are those day-planners you can purchase at any office supply company. Make sure those you choose have plenty of space in which to write. Your journal will be a record of the types and amounts of food you ate and at what times, beverages consumed, type and duration of exercise, and your mind exercises and when you did them. You will treat the journal like a diary; recording events that you feel had an impact on either your emotional or physical well-being. In addition, you will also record illnesses and stresses, and evaluate how you are feeling each day. Think of yourself as a scientist compiling important data about yourself. This journal will be invaluable in precisely pinpointing your weight-gain triggers, providing insights for the formulation of strategies to control and/or eliminate them. The journal also helps you to reinforce the treatment program and to make sure you are not making mistakes.

30. Succumbing to Weight-Gain Triggers

Horrors! What if you inadvertently succumb to a weight-gain trigger because of a momentary indiscretion or memory lapse? Simple. *No damage is done if you go right back on your program.* Adopting the attitude

"I blew it so I might as well blow it the rest of the weekend or day" will cause unwanted pounds to come back and stick tenaciously. w

Modification to the Core Diet

There are any number of reasons that you may not be able to follow the Core Diet exactly.

For example, you may not be able to eat the minimum amounts. Because some longtime dieters have developed sluggish metabolisms and/or may be very short in stature, they can't always consume the minimum amounts suggested in the Core Diet. Although individual helpings may be small, the combined helpings for any single day may be too large. Rather than eliminating entire food categories, continue to eat from each category as directed, but just eat smaller portions. For example, rather than eliminate a cup of skim milk with a meal, drink half a cup.

What is important is that *all* the foods be included in your diet, even if recommended quantities must be slightly adjusted. You will find that as you eat nutritiously and exercise conscientiously, your metabolism will gradually speed up and you will be able to eat at a higher caloric level without weight gain. Also, remember that it is acceptable to eat more than the minimum amounts. If you are especially tall, are physically fit, very young, or your metabolism has not been damaged by inappropriate dieting, you can eat more than people who are smaller, older, or less fit than you, or who have damaged metabolisms. Just follow the guidelines in the Core Diet. Most people will adjust the amount they eat according to how much energy they are expending.

At one time, I consumed 500 calories a day and fasted one to two days a week just to *maintain* my weight! Now I eat over three times that and am fifteen pounds lighter. I have changed my metabolism from that of a fat person to that of a thin person. You can do this too!

As always, before embarking on any diet or exercise program, consult with your doctor, especially if you are pregnant, nursing, or have a chronic or acute illness.

Chapter Nine

Right Bites for Life

Phase II

There is an applause superior to that
of the multitude—one's own.
—Elizabeth Elton Smith

Several years ago, a client named Jack called my office in a frenzy. He and his wife had been on my Right Bite Program for three months. Both were delighted with the program and with their progress losing weight on it. "But you've got to talk with Vanessa," Jack implored. "She's carrying this diet thing too far."

He explained that at a dinner party with friends the night before, Vanessa had hauled a food scale out of her purse, placed it on the dinner table in front of all the other guests and carefully weighed each portion before eating. The hostess had nearly come unglued, and Jack was mortified. He begged me to tell Vanessa she was going too far. I did as he requested of course, since I totally agreed with his assessment. Thankfully, it was time for Vanessa to loosen restrictions on her eating by initiating Phase II of the Core Diet. I reminded her that there is more to life than rigidly following a diet plan and that we should be discreet about our eating regimens when we're in public situations.

The Right Bite Program is intended to be a total program, and a way of eating for life. It is not a quick fix to be used only when you've noticed you want to lose a few pounds. For any long-term weight-loss program to be effective, the complete person must be considered. It is for this reason that the Right Bite Program has been so carefully and comprehensively designed, taking into account that each person will want to tailor it to fit their unique lifestyle and tastes. In this way, you can successfully integrate the Right Bite principles into your life for the long-term, not just until some magic number turns up on your scale. When Vanessa started incorporating the concepts and food selections of Phase II into her life, she achieved a higher level of fulfillment than she had experienced before embarking on the program. She now enjoys life free of weight-control problems, yet relishes eating a great variety of delicious foods . . . and her husband John no longer worries about her stuffing a food scale into her purse wherever they go!

Phase II Expands Your Diversity

In Phase II of the Right Bite Program, you will continue to drop pounds and attain your ideal, healthy weight while exploring and expanding your program with medium- and high-pleasure foods. This can be done without detonating any appetite and weight-gain triggers. We will also be learning about deviation foods—such as chocolate amaretto truffles—whose flavors are so exciting for most people that the tastes themselves become weight-gain triggers. As you develop and customize your program you will be satisfying sensory and social pleasures while managing your ideal weight and nurturing your body for optimal health.

Phase II is an important part of the Right Bite Program. In addition to broadening and customizing your program, you will be pinpointing precise trouble-making triggers that disrupted your previous diets. If you are concerned that these new foods are going to set off all the weight-gain triggers that you've worked so hard to get rid of in Phase I, be assured that I will guide you though this new territory.

Is it necessary to embrace this part of the Right Bite program? You'd be surprised how many people ask that question. So many men and women who have tried a lot of diets feel that if they are doing well with Phase I, they don't want to disturb anything. They don't want to risk going off the plan and possibly backsliding into the old routine where they were the captive of their weight-gain triggers. Believe me, I understand this concern! That's why I put so many years into researching this material.

Why is it necessary to integrate these new foods into our lives? Because there are two elements in a food that make it attractive to us: its nutritive value and its palatability. Integrating new foods to enlarge your nutritional range and tastes results in increased health benefits and more enjoyment. If we fail to honor the pleasures of our lives, we eventually start feeling deprived both physically and emotionally. That's when food cravings will take over again, and you may find yourself binging.

With all that in mind, let's turn our attention to the medium-pleasure foods and see how to introduce them into the Basic Core Diet.

MEDIUM-PLEASURE FOODS

What is a medium-pleasure food for one person may not please another. For that reason, it's important when choosing medium-pleasure foods that you make up your own list. I'll help you with this as we go along. But do respect your own tastes! Keep the list personal and remember that you are the one whose senses need to be delighted.

Pleasure Foods Defined

Standard pleasure foods have appealing tastes and satisfy your hunger but don't stimulate your appetite for more and more of them. For example, most people probably won't find themselves sitting at their desks at work daydreaming about the wonderful bowl of plain, unadulterated oatmeal they are going to have when they get home at the end of the day or dreaming about a helping of steamed green beans. I think it safe to assume that, for most people, plain oatmeal—no sugar, milk, raisins, or honey—will be a standard-pleasure food. Add half cup of skim milk and a little cinnamon with an artificial sweetener, however, and you are moving into the realm of medium-pleasure foods, that is, if you happen to be an oatmeal fan like me. Okay, maybe you still won't daydream about it as you sit at your desk, but you might look forward to it.

The medium-pleasure food is often a standard-pleasure food that, with a little doctoring up, can sound pretty good if you are hungry, or even if you are looking for a little treat. In general, these are foods that start out pretty basic but can be made to taste more interesting with the addition of a simple ingredient that may or may not contribute moderate calories.

Medium-pleasure foods are also ones that in the gastronomical opinion of the person eating them are more appealing than their standard-pleasure counterpart. By most people's reckoning, medium-pleasure foods are ones you could possibly continue to eat after getting full on standard-pleasure foods but refrain from doing so because your appetite is not highly excited by them.

Some medium-pleasure foods are calorically dense. Raisins, for example, which many people nibble on because they are sweet and because the nibblers believe they are low in calories, are actually pretty high in calories—30 per tablespoon in fact. All things considered, that's pretty high for such an innocent-looking food. By contrast, fresh grapes, which might be described as raisins with the water still in them, are calorically sparse. You can eat half a cup of them and only be taking in about thirty calories.

Medium-pleasure foods should be eaten with standard-pleasure foods. Supplementing our diet with medium-pleasure foods should never cause your total caloric level to exceed the healthy caloric values you attained during Phase I; otherwise, the food cannot be considered medium-pleasure. Medium-pleasure foods, like standard-pleasure foods are low in fat, sugarless, (with one exception, see below), nutritious, whole grain (when applicable), MSG free, caffeine free, and alcohol free. "No smoking" continues to be a lifetime requirement. The exception to "sugarless" is that you may select foods that contain two grams or less of sugar per serving. Cheerios, that old favorite breakfast cereal, meets this requirement.

If you cannot recognize all the ingredients in a meal or dish, classify it as a "deviation food." An example might be a casserole that you did not make yourself, and so cannot identify everything in it. In short, you must know what you are putting into your mouth before deciding whether or not it is a medium-pleasure or deviation food.

The key word here is control. No medium-pleasure food should threaten your control of weight or appetite, otherwise you need to classify it as a subversive weight-gain trigger or deviation food. Also, no medium-pleasure core foods are by definition "bad." That is, they are part of a nutritious diet and not considered junk food. This is why they are so named.

CORE MEDIUM-PLEASURE FOODS

I have compiled a partial list of medium-pleasure foods based upon my work with hundreds of clients. These are foods that almost everyone agrees offer medium eating pleasure and taste-wise are a "step up" from most of the more moderate, Phase I foods. The list I offer here is not iron clad. There is a certain amount of overlap that occurs between standard-, medium-, and high-pleasure foods, and even deviation foods, depending on your individual tastes and calculated reactions to these foods. This is what tailoring and customizing your program is all about. Depending on your tastes, or trigger reactions, you may decide to take some food items off the Basic Core or Medium-Pleasure List and add them to high pleasure foods or deviation foods. Medium-Pleasure foods can never be considered standard-pleasure foods.

Examples of Basic Core Medium-Pleasure Foods

Not all items have calories listed because of the variability of the products. Read labels of any foods you purchase for the manufacturer's portion sizes and nutritional facts that are pertinent to this program.

Cheerios: 1 cup 90
Shredded Wheat: 1 biscuit 90
Whole grain bread: 1 slice 80
Whole grain muffin: 1/2 80
Whole grain crackers: 3 crackers 90
Whole grain roll: 1/2 70
Whole wheat hot dog bun 114
6" corn tortilla fat free 70
4 cups air-popped popcorn (with or without
    no-calorie spray-on butter flavor) 50
Whole grain sugar-free waffle: 1 106
Whole grain sugar-free pancake: 1 100
Whole wheat or oat bran English muffin: 1 . .110
Ploy . . . . .see container for calories
Raisins: Limit to 1 tablespoon per meal 30
Figs: Limit to 1 per meal 47
Apricot, dried: limit to 5 halves per meal 41
Applesauce: 1/2 cup .50
Sugar-free jams or jellies—1 tablespoon— see jar for calories.
No-fat hot dog
Vegetarian no-fat hot dogs
No-fat, no-MSG, sandwich meats: see package—calories should be no more than 30–35 calories per slice.
Artificial sweeteners
Artificially sweetened sodas
No-fat mayonnaise with no or low sugar
Veggie sub on whole wheat bun (no mayo!) . .225
Kraft® Reduced Fat Grated Topping,
    2 teaspoons 20
Low-fat shredded cheese (1/4 cup) or
    2 slices low fat cheese 50
(Some people put low-fat cheese into the high-pleasure category)
Low-fat sour cream
Low-fat, sugar-free salad dressings
Sugar-free cocoa (some individuals put this in the basic
core high-pleasure foods) 1 tsp 6

If you like to bake, try making your own breads, rolls, or muffins using whole grain flour. Being a fan of the Hodgson Mill products, I particularly like the following: oat bran flour, buckwheat flour, whole wheat pastry flour, brown rice flour, soy flour, and whole grain rye flour.

1. Continue to follow the entire Right Bite Program and all rules and guidelines but now incorporate those dealing with the addition of medium-pleasure foods.

2. Add a medium-pleasure food once every four days. Please note your reaction to the food. If you do not experience any adverse reactions, such as food cravings or hunger pangs, you may wish to include it more frequently. For example, almost daily I enjoy oatmeal with a tablespoon of raisins sprinkled on top.

3. Never consume a medium-pleasure food on an empty stomach.

4. When you eat a medium-pleasure food, always combine it with a standard-pleasure food. For example, Cheerios plus milk is acceptable. Cheerios alone is not acceptable.

5. The addition of medium-pleasure foods should not raise your daily total caloric consumption. If the daily calorie level begins to rise, then the new foods incorporated into your diet must be eliminated or classified as high-pleasure or deviation foods.

6. If a medium-pleasure food causes a reaction—weight gain, or increased or excessive appetite—remove it from your diet. Clearly, it is a weight-gain trigger. You may wish to reevaluate this food when you are ready to study the instructions for adding high-pleasure or deviation foods.

7. If you are extremely hungry and are about to commence with a meal that includes standard-pleasure foods and a medium-pleasure food, always begin your meal with the standard-pleasure food when possible. I realize this is not easy to do when the combined foods are smashed together in a sandwich. The reason for trying to eat standard-pleasure foods first is that the less-filling medium-pleasure foods can stimulate you to overeat. For example, I have seen people consume six to eight slices of whole grain toast (medium-pleasure) at breakfast, but barely be able to finish a bowl of oatmeal (standard-pleasure).

8. The majority of each meal should consist of standard-pleasure foods.

All right. Let us assume that you have now incorporated all the medium-pleasure foods of your choice into your diet. Now you are ready to move on. It is interesting to note that in Phase II most people choose to include only a few of the new medium-pleasure foods. The most popular food is bread.

BASIC CORE HIGH-PLEASURE FOODS

Make a list of basic core high-pleasure foods exactly following the criteria of the following definition:

- ✓ Basic core high-pleasure foods are tastier to you than basic core medium-pleasure foods. In fact, they are often "indescribably delicious."

- ✓ When a high-pleasure food passes under your nose, it is almost beyond temptation.

- ✓ A high pleasure food under certain circumstances can cause you to *moderately* overeat that food. (You can call this the "try-to-eat-just-one syndrome.")

- ✓ High-pleasure foods are usually nutrient sparse and/or calorically dense and have the potential to wreak havoc with your blood sugar levels.

- ✓ Tolerance for high-pleasure foods will differ from person to person.

- ✓ Because they stimulate your appetite and cause you to overeat, high-pleasure foods can raise your daily calories too high.

- ✓ If eaten in moderation, high-pleasure foods push our calories only *slightly* higher than allowed under Basic Core conditions. Do keep in mind that if you eat the high-pleasure foods daily you'll be increasing your calorie consumption by small but definitely significant increments, which can cause monumental weight gain over time.

    It's easy to overeat high-pleasure foods without realizing it. These food are sneaky. One day we struggle into our jeans, and there is no way we can button them up. Or we step on the scale and are just certain someone has been tampering with the dial.

    High-pleasure foods are not junk foods or deviation foods. Like medium-pleasure foods they are not inherently bad for you, so you may feel pretty virtuous eating them. Even so, don't deceive yourself. Enjoy them with moderation and exercise your good sense. As a client of mine remarked one day, "I never enter into a liaison with a high-pleasure food lightly."

✓ In comparison to a medium-pleasure food, a high-pleasure food can be slightly higher in fat, but it must be a low- or no-sugar selection. Avoid MSG, alcohol, and caffeine. Also, a high-pleasure food can be slightly more "processed," as in white flour.

✓ In general, think of high-pleasure foods as special occasion foods and accept them only as a last option, such as in a social situation or if your plane is hijacked, and you are forced to eat pretzels left over from the last flight.

In social situations, with a planned menu—such as a pancake and sausage breakfast or a dinner of prime rib, mashed potatoes, and gravy, with chocolate fudge cake a la mode, you will want to avoid the menu at all costs. I describe tips for eating out in Chapter 12.

Last, be sure you know what's in any food you put into your mouth. If you do not know all the ingredients, classify the food as a deviation food.

From Standard-Pleasure to High-Pleasure Food in One Easy Step

To illustrate how a food can move from a standard-pleasure food to a medium-pleasure food to a high-pleasure food, I will use oatmeal again as an example.

Oatmeal by itself is pretty bland and would be classified as a standard-pleasure food—nearly impossible to eat more of than to quell your hunger pangs. However, the addition of cinnamon and artificial sweetener moves it into the range of a medium-pleasure food but does not increase its calories. You will certainly enjoy your cereal more, but you will still not be tempted to overeat this treat. When I also add three tablespoons of thick cream to my oatmeal and dot some sugar-free jam over the top, it becomes like a dessert—a high-pleasure food and indescribably delicious! I could eat more oatmeal prepared this way, but I do not. However, I know that in making oatmeal a high-pleasure food I have raised my breakfast's caloric total by 150 calories, even though I don't feel 150 calories fuller! If every day I similarly embellished every meal, I would soon be packing on the pounds.

Here is a partial list of basic core, high-pleasure foods compiled from the menus of different clients. As in the medium-pleasure list, it is not iron clad and you may need to reclassify some of these items as deviation foods.

BASIC CORE HIGH-PLEASURE FOODS	CALORIES
Cream: 1 tablespoon	50
Half 'n half: 1 tablespoon	20
Unsweetened fruit juice: apple: 1 cup	116
grapefruit: 1 cup	96
orange juice: 1 cup	110
grape: 1/2 cup	77
prune: 1/2 cup	90
pineapple: 1/2 cup	70
Peanut butter, natural: 1 tablespoon/day	90
Egg: 1 (2/week)	80
White bread: 1 slice	80
White pasta products: 1/2 cup	100
Pretzels: 14 midget-sized	50
White rice: 1/2 cup	133
Margarine or butter: 1 tsp	30
Sugar-free ice cream: 1/2 cup	see label
Sugar-free pudding: 1 serving	see label
Fat-free chips (potato, taco, Doritios®) 1 oz	70
Beef, pork, veal, lamb 2–3 oz portion	180–400

INSTRUCTIONS FOR ADDING HIGH-PLEASURE FOODS

1. Follow the entire Right Bite Program and all rules and guidelines but now incorporate the rules for the addition of high-pleasure foods.

2. Never add a medium-pleasure and high-pleasure food at the same time.

3. Add a high-pleasure food no more than once a week! Please note your reaction to the food. If it causes you to overeat or binge, it is a weight-gain trigger for you and you need to eliminate it from your diet. If it causes you to gain weight, you will obviously want to avoid it in the future.

4. Never eat a high-pleasure food on an empty stomach or under stress.

5. Never eat a high-pleasure food when you are ravenous.

6. Never eat a high-pleasure food during your preperiod week.

7. When you eat a high-pleasure food, always combine it with a standard-pleasure food.

8. Your daily caloric consumption should be the same or only *moderately* higher when you add a high-pleasure food. When the caloric total is moderately higher, you can undo the weight gain damage as the week progresses and continue to lose weight. However, be forewarned: The addition of high-pleasure foods will slow steady weight loss significantly.

9. For those wanting to lose weight consistently and quickly, stick with standard- and medium-pleasure foods.

10. For those who want to lose weight at a snail's pace or who are just interested in maintaining their present weight, the addition of high-pleasure food once a week will accomplish just that.

11. When a meal consists of standard-, medium-, and high-pleasure foods, begin your meal with the standard-pleasure foods.

12. The majority of each meal should consist of standard-pleasure foods.

13. Try not to consume white steamed rice, white flour products such as white bread, or white pasta products except on those occasions when you cannot escape from a social dining situation.When you are at home, enjoy only the whole grain varieties.

I am going to use myself to illustrate how I incorporate high-pleasure foods into my diet. During the weekdays I eat standard-pleasure foods with some medium-pleasure ones. Once a week, usually on Saturday evening, my husband and I visit our favorite Italian restaurant, Gavi's. I always order the same meal: penne pasta with marinara sauce with a side order of a grilled chicken breast. And no, I don't weigh or measure any of the portions! The meal comes with white bread and an incredible salad tossed in an oil and vinegar dressing. For my beverage I drink decaf with four tablespoons of half 'n half. The pasta is white, and god only knows what's in the marinara sauce, but it is out of this world. I enjoy every bite of that meal, including several slices of hard-crusted white bread topped with a scant teaspoon of butter. For dessert, my husband and I usually stop for an ice cream cone. I choose a sugar-free, fat-free flavor. Although the major portion of my meal consists of high-pleasure foods, and I realize I have bent my own rule #13, I have had twenty years experience tailoring my diet to fit my needs and lifestyle, and I have learned that I can consume spaced meals like this one without repercussions. You too will discover how to successfully tailor your diet to include special foods as you progress with this program.

You may wish to incorporate deviation foods into your diet when you have accomplished all the following:

1. Mastered the Right Bite Program's basic core, standard-pleasure program with all its relevant guidelines.

2. Mastered the ability to add Basic Core medium-pleasure foods to your diet using relevant guidelines.

3. Mastered the addition of Basic Core high-pleasure foods to your diet using relevant guidelines.

4. Become fully knowledgeable about your weight-gain triggers, having assimilated this information from Chapter 7's instructions for isolating and analyzing these diet troublemakers.

5. Learned how to control and/or eliminate your weight-gain triggers.

6. Formulated strategies to control and/or eliminate any new weight-gain trigger that you may discover.

7. Learned to handle slip-ups successfully and been able to get back on track again.

8. Continued to lose weight if you are overweight, or if you have reached your slimmest healthy weight, been able to maintain it without a struggle.

Deviation Foods

I call some of the health-sabotaging, adulterated substances that people ingest deviation foods because they "deviate" from the nutritious, calorically and nutrient dense foods of the Core Diet. I also think of them as subversive, for they are usually fattening and trigger-laden. Unfortunately, many of our commercial food products fall into this category. These foods deviate from that which is pure and natural. They are foods I do not include in the acceptable lists found in the previous three sections. They are the "Not Allowed Foods."

I realize that in the course of living not all of us are doggedly content to eat nutritiously day in and day out. Sometimes we crave to abandon our constraints, throw caution to the winds, and whoop it up. The usual time for this is when celebrating special holidays, birthdays, and anniversaries, or when we are on vacations. Therefore, when you consciously give yourself *license* to have a fling, these guidelines will give you a modicum of help for keeping your waistline from expanding beyond an easy recovery. Deviation foods are generally high fat, high sugar, nutrient sparse, calorically dense, additive riddled, processed, MSG enhanced and overly salty. Yes, they include most junk food! As a deviation food, alcohol in moderation is allowed even though it is a subversive substance. Nicotine and caffeine continue to be prohibited.

RULES FOR TRYING DEVIATION FOODS

1. Follow the entire Right Bite Program and all rules and guidelines up to but not including deviation foods.

2. Try one deviation food a maximum of once a week and at only one meal. Why? Because deviation foods are characteristically high in fat, calories, and/or cholesterol, nutrient-sparse, and/or high in sugar and additives, all of which can all too rapidly add ounces and pounds.

3. Always try a deviation food after first consuming Basic Core, standard-pleasure foods.

4. When you have determined that a deviation food is safe for you to try—i.e. you don't go bonkers and binge—you may wish to include that specific deviation food at one meal, once per week. Most people who choose to deviate do so on a weekend night.

5. Don't ever have a whole day of deviation eating. If you need something to deter you from this, just remind yourself of how long it may take you to get back on track and get your weight back to where you wanted it.

6. You may schedule your deviation foods for special occasions and holidays. Warning! Don't ferret out or start inventing bizarre holidays to celebrate, such as National Love a Potato Day, or Glasses Awareness Week. Stick to the customary holidays or special occasions. Don't allow yourself to indulge in champagne bubbly every time you attend an obscure birthday, wedding, or funeral. The

deviation day must be significantly special to you—your wedding, your birthday, Christmas, Hanukkah.

7. If you should "slip" because a deviation food acts as a weight-gain trigger for you and you overeat, binge, or gain unwanted pounds, return to the Basic Core, standard-pleasure phase of the diet *until the newly gained pounds are lost* and you have regained control. Place the harmful deviation food on your sensitivity list for appetite/weight-gain triggers and avoid it in the future.

8. Be aware that although a deviation food may not cause an immediate triggering effect, it will eventually have a negative effect on you because it generally is nutrient-sparse, high calorie, high in fat, and high in sugar, with a high glycemic index, and full of camouflaged additives. Deviation foods are also usually cumulative in their effect. Be careful!

9. You may not have illegal drugs. Ever! Many of the more common ones, such as marijuana, can immensely disrupt your appetite triggers.

10. Categorize all food you eat as standard-, medium-, or high-pleasure foods. The majority of your diet should consist of standard-pleasure foods and medium-pleasure foods. A fraction of your diet may consist of high-pleasure and occasional deviation foods *only as long as they do not act as weight-gain triggers.*

12. Never consume a deviation food on an empty stomach.

13. Never consume a deviation food after exercise.

14. Never consume a deviation food or sugar during your preperiod time.

15. Never consume a deviation food or sugar during episodes of stress or during a disruptive change in routine. For example, the week your mother-in-law comes for her annual visit is not the time to experiment with your favorite cookie recipe. Remember, that a change in routine can be good or bad. New foods or deviation foods should be consumed when you are in optimal health, and your life is chugging along in a contented normal routine.

16. Take only a small serving of any deviation food.

17. Be aware of cumulative reactions. For example, one woman found that she could successfully sip a glass of red wine with her meal on one day, and enjoy a dish of ice cream the following week. However, she soon found that if she consumed both wine and ice cream at the same meal, the combination became a compelling weight-gain trigger for her. Sometimes a deviation food may not cause an adverse reaction by itself but when combined with another or eaten to excess, look out! Also, a reaction does not refer just to overeating or binging. It can consist of any physical or mental discomfort, such as malaise, headaches, or upset stomach.

I once had a client who, six months into the program, yearned for a candy treat once a week. The first test went well. She remained in control of her eating and her weight held steady. Because she detected no sinister reaction, she argued that she would be able to handle a sweet treat daily. "Just one," she promised herself. Soon after she did this her weight began to increase. Though she had started out only wanting to satisfy her sweet-tooth, she found that her one-a-day sweetness fix had become two, three, and sometimes four a day. She had a great deal of difficulty getting back on track and did so only after regaining nearly twenty-five pounds, insisting she was not out-of-control until she could no longer get into her favorite clothes. Ultimately she returned to Basic Core foods, lost the unwanted weight and has held her weight steady ever since. She no longer eats candy daily but is able to enjoy her once a week deviation.

Slimmest Healthiest Weight

At some time during the Phase II program, each of you will reach your slimmest healthy weight, your true *set point weight*, and you will begin exploring ways to maintain this ideal. True set point weight is the lowest weight at which your good health is ensured. Should you intentionally continue to lose weight below this mark, many problems will begin to manifest themselves. For example, you may find that for the past two years on other diets you weighed 125 pounds but had great difficulty controlling your weight fluctuations. Every time you dieted below that weight you found that you consistently overate, and you rarely felt your best. After following the Right Bite Program your weight may gradually decrease to 118 or less as you become fitter and leaner. There will come a point where no matter how nutritiously you are eating and how much you are exercising, your weight loss will cease.

You have arrived at your true set point weight—your slimmest, healthy weight.

While it is possible to get your weight down to less than your set point, you will then be forcing your body to reduce its weight to a point of compromising your health and feeling awful. At your set point, you should feel mentally alert and physically vigorous without the urge to overeat or binge. If you are a woman, and if you diet below your set point, menstruation often becomes irregular or ceases. At your slimmest healthy weight, you will not experience unpleasant symptoms associated with insufficient calories such as fatigue, lethargy, headaches, swollen lymph nodes, susceptibility to infection, abnormal cravings for sweets, constant hunger, and insomnia, to name a few. This is not to say you will never experience the above symptoms for other reasons, but I commonly observe them in overzealous dieters who attempt to reduce below their set point.

Guidelines for maintaining your ideal weight can be found in the concluding chapter.

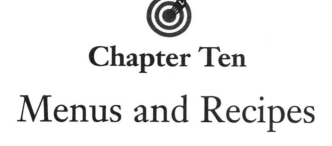

Chapter Ten

Menus and Recipes

The discovery of a new dish does more for the happiness of mankind than the discovery of a star.
Anthelme Brillat-Savarin

With the proliferation of cookbooks and TV cooking shows today, one would think the whole world was at home preparing complex and time-consuming gourmet meals. However, what I present in these pages are delicious recipes that are easy to prepare and Right-Bite-approved. After trying some of these you'll quickly see the basic principles of cooking this way and will find that you can adapt recipes you are already familiar with so that they meet the Right Bite requirements.

The recipe we are going to start with is one of the most important and also one of my favorites:

Stephanie's Super Lentil Soup

INGREDIENTS
Salt Substitute (potassium choloride) (to taste)
Lemon Mrs. Dash® (to taste)
10 cups low-sodium chicken broth (*if you are a vegetarian, substitute the same amount of vegetable stock. There are many delicious prepared vegetable stocks available these days, either at better supermarkets or in health food stores.*)
1 can low-sodium stewed tomatoes
1 cup shredded cabbage
3/4 cup dried lentils
1/2 cup pearl barley
1/2 cup dried whole wheat elbow macaroni
1 cup onions diced (packaged or fresh)
1/2 cup carrots diced
1 cup diced celery
1/2 cup frozen Italian green beans (cut in approximately 1" lengths)
1/2 cup frozen peas
1/2 cup frozen lima beans
1/2 cup mushrooms
1 cup diced zucchini

PREPARATION
Use a 5-quart stock pot, combine the chicken or vegetable broth, tomatoes, onion, celery, potatoes, lentils, carrots, green beans, peas, lima beans, and barley. Cook uncovered over a moderate heat, then adjust the heat to a slow simmer, cover, and cook for 30 minutes. Now add the zucchini and whole wheat macaroni. Cook uncovered until the macaroni is done, usually between 10 and 15 minutes. As the dry ingredients cook, you may wish to add more chicken or vegetable stock, keeping in mind that this is a very thick soup. Now add the mushrooms, which will be cooked within a couple minutes. Finally, season to taste with Mrs. Dash® and a salt substitute.

This soup is best when the consistency is somewhere between a soup and a stew, or thick minestrone. After you have prepared the soup, as described above, experiment with adding other ingredients, both as flavor and to thicken it. You may wish to use frozen, presliced ingredients to save time. Here are some suggestions for ingredients to add. Experiment with quantities. If the soup gets too thick while you are experimenting, add more broth or tomato juice rather than water. If you add plain water it will compromise the taste. Try adding things like yellow squash, chopped spinach or chard, chopped cauliflower, or broccoli.

Or try bok choy, snow pea pods, Brussels sprouts (which make the soup much stronger tasting, so make sure you like them before adding them), rutabaga, and so on.

As you get up your courage to make the recipe even more interesting, try adding grains such as wild rice, brown rice, millet, oatmeal, and/or kasha. Now this is *important!* Cook these *separately*, because each of these requires a different cooking time. Wild rice and brown rice, however, can be cooked together to save time. Similarly, millet and barley can be cooked together, cook oatmeal and kasha separately from the others, setting them aside to add later if you use them.

More suggestions: I occasionally add other legumes, such as canned, precooked kidney, pinto, and garbanzo beans. Be sure to strain off all the liquid by pouring them into a strainer and then rinsing them off with water to get rid of the salt with which they are usually cooked. And be sure to add these only after the soup is cooked. You should only be heating these. If you add them before the soup is cooked they will get too mushy and may even cause the soup to burn. There are also other beans you may wish to try: black-eyed peas, Great Northern beans (they are white), or black beans. You can add all six varieties, and I sometimes do.

When the soup is completed, it should be so thick you can eat it with a fork—no commercial intended here—with minimal liquid. One cup is about 200 calories and will be the most filling 200 calories you've ever eaten! My children will eat the vegetables camouflaged in the soup, whereas if they saw spinach on their plate they would turn their noses up at it. So, this soup is great for picky eaters. (lentil soup is a Phase I recipe.)

As you become really comfortable preparing this soup—and hopefully become as fond of it as my own family is—do what I do. Make huge quantities of it at a time and freeze it in quart-sized containers. I often make batches two to four times the above recipe. Expand the recipe simply by doubling or tripling it. It's a very forgiving recipe, as you'll discover, and a great quick meal in itself. Once you have your stock of soup in the freezer, all you have to do is pop a container into a pot, simmer over low heat, and dinner (or lunch) is ready! If you are really in a hurry, defrost it in your microwave first, then heat it to your desired temperature over your conventional stove.

Ideas for Phase I Core Diet Meal Combinations

In this section, I will provide a series of favorite Phase I Core Diet breakfasts and lunch/dinner combinations. *You may need to increase or decrease quantities depending on your hunger.*

PHASE I CORE DIET BREAKFAST COMBINATIONS

#1. 1/3 cup (precooked, dry measurement) multigrain oatmeal or regular oat meal
1/4 cup bran
1/2 cup fresh strawberries
1/2 cup cottage cheese
1 tsp flax seed oil

#2. 1 serving Wheatena®
1/2 cantaloupe
1/2 cup cottage cheese
1 tsp flax seed oil

#3. Egg Beater® veggie omelet (see Minute Menus)
1 serving corn grits
1 orange
1 tsp flax seed oil

#4. 1 serving oat bran
2 tablespoons wheat germ
1 cup raspberries
1 cup plain unsweetened yogurt
1 tsp flax seed oil

#5. 1 serving 7-grain cereal
two peaches
1/2 cup cottage cheese
1 tsp flax seed oil

#6. 1 serving shredded wheat and bran
1 cup skim milk
1 grapefruit
1 tsp flax seed oil

#7. 1 serving Red River® Cereal
1/2–1 cup blueberries
1/2 cup cottage cheese
1 tsp oil

PHASE I CORE DIET LUNCH OR DINNER COMBINATIONS

#1. 1 cup lentil soup
2 oz chicken diced on top of soup or
3 oz can Swanson® chicken in water or

1/2 cup cottage cheese
1 tsp flax seed oil
1/2 cantaloupe

#2. The following meal sounds unappealing but this is a very useful selection when you are in a rush.
1-1/2 cups low-sodium canned peas
1–2 tsp olive oil mixed in peas
balsamic vinegar mixed into peas
onion powder and salt substitute to taste
1/2 cup cottage cheese (on top of peas)
2 peaches

#3. 3 oz cod
5–10 oz baked potato (depending on hunger)
steamed broccoli
1 tsp canola oil
1 cup skim milk

#4. 1 cup cooked whole-wheat pasta
Hal's Spaghetti Sauce (see recipes) or some other plain, sugar-free, low-calorie sauce
1/2 cup cottage cheese
1–2 tsp canola or olive oil with vinegar for dressing
salad
yellow squash

#5. 1/2 cup brown rice with 1/2 cup kidney beans on top seasoned with salsa
1/2 cup corn
1/2 cup cottage cheese
1 tsp flax seed or canola oil
sliced steamed zucchini
sliced tomato

#6. 3 oz can water-packed tuna
1/4 cup dry millet cooked
1 cup asparagus
1/2 cup cooked carrots
1 cup raspberries
1 tsp canola or olive oil

#7. tofu-veggie egg omelet (see Minute Menus)
    sliced tomatoes
    snap beans
    1 tsp canola oil
    2/3 cup mango

#8. 1 cup lentils
    1/2 cup cottage cheese
    spinach salad with tomatoes and mushrooms
    1–2 tsp olive or canola oil with vinegar for dressing

By now, you should be seeing a pattern of a whopping-size carbohydrate with a protein, oil, and vegetables and/or fruit. There are hundreds of ways to combine these. I have found that those on the go, who must pack lunches, frequently take a thermos of lentil soup with a teaspoon of oil added to it and with a fruit that carries easily like an orange or peach.

Ideas for Phase II Core Diet Meals

MEDIUM CORE BREAKFAST COMBINATIONS

#1. 1 serving Wheatena®
    sliced banana
    1 tsp flax seed oil
    1 cup skim milk
    1/2 cup cottage cheese

#2. low-fat cheese omelet (see Minute Menus)
    1 slice whole grain toast
    1 tsp flax seed oil
    1 cup strawberries

#3. 1 serving oatmeal or multigrain oatmeal
    cinnamon and artificial sweetener
    1/2 cup cottage cheese
    1 cup blueberries
    1 tsp flax seed oil

#4. 1–2 slices French toast (see Minute Menus)
    scrambled Egg Beaters®
    orange slices
    1 tsp flax seed oil

#5. 1 serving oat bran
    1 tablespoon raisins stirred into oat bran

cinnamon and artificial sweetener
dot sugar-free jelly on top
1/2 cup cottage cheese
1 tsp flax seed oil

#6. 1–2 shredded wheat biscuits with artificial sweetener
1 cup skim milk
2 peaches sliced on top of biscuits
1/2 cup cottage cheese
1 tsp flax seed oil

#7. whole wheat or oat bran English muffin
veggie omelet (see Minute Menus)
1 tsp flax seed oil
1/2 cantaloupe

MEDIUM CORE LUNCH OR DINNER COMBINATIONS
#1. Chicken or turkey sandwich:
2–3 ounces chicken or turkey
2 slices whole grain bread
sliced tomatoes and lettuce
low-fat mayonnaise
1 apple
1 cup skim milk

#2. Hot dog:
1 low-fat hot dog
whole wheat hot dog bun
1-1/2 cups watermelon
1 cup skim milk

#3. 1 cup whole grain pasta
1/2 cup cottage cheese or other protein selection
1/4 cup plain spaghetti sauce or Hal's Spaghetti Sauce (see recipes)
Kraft Reduced Fat Grated Topping® lightly sprinkled on top
Italian green beans
1 tsp flax seed oil

#4. On the go:
veggie sub on whole wheat bread with mustard (without cheese)
1 apple (which you will have brought with you)

#5. 1 cup macaroni and cheese* (see Minute Menus)
   1 cup skim milk with 1 tsp sugar-free cocoa
   1 cup raspberries
   1 tsp flax seed oil
   * Hodgson Mills has an excellent packaged macaroni and cheese.

#6. 5–10 oz baked potato
   1 tablespoon low-fat sour cream
   1/4 cup shredded low-fat cheese
   1/2 cup cottage cheese
   steamed broccoli
   spinach salad with sliced tomatoes
   1 tsp olive oil and vinegar for dressing

#7. Fruit salad (see Minute Menus)
   1/2 cup cottage cheese
   green beans
   sliced tomatoes
   1 tsp oil

#8. Steffy's Stomach Stuffer (guaranteed to fill you up)
   1/2 cup lentils
   1/2 cup brown rice
   1/2 cup cottage cheese
   sliced steamed zucchini
   sliced steamed yellow squash
   sliced tomato
   large serving cooked spinach
   Italian green beans or green beans
   Spray-on butter flavor with a sprinkle of reduced-fat parmesan cheese
   1 tsp oil

MINUTE MENUS
   The following are all one serving unless indicated.

Pita Pizza
   1 piece whole wheat mini pita
   1 tablespoon tomato sauce seasoned with Italian herbs
   sprinkle with reduced-fat mozzarella shredded cheese
Warm in microwave for 15 seconds. (Phase II Medium Core)

Tuna Patties
> 1 three-ounce can water-packed tuna
> 1/4 cup Egg Beaters® or 2 egg whites
> mixture of chopped onions, mushrooms

Blend all ingredients in a bowl. Saute in a nonstick pan with a nonstick spray. (Phase I Core; Phase II Medium Core if you top with 1/4 cup low-fat grated or shredded cheese)

Spanish Brown Rice
> 1 cup uncooked brown rice
> 2 cups water
> chopped green pepper
> 1 chopped tomato
> 1/2 tsp cumin
> onion or garlic powder

In a large saucepan, add all ingredients and cook until rice is tender and water is absorbed, about 25 minutes. Another way to make Spanish rice is to just take a can of stewed tomatoes and substitute it for 1 cup of water. (Phase I Core)

Veggie Omelet
Basic Omelet Mix: 1/2 cup Egg Beaters® with 2 tablespoons skim milk and your favorite veggies—green peppers sliced, mushrooms, sprouts, and so on.

Blend Egg Beaters® and milk, pour into nonstick pan sprayed with nonstick spray, and cook until firm. Put veggies on one side of the omlet and flip the other side of omelet over the veggies. Cover, turn off heat, and wait until veggies are warmed through. Some individuals like to cook the omelet with the vegetables stirred in the mix. (Phase I Core; Phase II Medium Core if you add cheese)

Omelet Variations
PIZZA OMELET: Cook with mushrooms and onions and top with tomato sauce, Italian seasoning, and low-fat cheese. (Medium Core)

BROCCOLI OMELET: Add steamed broccoli to cooked omelet. (Phase I Core, or with broccoli and cheese, Medium Core)

COTTAGE CHEESE OMELET: Add chives and cottage cheese. (Phase I Core)

SHRIMP OMELET: Add 2–3 chopped shrimp to mix. (Phase I Core)

Veggie-Tofu Omelet: Mash one quarter cube of tofu in basic omelet mix with your favorite veggies, or add diced tofu.

Tater Toppings
   Baked potato and:
   broccoli and low-fat cheese (Phase II Medium Core)
   1/2 cup cottage cheese and chives (Phase I Core)
   mustard (Phase I Core)
   salt substitute and vinegar (Phase I Core)
   1 tablespoon low-fat sour cream (Phase II Medium Core)
   spray-on butter flavor (Phase I Core)
   salsa (Phase I Core)

French Toast
   1–2 slices whole grain bread
   1/2 cup Egg Beaters® and 2 tablespoons skim milk
Mix Egg Beaters® and milk, and put the bread in mix until the bread is soaked through. Cook in a nonstick pan coated with nonstick spray until done. Sprinkle with cinnamon. (Phase II Medium Core)

Chicken Cacciatore
   2–3 oz cooked white meat sliced in strips
   green peppers, mushrooms, onions
   1/4 cup sugar-free spaghetti sauce
Chop peppers, mushrooms, and onions. Place in bowl with small amount of water, cover and microwave until soft. Pour out liquid, add chicken and sauce, stir, heat, and eat. (Phase I Core; with low-fat parmesan and/or low-fat mozzarella sprinkled on top, Phase II Medium Core)

Macaroni and Cheese
   1 cup cooked whole wheat elbow macaroni
   shredded reduced-fat cheddar cheese
Heat macaroni until tender and add a serving of reduced-fat cheese and stir. (Phase II Medium Core)

Festive Fish
   1 serving fish: your choice
   salt substitute
   pepper
   1 thinly sliced onion
   1 tomato thinly sliced
   1 tsp lime juice

Place fish in ungreased glass baking dish; sprinkle with salt substitute and pepper and lime. Top with onions and tomato. Cover and microwave until fish is done. (Phase I Core)

Grilled Cheese—Crispy or Soft
2 slices whole grain bread
1/4 cup reduced- or low-fat cheese or two slices low-fat cheese

Put cheese between bread and grill on nonstick pan sprayed with non-stick spray very slowly on moderate heat for a crispy texture. Microwave for 20–30 seconds for soft. (Phase II Medium Core)

Cranapple Sauce
1 bag fresh cranberries
23 oz jar sugar-free applesauce, smooth or chunky
1–2 boxes cherry or strawberry sugar-free gelatin

Cook cranberries in 1/2 cup boiling water until all berries pop open. In a separate pan dissolve gelatin mixes in 1/2 cup of almost boiling water. Pour cranberries into gelatin mix. Add jar of applesauce and stir. Pour into a dish, cover, and refrigerate. Delicious. Serves 12. (Phase II Medium Core)

Bean Salad
1 can (15–16 ounces) of Great Northern beans
1 can kidney or pinto beans
1 can garbanzo beans rinsed and drained.
1 cup fresh green beans or Italian green beans steamed
1/2 cup water
1/4 cup balsamic vinegar
3 tablespoons red wine vinegar
3 tablespoons chopped shallots
3 tablespoons minced fresh parsley
black pepper and salt substitute to taste
olive oil

In a shallow, wide bowl layer kidney or pinto beans, Great Northern beans, garbanzos, and green beans. Set aside. Mix remaining ingredients together in a separate bowl and pour over the beans. Tastes best if marinated over night. Makes 8 one-cup servings. Many add 1 tsp olive oil to the serving if you need to satisfy an oil requirement. The olive oil, with its unique taste, adds extra flavor as well. (Phase I Core)

Coleslaw
3/4 cup finely shredded cabbage
1/4 cup finely shredded red cabbage

1 tablespoon low-fat mayonnaise
juice of 1/4 lemon
1/2 carrot chopped
1 pack sugar substitute
pepper and no-salt to taste

Mix together all ingredients and chill. Makes one serving. (Phase II Medium Core)

Sugar-Free Whipped Cream
1/3 cup nonfat dry milk
1 tsp lemon juice
1/3 to 1/2 cup cold water
1 tsp vanilla extract

Combine all ingredients except vanilla in a glass bowl and put in freezer. Put electric beaters in freezer also. When ice crystals begin to form, beat mixture thoroughly and put back in freezer until ice crystals form again. Repeat procedure until mixture is slushy. When mixture is slushy, whip the mixture until it's the consistency of whipped cream, add vanilla and whip again. Eat as soon as it reaches a whipped cream consistency, because it will not hold its form long. Makes a lot and is delicious with fresh fruit. Tastes like a million calories. One serving. (Phase II Medium Core)

Fruit Salad and Cottage Cheese
3 cups of a mix of your favorite fruit
Top with 1/2 cup cottage cheese.

Hal's Spaghetti Sauce
1 teaspoon virgin olive oil
2 diced, fresh tomatoes
2 medium-sized finely diced onions
4–5 tsp of freshly diced sweet red bell peppers
or fresh pimento or green bell pepper
1/2 cup fresh mushrooms—shiitake are preferred—
sliced as thin as you can
1 tablespoon balsamic vinegar
2–10 cloves fresh garlic—use a garlic press
1/2 tsp thyme, basil, rosemary

Start with a large frying pan on medium heat, add 1 tsp olive oil, add the onions and sauté until they are just beginning to look transparent, add two finely diced tomatoes. If pan is sizzling, turn down the heat. Now add pepper or pimento. By now the mix in the pan should be pretty liquefied with a bit of steam rising from the pan. The mixture can bubble gently but don't boil the life out of it. Controlling the heat helps to keep the natural tastes. Add balsamic vinegar. Add sliced mushrooms to the top of the sauce, allowing them to just absorb the tastes in the moisture for a minute or so. Add the juice of the garlic cloves to the mix. Sprinkle with thyme, basil, and rosemary, and give the whole thing a gentle toss. Add a little water if it looks dry, cover and remove from heat.

HOW TO MAKE SUBSTITUTIONS IN RECIPES

I have made the observation that most single-strategy books have recipe sections that comprise anywhere from one quarter to one half of the book as well as several "filler" chapters to help bulk up the book. After all, there is only so much you can say about one strategy in 300-plus pages. Although it is important to get ideas on food combining and menus, it is equally important to learn how trigger-free recipes are created, so you can make and enjoy all your favorite dishes. I feel it is superfluous to go on listing page after page of recipes, because all I am doing is taking my favorite recipes, eliminating any item that is a trigger and making simple substitutions. You can also learn to do this. The following list will give you some basic ideas on how substitutes can render any recipe completely nutritious and trigger-free.

Original	Substitute
mayonnaise	low-fat or reduced-fat mayonnaise
sour cream	low-fat sour cream, low-fat yogurt
1/2 cup heavy cream	1/2 cup evaporated skim milk
ricotta cheese	low-fat cottage cheese
cheese	reduced-fat cheese
whole milk	skim milk
1 egg	2 egg whites or 1/4 cup Egg Beaters®
ground beef	ground turkey or chicken breast
oil for frying	nonstick spray
butter or margarine	butter-flavored sprays
1/4 cup granulated sugar	6 packets or 2 tsp sugar substitute
Large quantity sugar	Many people use applesauce.
ketchup	tomato sauce or tomato paste
white rice	brown rice
white flour	whole grain flour
white pasta	whole grain pasta

Now, let's modify a recipe.

Original Recipe	Right Bite Recipe
1 pound Italian sausage	Eliminate! Let's replace the meat with mushrooms, spinach, and carrots or mushrooms, eggplant, and carrots.
1 medium onion	
1 clove garlic	
1 can whole tomatoes	low-sodium tomatoes
1 can tomato sauce	
2 tablespoons dried parsley flakes	
1 tsp sugar	1 pack artificial sweetener
1/2 tsp salt	1/2 tsp salt substitute
9 uncooked lasagna noodles	9 whole wheat lasagna noodles
1 carton ricotta cheese	1 carton low-fat cottage cheese
1/4 cup grated parmesan cheese	1/4 cup reduced-fat parmesan cheese
1 tablespoon dried parsley flakes	
1-1/2 tsp dried oregano	
2 cups shredded mozzarella cheese	2 cups reduced-fat mozzarella cheese

Modifying recipes is easy. With just minor alterations and a little imagination you can enjoy almost all of your favorite foods. For many recipes you can totally eliminate oil without compromising taste. For example, macaroni and cheese tastes just as good without the added margarine. If the addition of a larger amount of oil is essential to the recipe, think in terms of serving size. For example, if a recipe that makes 16 servings calls for 1/4 cup oil (12 teaspoons) you would be getting less than a teaspoon per serving. Take this into consideration when you are adding oils to your diet.

When you create lower- or no-fat versions of your favorite recipes, choose an alternative to fat that is compatible with the other ingredients. For example, if the recipe already has buttermilk or yogurt as an ingredient, just increase these as you reduce the fat.

Going Further

Before going on to the next chapter, where I describe the role of physical exercise in the Right Bite Program, I have to confess to you that I am a former exercise dropout. Yes, I know that physical exercise is an important part of any respectable weight-control program. And I know about all the health benefits to be derived. No matter! Try as I might, I just wasn't able to endure the rigors of jogging five miles every day or slogging to the gym for a workout every night after work.

I finally discovered a great exercise program that works for me personally, as well as for those I counsel. The best part is that it perfectly complements the Right Bite Program. You will be amazed at how easily you can incorporate it into your life and even more amazed by how much better you will look and feel once you get started. The exercise program described in the next chapter is effective, extremely easy, of short duration, and can be accomplished under any circumstance.

Chapter Eleven

Fat to Fit, Fast— Physical Exercise for a Lifetime

My grandmother started walking five miles a day
when she was sixty—she's ninety-seven today
and we don't know where the hell she is.
—Ellen DeGeneres

There are endless stories about people who exercise to extremes. But none compare with the one I am going to tell you. One hot summer morning, after her husband left for work, my client decided to do her exercises indoors instead of jogging outside in ninety-degree heat. After a few moments she was perspiring, so she stepped out of her nightgown, took off her thick glasses, and proceeded to jog around in the house nude as she did her housework.

In the kitchen, she scooped up the plastic bag full of garbage and jogged outside the back door to toss it in the garbage can. But the can was full, so without missing a beat, she jumped on the top end and with great rhythmic vigor began to stomp the garbage down. Determined to keep her heart rate steady, she was merrily bouncing up and down, naked, kicking garbage packets here and there, when a slightly apologetic masculine voice greeted her: "Good morning."

She managed to make out the outline of one of the three brothers who farmed the alfalfa fields next door. Without her glasses she couldn't tell which one it was. With a regal nod of her head, and hoping his eyesight was at least as bad as hers, she returned his morning greeting. Then summoning all the dignity she could muster, and blushing all over, she stepped to the ground and with queenly composure turned and walked into the house. Given what she'd been through, she felt she could be forgiven for not completing her Right Bite exercises that morning.

To this day, she cannot pass any of the three brothers without wondering if he is the one who watched her dance naked on the garbage can.

Establishing a healthy lifelong exercise program is essential for those of us who wish to lose weight successfully and maintain the loss, or fashion for ourselves as attractive a figure as possible given our inherited arrangement of bones.

Many people who are trying to lose weight would prefer to ignore this fact, and I confess that for an embarrassing number of years I searched in vain for an exercise substitute. I was your classic exercise avoider, endlessly championing different slow-or-no-progress diets until I finally realized I could no longer sidestep the issue. I discovered through trial and much error that programs that leave out exercise simply do not work, and ultimately I had to acknowledge that for health and good looks exercise must be a priority each day.

In the past, even thinking about rigorous physical activity filled me with dread. Exercise exhausted me, bored me, took too much valuable time, and gave me sore hamstrings. Surely, I thought, there must be an easier way to slim down and become reasonably presentable than by sweating away half my life in a smelly gym.

Well, take heart, my friends, and read on. There *is* an easier way, and it works! Twenty years ago, my outlook on the importance of exercise changed significantly after reading the bestselling book *Fit or Fat* by Covert Bailey. Although I was impressed with the material he presented, I forced myself to temper my enthusiasm with a bit of skepticism. The book seemed too good to be true. However, I decided to establish an exercise regimen according to the book's guidelines with an eye to measuring scientifically whether or not I was obtaining the fitness Bailey claims is achieved by following his program.

At that time, I was already slim, but it was a daily struggle to keep my weight from fluctuating widely. I was particularly interested in Bailey's assertion that on his program one will gain *lean* body mass and *lose fat* as fitness is achieved even if the scale weight reflects no loss of pounds, as is more often the case when one is already slender. In fact, he says, one may even gain scale weight.

Acting on Bailey's suggestion, I decided to have myself water-weighed at the beginning and again at the conclusion of the experiment to determine if any changes had taken place in my body's composition over a twelve-month period. With water weighing, measurements are taken while you are immersed in a tank of water, and this tells you precisely the percentage of fat on your body. The end result is that you have an objective way of measuring how much fat has been replaced with lean tissue.

Consistent with my personal revulsion for physical exertion, I was careful to start my own exercise program, designed specifically for novices, which allowed me to do a minimum amount of recommended exercise several times a day. Because I was very unfit I chose twelve minutes of chair stepping, sandwiched into my day, three times a week. I found to my immediate pleasure that I was almost able to exercise with enthusiasm, and after following this painless exercise program, the svelte, well-toned body I had always envisioned as my ideal gradually began to take shape in my mirror. My enthusiasm for exercise moved from "tolerance" to absolute delight. Not only that, I was getting to look forward to every exercise session because during and after them I felt wonderful, with more energy and stamina than I'd ever had in my life. It was an added bonus to find that although I was enjoying much larger portions of food than ever before in my dieting life, I no longer had a problem stabilizing my weight.

There are three great things about this exercise program: (1) it is totally compatible with everything about the Right Bite Program, (2) it helps you lose weight faster, while toning your body (remember, that's lean body mass!), and (3) it only takes twelve minutes a day! If you are one of those people who simply doesn't have the time to exercise, this program is definitely for you.

After exercising this way for almost twenty years now, it is difficult for me to imagine that there isn't a way to slot this program into even the most pressured lifestyle. For instance, you can exercise while tethered to the telephone, taking advantage of those times when you are put on hold. You can do it while waiting for the bathtub to fill or while engrossed in watching a gall bladder operation on television. My violist mother, also an enthusiast of this program, finds the time to exercise and simultaneously relieve travel boredom, by climbing up and down on the inside entrance step of a moving tour bus, much to the amusement of her fellow orchestra members.

When I first started, I followed this minimal, twelve-minute exercise regimen for approximately two months. Then the routine became so habitual and even pleasurable to do that one day I found that I'd automatically extended it to fifteen minutes, four times a week. Once my body had tasted exercise on a regular basis, it increasingly craved more. Eventually I was happily exercising five times a week and had switched from chair stepping to jogging. At the end of twelve months,

I was jogging thirty minutes five days a week—and absolutely loving every minute of it!

At the end of the trial year, my home scale registered that I was no heavier or lighter than I had been at the beginning of the experiment. There was not even a quarter pound difference. With mounting curiosity, I dug out my stored "reference jeans" and eyed them apprehensively. In case you do not know what reference jeans are, they are denim pants that many women buy and wear when they feel they are at their slimmest weight. When reference jeans are too tight, we know we have gained weight, and when they're loose, we have lost weight. I had purposely not worn my reference jeans for one year, and having already discovered that I had not lost or gained scale weight during that time, I was understandably hesitant to slip them on. I needn't have worried, for it was immediately apparent that the jeans no longer fit me! They were much too loose! They hung limply around my hips with at least a couple of inches to spare at the waist. I was elated.

I returned to the spa to have my body composition analyzed a second time by water weighing. These results confirmed that my scale weight had indeed remained the same as the previous year, but the ratio of fat to muscle had changed dramatically. Excess fat had melted from my frame and had been replaced with almost seven pounds of lithe muscle! Not only had my body become harder and leaner, but also my body's metabolism had sped up, enabling me to burn away calories more quickly and more efficiently than before. Consequently, I was able to increase my daily number of calories without gaining any fat weight, a gastronomic reward that reflected a remarkable metabolic change in my body.

In case you are wondering how to have your body composition analyzed, there are now many inexpensive scales on the market that analyze your body composition. You no longer have to almost drown yourself with underwater weighing, which was all I had available at the time *Fit or Fat* first appeared on the market. Although there are skin fold calipers that one can use to pinch and measure your fat in various places, they are difficult to use and require a professional who knows how to grasp your fat correctly with the calipers and take valid measurements. Also, it is easy to cheat and make yourself thinner than you are just by the way you pinch your flesh.

The body fat scales, which are available at some gyms and spas, use the *bioelectrical impedance analysis* technique. In this method, a low-frequency electrical current—so low you can't even feel it, by the way—is passed through you body when you step on the scale. It is difficult for a current to flow through fat in the human body, but easy for it to flow through moisture in the muscle. The difficulty with which a current flows through a substance is called "electrical resistance." Therefore, the amount of fat in your body can be estimated by measuring the electrical resistance. The current used for measurement is very low, so it is safe and imperceptible. Rest assured that your feet will not tingle or burn, nor will your hair singe, stand on end, and then spring into tight little curls.

Body fat readings fluctuate throughout the day, so for the most accurate reading you should measure body fat in the evening before sleeping because electrical resistance increases during sleep and decreases when you are awake and active. If you are overhydrated, body fat readings will be unusually low, and if you are dehydrated or have just exercised, your readings may be high. I have compared underwater weighing, skin fold calipers, and bioelectrical impedance and have obtained body fat readings within one to two percentage points of each other. Because of their simplicity, I like the scales best. Also, they are inexpensive, fast, and, best of all, private. Because the cost is comparable to a good-quality bathroom scale, I recommend that everyone reading this book seriously consider investing in one.

It is not difficult to see why I have remained a Covert Bailey devotee and why I have incorporated his teachings into my own Right Bite Program. His in-depth instructions that help each person choose the best exercises, as well as his explanations about how long and how hard to perform them for maximum long-range effectiveness are perfect. I have seen the extraordinary results, both in my own life and in the lives of my clients. Within weeks, in most cases, you will be the proud owner of an extraefficient fat-burning metabolism, which will make controlling your weight easier, faster, and more pleasurable than you have ever dreamed. I generally consume between 2000 and 2500 calories each day and presently weigh in at a shapely 100 pounds, thanks in great part to Covert Bailey's scientific exercise program.

One client, who has now been on the Right Bite Program for three years, and who exercises at about the same rate that I do, recently told me: "I'm down to 124, which is great for me. When people see the heaping piles of food I am able to wolf down while still remaining slender, they are incredulous and want to know how I do it."

PHYSIOLOGICAL REASONS WE LOSE WEIGHT WITH EXERCISE

Why is exercise so important to human health? How does it help us to lose body fat? We all vaguely suspect that it is good for us, and we feel guilty when we don't do any, but few of us know very much about the healthful physiological processes that regular exercise puts into motion. Consider the following:

People who are active and slender burn more calories then people who are sedentary. That's just a physiological fact of life. Even when not deliberately exercising, they steadily expend more calories than do unfit people, whether they are at rest or involved in a daily physical routine. Why? In part because they move about more energetically than people who are lethargic and unfit. They are the people who climb stairs or run up escalators rather than wait for the elevator. They are the ones who belly surf or play volleyball at the beach, and they are the ones who rush hither and thither getting little things done as they watch TV programs, listen to the radio, or listen to their favorite CDs. Even when they claim to be resting, they still seem to be moving. Some of them jiggle, shift positions, and bounce around for no discernable reason. I have an idea that their incessant activity often drives sedentary souls to sheer distraction.

I suspect Covert Bailey would observe that these always-in-motion types are indulging in what he calls "insensible exercise," that is, they are largely unaware of their ongoing motion. But all their little movements added together help them burn a greater number of calories in an hour than your average couch potato might burn in a week.

You may be happy to learn that there are benefits from this constant physical activity. A study from the National Institute of Health has shown that those who continually cross and uncross their legs when sitting, pace restlessly about, or fidget continuously, burn up to 685 more calories per day than those who spend most of their waking moments quietly vegetating.

In other studies, scientists have determined that active slender people generally consume an average of 600 calories more a day than fat persons. Even so, their exercised bodies remain slender. Not only do they burn more calories, but they automatically increase muscle mass, tone their bodies overall, alter their biochemistry, and just generally enhance their fat-burning ability by increasing their metabolic rates. With all this, these people burn more calories even when they are asleep.

Exercise Encourages Brown Fat Activity

We have two kinds of fat in our bodies: yellow and brown. Yellow fat is visible fat, the obvious kind that hangs over one's belt. Brown fat is more inconspicuous, and there is less of it than yellow fat. It is located near your heart, under armpits, between the shoulder blades, and around the kidneys, and its sole purpose is to warm vital organs by producing heat. Brown fat requires and expends a large load of calories in order to produce this protective heat. It is a scientific fact that the brown fat of slender, active people works harder and consumes more calories than the brown fat of the inactive or obese. Because the rise in heat production after exercise is greater than can be accounted for, researchers suspect that our brown fat, in response to exercise, is continuing to burn calories for hours after the exercise is discontinued.

Exercise Decreases Insulin

As you've already learned, insulin becomes a weight-gain trigger because it stimulates our cells to take up glucose when glucose concentrations in the blood rise too high. Most of our body's cells can use glucose only for immediate energy needs, but the liver and muscle cells are an exception. They can convert glucose into a stored form of sugar, called glycogen, which can be used by the body as needed. The liver can also seize incoming glucose, such as that from candy, for instance, and convert it into fat for export to other parts of your body, such as your thighs or belly. Our versatile fat cells not only pick up this ready-made fat from the liver, but they can also make their very own fat from the excess glucose that insulin has been pushing into their cells.

One reason that weight loss can seem to stall interminably after a dieter has consumed unusually large amounts of food is that these sudden abnormal influxes of food precipitate a correspondingly large insulin response. This response sends the extra glucose into fat cells where it is converted to fatty tissue, or to liver cells where it is first converted into fat, then routed to the waiting fat cells. After excess glucose has been converted to fat and stored in fat cells, it can be trapped there for a long time. Logically, it follows that the less insulin you have careering around in your system, the less likely you are to gain unwanted pounds.

You will be happy to learn that it is entirely within your power to do something about this—to decrease your body's excess insulin. You can do it by:

✓ Reducing body fat through exercise;

✓ Eating fewer fatty and sugary foods;

✓ Including more high-fiber foods in your diet.

Simply eating several small meals a day instead of three large ones can keep insulin responses to a minimum, thereby more easily balancing your glucose and insulin levels. By keeping insulin levels low, you can help prevent the conversion of sugar to fat and its subsequent storage. In addition, a stabilized blood sugar level can virtually stop erratic blood sugar plunges and the accompanying hunger precipitated by these sudden drops.

Studies have shown that the unfit body burns more carbohydrates than does the fit body. Consequently, after eating, unfit persons will become hungry sooner than fit persons, due to the more rapid lowering of their blood sugar, which you'll recall acts as a weight-gain trigger. One reason athletes burn more fat than carbohydrate is that they maintain lower insulin levels than sedentary people. These low insulin levels enhance the burning of fat, not glucose.

Aerobic Exercise Increases Fat-Burning Enzymes

Aerobic exercise, combined with adequate calories, increases the number of fat-burning enzymes in the body, allowing you to burn fat while you exercise.

There are no two ways around it, if you lack fat-burning enzymes, you are going to get fat. But here's the good news: If you exercise regularly, you increase these enzymes in your muscles.

When you start an exercise program, make certain you are getting enough calories, however, or your body won't be able to synthesize these enzymes. (Too few calories = weight-gain trigger.) The calories are also necessary to give you the stamina to exercise. So, the bottom line is that if you want to lose weight you've got to provide your body with enough calories to make enzymes and to lose weight. Your body needs calories both to provide you with the energy to exercise and to make fat-burning enzymes.

Exercise Builds Valuable Muscle Protein When We Eat Healthily

Eating a healthy diet, one that provides sufficient calories, is the key to building valuable, fat-burning muscle tissue. The truth is that you will lose this valuable lean tissue if you don't exercise—no matter how healthy your diet. Also, an inadequate diet when you are exercising can destroy valuable muscle protein. (Loss of lean body mass = weight-gain trigger.)

If you are on a diet program that doesn't include physical exercise, your scale may tell you that you are losing weight, but what are you actually losing? For every three pounds of fat you lose, you could be losing up to a pound of muscle. If you are eating a healthy, adequate diet but still not exercising, you'll also lose muscle protein along with the fat—just not as fast as when you are exercising and eating a poor diet. For anyone aiming to become thinner, the loss of precious lean-muscle tissue is hardly a loss to be celebrated, because it retards your calorie- and fat-burning capacity. This partly explains why for years, even though I was following a nutritious diet, I still had difficulty controlling my weight—I was not building valuable muscle protein that burns calories.

Muscle tissue constitutes between 30 and 50 percent of the healthy body. By preserving the health of this tissue you optimize your ability to get and stay thin, both because of the way muscles make use of calories and because fat-burning enzymes created here can increase your calorie-burning capacity by fiftyfold during exercise.

Exercise Increases Endogenous Opiates

Endogenous opiates are hormones created in the brain. Neurophysiologists believe that they play a significant role in affecting our appetites. These opiates act like analgesics, reducing or even deadening pain. When your body is under stress, these natural analgesics become depleted. By eating, you raise the production of these opiates to a level that makes stress more tolerable. You can see from this why many people use food as a way of relieving stress; when stressed, our brains may actually be sending out an SOS for food to increase endogenous opiates. (Stress = weight-gain trigger)

These hormones can also be increased by means other than eating. Yes, you have guessed correctly. They can also be increased by exercise! So here is another good reason why exercise is an important part of any weight-reduction program. If an ounce of prevention truly is worth a pound of cure, then anyone who is overweight would be wise to guard against depleted endogenous opiate hunger through regular exercise and by eating healthily.

Aerobic Exercise Increases Fat Breakdown

Aerobic exercise increases the capacity of the aerobic pathway within the cells' mitochondria to break down fat for energy.

Mitochondria are tiny structures within each cell that extract energy from the nutrients and oxygen, to allow the cell to perform its various functions. With aerobic exercise, more oxygen is available to the mitochondria, allowing them to more efficiently burn the fat contained in the cells. When more fat is burned, less muscle glycogen is used. The benefits of this "glycogen sparing" system include added endurance and more stable blood sugar levels.

Aerobic Exercise Reduces Lactic Acid Build-up

Those who exercise aerobically do not start to accumulate lactic acid in their blood until they are exercising at 70 percent of their aerobic capacity. The unfit start to accumulate lactic acid at 50 percent of aerobic capacity.

The point at which lactic acid accumulates is called the "anaerobic threshold." This is important because lactic acid speeds up the rate of muscle glycogen breakdown by interfering with the use of fat as a fuel. People who are unfit begin to accumulate lactic acid with less effort than fit people, and burn less fat as a consequence. People who are physically fit are able to exercise at a higher intensity and burn more fat in the process.

When you are physically fit, you have roughly a third more capacity for storing glycogen than when you are not fit. Thus, exercise confers a double advantage—muscle glycogen stores are higher at the outset and are also depleted more slowly. This translates into less hunger and more sustained energy.

OTHER BENEFITS OF EXERCISE

The benefits of an active physical life go beyond weight loss, and these benefits are particularly important for anyone who wants to lose weight. Physical exercise can delay or prevent osteoporosis by helping to keep your bones strong. It lowers your resting pulse rate so that your heart won't have to work so hard. It induces capillary growth in heart muscle, as well as in every other muscle in your body, and lowers blood pressure. It can raise the level of "good" cholesterol HDL, which lowers the risk of heart disease. It lowers LDL (bad cholesterol) and helps prevent the formation of blood clots. Exercise reduces the chances of colon cancer, improves resistance to infections of all kinds, and improves tissue repair. It also reduces the hours of sleep we need and can alleviate depression and anxiety. And it improves brain function. Last, if this isn't enough, exercise improves our sense of balance and coordination.

These are just a few of the many healthful benefits attributed to exercise. In addition, I do not think it can be denied that people who exercise look better than those who do not. Their skin tones are healthier, their muscles are firmer, and their clothes look better on their exercised bodies. Active people exude a certain confidence, and they are more graceful in the way they move. Most men and women who exercise regularly seem to be more animated and energetic than their underexercised counterparts, and many studies suggest that it may be one of the best ways to prevent and get over depression, helping you to maintain a positive and upbeat look on life. Surely, exercising is an investment in health and appearance that will pay you back for the rest of your life.

Covert Bailey: The Ultimate Fit or Fat

I have been a devotee of Covert Bailey's for many years, and because of this I highly recommend every one of his books, but in particular his latest, *The Ultimate Fit or Fat.* For anyone wishing to successfully lose weight and maintain his or her ideal weight, I believe this author's books are "must reads."

Bailey maintains that dieting alone is only a superficial solution for weight control and points out that most fat people eat less than skinny people. In my case this was certainly true. Throughout my teens, while going through frustrating periods in my quest for answers to weight problems, I observed that even during periods when I ate normally, or very little, my body was still mysteriously triggering my body's fat-making mechanisms.

The reason for this, as we've already explored, is that the biochemistry of the fat person's body has adapted to a low-calorie intake, so when fat people overeat occasionally—and who doesn't?—they gain weight, while their thin friends stay the same or gain so little weight that it is invisible on them. The more fat you have on your body, the more your biochemistry works to keep the fat on. Seems grossly unfair, doesn't it? You can stop this vicious cycle by changing your biochemistry so that your body automatically burns the calories you consume, instead of turning them in to fat. Happily, every one of us can be in control of this situation.

Every person? Yes, every one, and that means you and me. We do this through "aerobic exercise." This is an exercise that gets your heart and lungs working vigorously, pushing you just to the outer edge of your present physical capacities, and does so continuously, for a minimum of twelve minutes. That's not a lot a minutes, about what it takes you to brush your teeth and your hair in the morning. Yet this kind of exercise will increase your fitness more than other kinds of exercise because it promotes the growth of fat-burning enzymes, while helping to tone your body. And what's so magical about twelve minutes of this kind of exercise? The twelve-minute minimum seems to be the point at which the benefits begin to accrue.

There is a specific level of exertion that you need to maintain for this twelve-minute period. Think of "aerobic" as oxygenating your blood, since that is a big part of what's happening. To do this, you need to be pumping a lot more blood in that twelve-minute interval than you do watching quiz shows on TV. And along with your blood pumping through your body at a faster rate, you also want your lungs bringing in more oxygen to deliver to the blood. So you do need a certain level of physical exertion to get all this happening. There are formulas for doing this, measuring your heart rate and respiration rate as you exercise, but you don't really have to get that technical about it unless you have suddenly developed an ambition for becoming an exercise physiologist. Covert Bailey gives a very simple procedure for determining if you are exercising aerobically. He says, "if you are able to talk haltingly while breathing deeply but comfortably, you are almost certainly exercising aerobically."

Is there a general prescription for how much and how hard you should exercise? The best prescription I know is to simply get out there and start exercising as much as you possibly can without overexercising. It's best to begin with what is comfortable for you. Each of us is different, with different needs and different capabilities. Respect your own limits. If you are starting out feeling comfortable walking leisurely around the block, do that. Then gradually increase distance and speed, with the goal in mind of eventually getting up to a twelve-minute aerobic workout.

What if you are already fit? Then exercise for slightly longer durations than you are at present. And if you are fat and really unfit, exercise at short intervals of ten to fifteen minutes two to three times a day. The fatter you are the more often you should exercise.

Don't let anyone push you into exercising at their rate, unless the two of you are pretty closely matched. Age also affects how long you should exercise. The older you are, the longer you need to exercise, but you need to do it more *gently* and don't do the same exercise every day. Remember the old story of the Tortoise and the Hare: If you just steadily plod along, you will get there in your own good time.

As you embark on your exercise program make sure that you are eating a healthy diet with adequate caloric content. If you don't eat enough when exercising aerobically, your body registers this as stress and reacts by depositing more fat in your cells, using less stored fat and leaving you with hunger pangs. Undereating always encourages your body to become fatter, so don't make the mistake of fasting or eating just one meal a day when you start exercising aerobically.

With a combination of healthy eating and aerobic exercise, you are certain to change your body chemistry to that of a fat-burning machine, and as you lose body fat, you will replace it with handsome lean muscle. Since the biochemical replacement of flab with solid muscle reflects the efficiency of your new fat-burning metabolism, you will never have to be concerned about regaining unwanted pounds.

Your Ideal Weight

BODY FAT PERCENTAGES

As you are developing your new, thinner metabolism through exercising and healthy eating, how do you determine your ideal weight? While there are individual variations, it is sometimes helpful to have some approximate numbers to work with. I have looked at a great many different systems for doing this and favor Covert Bailey's methods, since he has based his calculations on metabolic needs, not just on how a person looks. He bases these calculations on percentage of body fat in our bodies, remembering that without some fat reserves no person can be considered completely healthy. Here are his basic recommendations:

✓ An adult woman's maximum weight should reflect a body fat percentage of no greater than 22 percent of her total body mass.

✓ Men's bodies, being generally more muscular than the average woman's should be no more than 15 percent fat.

MEASURING BODY COMPOSITION—RATIOS OF LEAN TO FAT TISSUE

While you can certainly start exercising whether or not you know your ratio of lean to fat tissue, I recommend that as soon as possible after starting the Right Bite Program, you have your body composition analyzed. If you belong to a gym or health spa where getting this measurement is a simple routine, that's ideal. If you don't have access to such a club, I believe that one of the new bioelectric scales (available in many discount stores for under $100) is a great asset, because it will allow you to get accurate calculations in the privacy of your own home. If you are not into bioelectrical devices, the next best and most accessible way of measuring body composition is with a cloth tape measure. This is a system Covert Bailey developed. He writes about it in his book, *Ultimate Fit or Fat.* You'll find it all in that book: his own formulas for calculating your body fat percentage, your lean body mass, and your ideal weight.

I'm going to assume that you will find out your percentage of fat by either having it measured by an outside source, getting yourself a bioelectric scale, or buying Covert Bailey's book and using his tape measuring method. Remember that as your metabolism is transformed from that of a fat person to that of a thin person, lean body tissue will replace fat. So it would not be unusual, particularly in the beginning, for your body weight to remain the same, even though you are making great progress in changing your composition. Your handy bioelectric scale will erase any confusion you might have about that.

Remember that your goal is not just to achieve a certain number on the standard weight scale. It is also to achieve a good ratio of lean tissue to fat since the more lean tissue you have, the more calories you will automatically burn and the easier it will be for you to maintain your idea weight and composition. For instance, you can be 5'5" and 125 pounds, but if your body fat percentage were 27 percent you would be fat and flabby. With the same height and weight but 18 percent body fat, you would be very lean and toned.

Pounds of Body Fat

Once you have determined your percentage of body fat, by any of the methods I've described, you can determine the total number of pounds of fat you have on your body by using this simple formula:

Your total weight times your percentage of body fat
equals the total pounds of fat you have on your body.

So let's say Johanna weighs 200 pounds and her percentage of body fat is 40 percent. (200 x .40 = 80). This means she is carrying around 80 pounds of body fat.

Does this mean that Johanna should lose 80 pounds? No. Remember that your body needs some fat to be healthy. Bailey tells us that the maximum amount of body fat should be 22 percent for women. So how do you figure that? Easy, start by figuring out what her lean body weight would be. You do that by subtracting the 80 pounds from Johanna's present total weight of 200 pounds. (200 minus 80 = 120).

But we're not there yet. Her maximum fat is 22 percent of her total weight, and this figure of 120 pounds is considerably less than that. So here's how you do it. First subtract .22 from 1. That gives you .78. Now divide 120, the lean body mass figure, by that number:

120 divided by .78 is 153.8. That would be Covert Bailey's recommendation for maximum weight for Johanna. Let's round that off to 154.

If that's the maximum Johanna should weigh, what's her ideal weight? According to the American Dietetic Association and the National Research Council, 16 to 19 percent body fat is rated as *good* for women, while 11 to 14 percent is rated as *good* for men. For an *excellent* rating, which is usually attained only by highly conditioned athletes, you'd strive for 10 to 15 percent for women, and 6 to 10 percent for men. Most of us will find our ideal weight in the good category. To calculate your ideal weight, figure 3 to 6 percent below the above maximums for the good category. So here are the calculations all in a row:

1. To determine the total number of pounds of fat you have on your body, take your present total body weight and multiply it by your percentage of body fat, as determined by your bioelectric scale, water weighing, or Bailey's tape measure method.

2. Get your lean body weight by subtracting the weight of your total fat from your total body weight.

3. Subtract your maximum percentage of fat (.22 for women; .15 for men) from 1. So that would be .78 for women, .85 for men.

4. Divide your lean body weight by that number. This gives you the maximum amount you should weigh, according to Bailey.

5. Your ideal weight should be 3 to 6 percent less than the 22 percent figure for women, and 1 to 4 percent less for men. In Johanna's case, she would divide her lean body weight of 120 pounds by .84 for 16 percent fat. That comes to 142.8 pounds. Or she'd divide her lean body mass by .81, which comes to 148 pounds. Therefore, her ideal weight range is from 142.8 to 148 pounds.

6. When you are all done with the numbers, you will have the healthy weight range for you, from lowest to highest.

Your Personalized Exercise Program

You are now ready to design your own exercise program. This begins by choosing a form of exercise that truly appeals to you. Keep in mind that having an exercise that you enjoy doing will be the best motivator you can have for sticking to a program. No matter how healthy an exercise might be said to be, it's not going to do you a lot of good if you dread getting out there and doing it. The more you enjoy your exercise, the more you're likely to do it—and that spells success in terms of your achieving your weight goals.

1. CHOOSE AN AEROBIC EXERCISE

Here is a list of suggestions:

Walking	Hiking
Running	Aerobics class
Elliptical trainer	Aerobic rider
Cross-country ski machine	Step/ladder climber
Jogging	Minitrampoline
Bicycling	Rowing
Cross-country skiing	Jumping rope
Roller skating, Ice skating	Health Rider
Stair-climber	Mountain biking

Do not choose for your "get-in-shape" exercise any of the following: downhill skiing, tennis, handball, racquetball, weight lifting, calisthenics, baseball, field/ice hockey, motorcycle riding, wind surfing, volleyball, dancing, soccer, horseback riding, water skiing, basketball, gymnastics, golf, or sprinting because they are not considered aerobic. They don't cause you to maintain a steady and consistent aerobic effect for the required twelve-minute duration. However, these are all activities you can enjoy in addition to your chosen aerobic exercises.

If you hate bicycling, for heaven's sake, don't buy a stationary bike. If you are the Greta Garbo type who "vants to be alone," there are many exercise options that ensure total privacy. For example, there are rowing machines that fold down and fit snugly under most beds when not in use. There are treadmills and stair steppers. So go to the nearest facility that sells exercise equipment and try out anything that appeals to you before you make a large investment. If you lack the nerve to sample these machines in full view of the display window, I'm sure an enterprising salesperson will be eager to demonstrate. If you don't want to invest in an exercise machine, then walk or jog outside, do chair stepping on steps or a low stool, or buy a two-dollar jump rope. You may also wish to jog in place to your favorite music or follow an aerobics video tape.

Those of you who don't mind an audience and want more support may choose to join a gym or other exercise facility; or if you don't care a fig what the neighbors think, exercise outside.

As mentioned earlier, I chose to step on and off a chair for my beginning exercise. I could do this in private, it did not take any financial investment, and it was a perfect exercise for someone who is always pressed for time. It also gave me a few minutes to catch up on my favorite soap opera that I taped earlier and saved to view when I was exercising. As my body's chemistry began to change, I found I wanted to exercise more vigorously, so I turned to jogging, which satisfied my desire to move my arms and legs to their fullest capacity.

I have not listed swimming as an exercise for fat loss, even though it is aerobic. It is great for increasing your fitness, but very poor for fat loss because your body wants to keep fat when it is in cold water—ask any whale. Also, If you are very heavy, do not pick jogging or running until you are leaner and fitter, even though the fat loss is rapid with these exercises. Running and jogging can put unhealthy stress on your bones and joints if you are seriously overweight, besides being too strenuous for the heart and lungs. Once you're in shape, of course, it's wonderful exercise. Walking and chair stepping are great beginning exercises if you weigh a lot.

2. Pick a Second Aerobic Exercise You Like

According to most exercise physiologists you can raise your fitness level more quickly by doing two different exercises rather than sticking to one. Because you are switching from one form of exercise to another, your muscles will react as if you are working harder—which is good—even though you are not increasing the intensity of your workouts. You'll also build extra fat burning enzymes more quickly. If you walk briskly for three days, you may want to ride a stationary bike on alternate days. If you jog three days you may want to use an elliptical trainer on alternate days. Varying your program in this way is like having your own "cross-training." Now doesn't that sound impressive! Also, by varying your exercises you reduce your chances of injury. For example, if you only jog all your life you'll most likely end up with some knee and ankle problems since the impact on your joints when you run, particularly on pavement or other compact surfaces, can be quite hard on them. Varying your exercises ensures that different parts of your body have a chance to rest and repair themselves even as you continue to get adequate aerobic workouts.

3. Decide on the Number of Days You Intend to Exercise and Work It into Your Schedule

Pick a minimum of three days and a maximum of six. If you have not been exercising regularly, it is a good idea to exercise one day, rest the next, always leaving a day between each session for your body to adjust to the new routine.

My recommendation is to make a conservative estimate of how many days per week you think you can exercise. If you are unfit or fat, make it a *low* number for your first week or two—a number you *know* you can stick with. Then if you do more than that, so much the better; you can cheerily congratulate yourself. Many people are very enthusiastic and excited when they embark on a new diet and exercise program. Unfortunately, they try to bite off more than they can chew. They do too much too soon, get tired, become discouraged, and lose their incentive. If you are not in the habit of regular exercise, begin your personal exercise program with a three-day week. In this way, you will feel successful when you match or exceed your goals. Once you are consistent about meeting your three-day week level of exercise, then increase it by one day. Executed properly, this minimal amount of exercise will begin the process of replacing fat with muscle tissue and give you the disciplined incentive to continue. Gradually increase your exercise to six days a week.

As you increase the days you exercise, give yourself at least one day of rest each week, free of any physical exercise. Rest and recovery are very important for improving your fitness. I love a statement that

Covert Bailey made, that exercise is worthless if you don't recover from it. Also, do not give up exercising for a longer duration than a week, unless you are ill, physically incapacitated, or are showing some of the symptoms associated with overtraining—muscle pain, fatigue, poor coordination, lethargy, and difficulty sleeping, for example. However, most people rarely if ever overtrain so when you take necessary rest time off from exercise, make sure you don't let days slip into weeks or into months. Any time you stop exercising, fitness is quickly lost.

4. DECIDE HOW LONG YOU ARE GOING TO EXERCISE AND PLAN IT INTO YOUR SCHEDULE

In the beginning, you can break your twelve-minute rule, being a little looser about how much you are exercising. For example, set your range at from ten to fifteen minutes, two to three times a day. Your maximum should be sixty minutes per day, even though you think you could do more.

If you are an aerobics beginner, unfit or fat, it would be wise to start your program with *short* frequent periods of exercise. Stick with ten to fifteen minutes, two to three times a day. After you have been performing your chosen aerobics exercise three to four days a week for several weeks, you will find yourself becoming fitter and leaner. As you see the new you emerging, you will love the way your body feels and want to exercise more.

As you become fitter, increase the length of time that you exercise. But don't exercise harder. This rule of thumb will help you get in shape faster. Over the years, I have increased my aerobic exercise from its initial ten to fifteen minutes, three times per week, to one hour a day six days a week. You will find that the more you exercise the more you will desire to exercise and the longer periods of time you will want to exercise.

5. INCORPORATE WIND SPRINTS

After you have been exercising regularly for at least four weeks start working "wind sprints" into your exercise routine once a week.

Wind sprints are short bursts of higher intensity exercise of between twenty and forty seconds during regular intervals of low intensity exercise. Wind sprints take place when you abruptly speed up within your normal exercise routine. For example, if your regular program is walking briskly, a wind sprint would be jogging for twenty to forty seconds, then returning to your usual pace. These little bursts of speed add intensity to your workout without injuring you. You don't have to go super fast or go superlong, and it is the recovery after the wind sprint that makes you get fit fast. I recommend incorporating a wind sprint after you have been exercising at your aerobic pace for five to ten minutes. Your aerobic pace is the speed at which you can perform your exercise for consecutive nonstop miles without getting out of breath. After your wind sprint, return to your usual aerobic pace. Eventually work up from one or two sprints per session—up to five sprints.

Most exercise physiologists maintain that if after four weeks you cannot walk a mile in twenty minutes without getting out of breath you should not add wind sprints or any other stressors to your program until you can.

For example, let us picture you ensconced on your stationary bike conscientiously pedaling away in your correct training zone. After five minutes, your jaw tenses; you grip the handlebars and squeeze your eyes shut. Suddenly, there is a frenzied burst of pedal activity, and your legs begin to rotate at an incredible speed. The A-flat murmur of your bike wheel shrieks to a high C, and all we can see is a cyclonic blur of whirling lean muscle tissue. That's a wind sprint in action! Then, just as suddenly as it began, this remarkable interlude has ceased. Once again, your countenance is placid, your shoulders are relaxed, and your legs are steadily pedaling in a rhythmic A flat. Except for the flying sweat, one could almost believe nothing extraordinary had happened.

But, no, we had truly witnessed a real Covert Bailey-style wind sprint, and I am certain that if we cared enough to stick around, we'd surely be treated to another one.

6. INCORPORATE WEIGHT LIFTING

After four weeks incorporate weight lifting into your program. Add a minimum of two days a week to a maximum of six days a week, making sure you rest weight-trained muscles 48 hours before the next work out, i.e., upper body Monday, Wednesday, and Friday and lower body Tuesday, Thursday, and Saturday.

Another weight schedule is to do both upper and lower body and skip a day in between. For example, Monday, Wednesday, and Friday or Tuesday, Thursday, and Saturday.

Start incorporating weight-lifting about the same time that you start wind sprints, but do both gradually. The increased strength you derive from weight lifting will make it easier to perform your aerobic exercise more intensely without becoming anaerobic. Lots of fat is burned during the recovery phase of weight lifting. Weight lifting will also contribute to muscle growth and as you have learned, the more muscle you have, the more calories you will burn.

There are many first-rate books you can consult on the "how to's" of weight lifting, or you may wish to get professional guidance at a gym or local spa.

Keep in mind that weight training does not necessarily mean that you must lift heavy bar bells or other massive equipment. Pushups, pullups, and situps are excellent forms of weight lifting you can do at home.

7. BEFORE YOU EXERCISE—WARM UP

A warmup is simply a gentler version of the exercise you are going to perform. If you like to jog, then jog very slowly before you go at your usual pace. If you walk, then walk more slowly first. According to Bailey, the harder the upcoming exercise, the longer your warmup should be. For example, the warmup before swimming an hour would be less than the warmup required for swimming fifteen minutes.

8. "RED X" YOUR CALENDAR

Mark a red X on your calendar for your start day and for every day that you exercise. It might sound a bit childlike to admit that seeing a red X on every successive day that you exercise can be such a source of pleasure and pride. But to people who have had trouble staying with health programs and exercise plans in the past, the red X plan is valuable reinforcement of one's commitment. You can actually see your progress, and what could be more satisfying than watching your calendar fill up month after month with vibrant red Xs?

By now, I hope that you have caught some of my enthusiasm for exercise and physical fitness as being vital for anyone interested in weight loss. In my own clinical practice, I have witnessed, time and again, how powerfully a well-integrated exercise program changed people's metabolism, their self-confidence, their endurance, and their strength, while speeding weight loss exponentially.

Mental Calisthenics

There is more to weight control than following a trigger-free diet and exercising properly. Take Marsha for example. When she came to me, she was ninety-three pounds overweight. She was filled with self-criticisms and her face was frozen in an expression of permanent pessimism, the result, in part, of too many failed diet efforts. I knew that with her failure-oriented attitude she'd likely sabotage her own efforts to follow the Right Bite Program. I started her out with *knee bends for her neocortex— mind exercises*. Before she did anything she needed to start building her self-esteem and a belief that she could succeed.

When she returned a month later she was a different person. A cheerful expression had replaced her furrowed brow. She confided that she was feeling a lot better about herself and about her prospect of succeeding on my program.

Marsha went on my weight-loss program, and two and a half years later she had lost 100 pounds. She never stopped believing in her ability to succeed, and she never stopped doing her mind exercises.

As Thomas Jefferson said, "Nothing can stop the man with the right mental attitude from achieving his goal; nothing on earth can help the man with the wrong mental attitude."

Don't ever think "I cannot" but instead think "I can." The pessimist is defeated before he even begins because he has put limitations on himself when there really are no limits. If your mind sometimes feels like a garden overgrown with weeds, then read on to learn how to practice positive mental calisthenics.

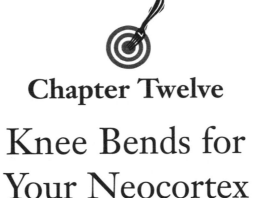

Chapter Twelve

Knee Bends for Your Neocortex

We are what we think about all day long.
—Ralph Waldo Emerson

Self-talk—how we talk to ourselves in the privacy of our minds—can make us either our own best friends or our own worst enemies. According to Cervantes, "our greatest foes, and whom we must chiefly combat, are within." Certain kinds of belittling or denigrating self-talk can imprint our brains and act as weight-gain triggers just as surely as a bowlful of greasy, salty chips.

We all indulge in self-talk, of course. When we make a mistake, we may say to ourselves, "Well, that was pretty stupid." When we are faced with a difficult challenge, we may coach ourselves: "Come on, you can do it." And when we accomplish something that particularly pleases us, we might say, "Ah, that was great! Good job!" Sometimes we actually tell ourselves these things out loud, but just as often we say them under our breath, or maybe only think them.

Self-talk can be a source of positive energy in your life, producing strength and enthusiasm for change and improvement. Or it can undermine your self-confidence, your willpower, or even your sanity. Which of these it will be depends on how you choose and direct your self-talk.

Sometimes our self-talk blinds us to larger truths that are obvious to everyone around us. Once, during a seminar I was giving, an extremely overweight woman began wildly waving her program to get my attention. I paused in mid-sentence to hear what she had to say. Breathlessly, she hove to her feet and bellowed, "I have a diet that really works! Every time I go on it I can lose at least 40–50 pounds. It's terrific!"

"But, Mary," I said, "If the diet is so wonderful, why are you still overweight? For heaven's sake, why do you keep going back to a diet that does not help you maintain a weight that is acceptable to you?"

Mary sank back onto her chair. After the lecture she thanked me for the rather embarrassing revelation. She had actually never thought about her weight problem in quite the light I had shed on it. Her little discourse about her "terrific diet" had prevented her from seeing that this same self-talk was keeping her fat.

While we don't always know the actual words of our own self-talk, we find the evidence in our actions: We start a diet every Monday, only to break it by Wednesday. We starve ourselves for two days, only to binge on the third. We experiment with still another quick-fix fad diet, intuitively knowing it's not going to work, and end up gaining rather than losing weight. We diet in an effort to change a specific area of our bodies—for example, trying to transform robust muscular legs into the willowy limbs of a ballerina. To cut calories, we skip breakfast; famished by ten o'clock, we end up overeating. More obvious are the times we tell ourselves "I can't," and block ourselves from even starting.

Let's face it, it takes a certain amount of skilled self-brainwashing to keep up these kinds of fallacious practices. But I'd like you to think about all this from a slightly different perspective. We know how successful we are at brainwashing ourselves into negative behaviors and habits. We know the power of talking ourselves into practices that in our more rational moments we know are questionable. But with the same mechanisms of self-talk, directed in a more conscious way, you can achieve your fondest goals. Instead of reinforcing self-defeating behaviors, you can reinforce thoughts, beliefs, and behaviors that fully support your most positive goals.

I began integrating conscious self-talk into the Right Bite Program over fifteen years ago after observing how much faster and easier the program worked for people who used these techniques. Conscious self-talk can even erase thought patterns that become weight-gain triggers. There are three key areas where positive self-talk is especially important for achieving weight loss. They are:

1. Self-perception: What we tell ourselves about ourselves

2. Body sensations: What we tell ourselves about certain physical sensations

3. Diet and food myths: What we tell ourselves about certain foods and diet plans

In the following pages, we'll explore each of these areas in detail.

Self-Talk #1: Self-Perceptions

The best example of self-talk affecting self-perception is found in the person who complains that she's "grossly fat," though her physician and everyone else sees her as only *moderately overweight*. It's clear that this person's self-perceptions are based on negative self-talk rather than on objective observation. Here's a good example:

Now in her late thirties Marguerite had gained twenty pounds in the past two years and wanted to get back to the weight she was as a teenager. At her present 132 pounds she was quite attractive. When she told me her weight goals—that she wanted to get down to 110 pounds!—I became concerned, because if she achieved that goal, she would be considerably underweight for her height and lean body mass.

Marguerite told me she recognized that most people thought she had an attractive figure, but she felt terrible about her weight and knew that she was putting herself down because of it. We started looking at how her self-perceptions had formed in her teen years. At the time, she said, she and her friends had admired a particular slender fashion model who was appearing on covers of magazines everywhere.

"I'd look in the mirror and think to myself that I was too fat compared to that model," Marguerite said. "I so wanted to look like her."

Marguerite had never thought of herself as fat until she started *comparing herself* to the fashion model. Soon, self-talk such as, "I am fat next to her" evolved into "I am just plain too fat!"

Marguerite began to see the basis of her negative self-talk and realized it had gotten quite extreme. As she expressed it: "I've started telling myself I'm a fat slob."

After she recognized how this negative self-talk was affecting her, she was able to be more objective and tell herself: "I have an attractive, healthy body and know for certain that I can maintain exactly the weight I want." It wasn't easy for her to tell herself this in the beginning because her self-judgments were deeply ingrained. She continued to say this five times a day, even when she felt she was lying to herself. And after a few weeks, she began to see measurable results. As she put it herself, "I've really gotten to love the way I look. I have a more attractive and sensual body than the skinny model I used to admire."

It was easy for me to sympathize with Marguerite because in high school nearly every girl in my class, including me, started dieting when the anorexic-looking model Twiggy made her appearance in the 1960s. At first, dieting was rather competitive fun—like a game. We idolized Twiggy and would never be good enough until we looked exactly like her. We just skipped breakfast and nibbled sparingly at lunch, but as the dieting craze gained momentum, some of us got carried away. Some of us began to binge after periods of starvation dieting. Even those who had been thin gained weight. Some became chubby. A few mature individuals (of which I was *not* one) stood back and said, "This is really stupid—I have had enough." However, after several weeks of the Twiggy-look brainwashing, most of us were sure we were unacceptably fat. Negative self-talk developed—"I'm way too fat!"—and quickly turned into self-fulfilling prophecies. In a single summer I found myself weighing far more than when I started on the Twiggy look-alike campaign. I was heartbroken.

Negative self-talk and misperceptions don't usually stop with weight. They expand into long lists of self-deprecations, including being ugly, weak, stupid, incapable, bad, depressed, introverted, hyper, weird, inattentive, a failure, unpopular, and shy, to name a few possibilities. After bombarding our brains with this kind of negative self-talk, is it any wonder that we evolve into the creatures we have been telling ourselves we are? Not only that, but when you reinforce false notions about yourself others start thinking of you the same way.

Learning to develop positive self-talk is far easier than you might imagine. It starts with looking at what you dislike about yourself, identifying your present self-talk that expresses that dislike, and then turning that statement around. In Marguerite's case, she changed her self-talk from "I'm getting to be a fat slob" into "I have an attractive, healthy body and know for certain that I can maintain exactly the weight I want."

With the Right Bite Core Diet supported by positive self-talk, Marguerite lost ten pounds. Her ten-year old son helped her with a bit of advice from his Little League coach: "You've got to fake it until you can make it." Marguerite did just that, and in time her positive self-talk became her truth.

Her whole attitude toward herself changed quickly as she made positive self-talk a daily habit, erasing her negative self-perceptions. She even readjusted her original weight goal to having a body that was as healthy as it was attractive, and for the first time in many years she felt content with her weight.

Self-Talk #2: Bodily Sensations

How we interpret certain bodily sensations, and what we tell ourselves about them through our habitual self-talk, frequently produces exactly the opposite of what we want; that is, our responses to the self-talk we create end up being weight-gain triggers rather than actions that will result in weight loss.

For example, Arlen interprets being full with being fat. This is not unusual, by the way. I have come to think of it as a key issue for many chronic dieters. This is not to say that everyone is aware of what they are telling themselves. The truth is that most people aren't. Self-talk can be quite insidious, a nagging little voice in the background.

Any time she felt full, Arlen immediately started a stream of self-talk that went something like this: "You are getting so fat! Feel your body swelling up! You're becoming a disgusting blimp."

Desperately trying to silence her self-talk, she skipped dinner, fasted, overexercised, cut calories drastically, and eliminated carbohydrates altogether. She spiraled into a cycle of starving herself and then binging, and felt increasingly bad about herself. Her negative self-talk escalated, as did her weight. And it all started with a normal and healthy feeling of having a full stomach, which disappears as food is digested.

The sensations of being fat themselves elicit negative self-talk, usually including harsh judgments about how one looks and feels. For Arlen, it escalated into self-talk enumerating supposed character defects that she associated with anyone who was unable to control her weight. She told herself how *weak willed* she was, with no discipline at all. And since this self-talk was painful, she searched for a way to dull the pain. One way to do that would be to lose weight. But that would take time. Another way was to . . . well, to eat! She had learned early in life that stuffing yourself helps to numb almost any pain.

A friend of Arlen's invited her to a party. Even though Arlen realized she should not tempt herself with party food, she accept the invitation. "No big deal," she told herself, "it is your friend's birthday. Surely we are all allowed a feast day occassionally." She shut out her self-talk—just long enough to pig out on ice cream and cake.

Next morning she dragged herself out of bed feeling bloated and stuffed. The bathroom scale said she'd gained three pounds. The nagging self-talk leapt to the fore: "You're a mess! Get the weight off!" So she fasted for two days and drank nothing but diet soft drinks. Three days into the fast she woke up feeling empty and weak. The scale said she had lost four pounds. With immense relief she told herself, "I will never let myself feel that full and fat again."

At breakfast she was preoccupied with the idea of fullness and anxious that if she ate until she felt satisfied she'd gain back the pounds she had lost. The little voice nagged, "Watch yourself carefully or you're going to blow it! You'll wipe out all the progress you have made." She ate even less than usual, determined to avoid feeling full. Her self-talk was now reinforcing the myth that having a full stomach is the same as being fat. She told herself, "this feeling of fullness is just the opposite of that concave feeling I have after starving myself for a few days—and that's the feeling of thinness I want." Although she pleaded and reasoned with herself, her body protested with cravings she couldn't ignore.

Arlen had forgotten how it feels to experience a full stomach without equating it to being fat. The empty feelings of a concave belly had become her perception of normality. From then on her self-talk reinforced feelings of guilt and fear any time she detected the sensations of feeling full. She had brainwashed herself through a misinterpretation of what feeling full really means. Her brain clung to this misperception, and continued issuing self-talk to reinforce it.

It did not take long to identify Arlen's negative self-talk. She admitted that she sometimes expressed this talk out loud, though always when she was alone, she assured me. Whenever she found herself doing this, she wrote down what she was saying so that she could recall it accurately. Soon she transformed her self-talk by correcting her misinterpretations of her feelings of fullness. She looked for phrases that were direct, logical, and to the point. For example, whenever she caught herself indulging in self-talk involving the fallacy about a full stomach, she now said, "Healthy feelings of having a full stomach are an important part of learning weight management. These sensations don't mean I am getting fat."

By changing this single self-talk theme, Arlen learned how to distinguish between eating to healthy fullness and eating until she was stuffed. Within weeks of starting our work together, she was halfway to her weight-loss goal. She was enjoying eating more than ever, no longer plagued by the confusing self-talk that had eroded her self-esteem.

Self-Talk #3: Diet and Food Myths

How many times have your read or heard it said that you should restrict your caloric intake drastically if you want to lose weight? As a teenager, I even had a doctor hand me a 900 calorie diet, recommending that I follow it for four weeks. Can you imagine any teenager trying to survive on a diet like that for a month?

Maybe you've read an article in a woman's magazine that told you how to quickly get rid of extra fat so that you would look great at the beach or for your next high school reunion. Recently I saw just such an article. I calculated the daily calories, which came out to less than 500 calories a day—about what you'd get as a prisoner of war in a Third World country! Theoretically, you could lose weight this way—if you were a robot with no feelings, no sensations, and no real interest in eating.

I sometimes wonder if these calorie-restricting diets aren't created on computers just for the sake of writing articles or books.

The trouble is that our brains record information like this without filtering it through greater reason. Even when we don't believe what we've read, such material is often converted into self-talk. We tell ourselves, "To lose two pounds a day, I need to take in no more than 600 calories!" Any time you get near food, that faint but powerful inner voice nags, "Think about the calories, now! That cookie is 100 calories at least. You've already had a club sandwich and a diet cola. Eat that cookie, and it will go straight to your fat hips." When approaching a diet like the Right Bite Program, your self-talk communicates the message that, "This can't possibly work because it tells me that I *must* eat more than 600 calories."

Remember that negative self-talk is often totally irrational, and even cruel. It can sound like a kindergarten bully or an insensitive parent badgering you for eating too much. Added to this, most of us with weight issues have learned that eating dulls the pain of hurt feelings and other discomforts, so we're tempted to use food to drown out the negative self-talk that is telling us we are getting fat and ugly from overeating.

Calories are not the only food issue that gets converted into negative self-talk. For example, although they are finally losing favor, thanks to the efforts of enlightened doctors, dieticians, and thousands of disillusioned dieters, high-protein diets have been very popular over the past few years. I have seen many people who, after being on these diets, have ended up gaining weight instead of losing it. Even these people, who are angry for buying into the high-protein diet fallacies, continue to hold onto self-talk associated with these programs. It takes them a while to erase the self-talk that in fact has gotten them to the sorry state they are now in. They have learned all the slogans of high-protein diets and have to unlearn them before they are able to totally commit themselves to the Right Bite Program. The most destructive self-talk they have adopted is that *carbohydrates are fattening*. The truth? Gram for gram carbohydrates have the same calories as protein.

If you have been on a fad diet, examine yourself for self-talk that may still be keeping you bound to those diet fallacies. Look for slogans that place heavy prohibitions on any groups of foods—such as eat only fresh fruits, only fresh vegetables, only protein, and so on—or that emphasize eating only a single kind of food. We've all seen these diets: Eat nothing but grapefruit for thirty days and lose thirty pounds. Avoid eating any kind of carbohydrate and lose ten pounds the first week.

When you start the Right Bite Program, you may at first find yourself in conflict with the old fad diet slogans and with the self-talk they have fostered. So you might look at the Right Bite Core Diet and think,

"Those veggies will just go straight to fat." Or, "Don't eat that soup; much better that you eat half a grapefruit." Be ready to remind yourself that you may have to transform negative self-talk associated with old diet programs to positive self-talk that supports your dedication to the Right Bite Program.

He will be the slave of many masters who is his body's slave. —Seneca

Temptations Aren't Always Sweet

Even when we have had bad experiences with a diet, we are often left with misinformation that stays with us. The problem comes when misinformation becomes self-talk that gets in the way of following a program that really works. Even well-meaning friends or relatives can pass on or reinforce misinformation about what you should and should not eat. How often have you heard the phrase "just eat less and you will lose weight?" But eat less of what? Often it is our elimination of the wrong thing that causes problems.

Dieters are famous for becoming nearly obsessive about certain foods, repulsed by the thought of eating a food deemed "hazardous" to their efforts to control their weight. The inner monologue of self-talk aimed at maligning potatoes, for example, deprives us of a food that is healthy, delicious, filling, and, if you don't load it down with butter and sour cream, slimming as well.

If you are told enough times that potatoes are fattening, pretty soon it becomes part of your self-talk, and you avoid not just potatoes but other carbohydrates besides. The trouble is that our bodies need and will eventually start craving carbohydrates, no matter how much your self-talk protests. At a dinner-dance recently, I was standing in a buffet line watching the woman in front of me as she served herself. The only foods she put on her plate were fish and salad without any dressing. It wasn't difficult to imagine her self-talk: "Don't eat those carbohydrates! They'll make you fat!" Without energy producing carbohydrates, was it any wonder that she sat like a rag-doll all evening? On the other hand, I loaded my buffet plate with carbohydrates and danced till dawn. I would not have had any energy to expend if I had eaten like the droopy carbohydrate-starved woman from the buffet line, nor would I have felt the least bit full. A dry salad and fish might be okay for a three-toed sloth but it's hardly the right diet for active people.

I have had clients with all sorts of strange beliefs about foods. One of them would only eat wheat bread if it was in the shape of a loaf—not the shape of a bun or muffin. Others ate only steak, avoiding fish and chicken, confident that steak was more slimming. Others were positive that all restaurant food would make them fat, and consequently never allowed themselves the pleasure of eating out. Still others loaded up on puffed cereals day in and day out, thinking they were consuming a nutritious diet. The truth is, they might as well have been scooping up spoonfuls of air!

While the above examples are extreme, they help make the point that the self-talk that monopolizes our thoughts throughout the day, can seriously influence our health, our weight, and our mental outlooks. All of us must feed our receptive brain cells healthy, truthful thoughts, just as we must feed our bodies healthy nutritious foods. To lose pounds permanently, it is essential to recognize and eliminate more than the physical triggers that can cause weight gain. It is equally important to address our fattitudes, the misconceptions and negativisms that keep us struggling with our weight, and through the Right Bite mind exercises erase these self-sabotaging habits from our brains. If we don't liberate ourselves from our fattitudes, we have about as much hope of successfully managing our weight as we would have trying to climb Mount Everest with a sack of rocks tied to each foot.

Creating Positive Self-Talk

Developing positive and supportive self-talk is a little like learning to ride a bicycle, ski, or play tennis. It takes practice and repetition to get good at it. And once you've learned the basics, that's about all there is to it. As our friend Arlen's son was quick to remind his mother, "You gotta fake it until you can make it." Positive self-talk works exactly like negative self-talk, only in reverse. Repetition imprints the thoughts in our minds, and then we echo those thoughts back in our behavior and in how we perceive ourselves. I have rarely met a person who wasn't already aware or well-practiced in self-talk of the negative kind, so it takes very little effort to turn this practice around to work in a beneficial way.

There are three steps for making self-talk work in your favor. They are:

1. Correct self-perceptions;
2. Separate truth from fiction;
3. Confront your fears.

Let's look at each one of these more fully.

1. CORRECT SELF-PERCEPTIONS

To change negative self-talk we first have to know what we are telling ourselves. Since self-talk often occurs on at a barely conscious level, this isn't always easy. But a good place to start is by asking yourself how you feel about yourself. Do you think of yourself as fat? If so, think of a phrase that describes that feeling. For example, "I am fatter than almost everyone I know." Chances are that the sentence or series of phrases you make up about yourself will be pretty close to the self-talk you engage in. If they are not quite on target, they are going to be close enough that they will lead you to your habitual, and maybe very old, self talk.

This is a good place to make use of your journal. On a left hand page of your journal, list your perceived, self-defeating thoughts, misconceptions, and denigrating self-talk, including any remarks you may make to others about yourself. Adjacent to each of these self-talk declarations (on the right hand page) place a positive statement to contradict or counteract its damaging effects.

In changing our mental attitudes, we must consistently nourish our brains with positive feedback, even though we are not yet emotionally ready to relinquish our old negative beliefs. Here are some examples:

Negative self-talk You tell yourself:	**Positive self-talk** You tell yourself:
"I can never stay on a diet."	"I can stay on a diet that is nutritious and well designed to satisfy my needs." (No one can stay on a nutrient-deficient diet.)
(While looking through your favorite magazine you see a picture of your favorite fashion model, who is skinny and tall.) "She is beautiful and thin. Next to her I am a fat cow."	"She is beautiful and thin. My body is beautiful, too. Although I perceive that there are those who are thinner than I am, just as there are those who weigh more than I, we all have a beauty that is uniquely our own."
"I am fat and ugly and will never lose weight."	"On the Right Bite Program, I am getting thinner every day. Not only that, I am a beautiful person." (Then smile confidently at yourself in the mirror.)

Negative self-talk	Positive self-talk
You tell yourself:	You tell yourself:
"I always feel depressed."	"I am happy. Today will be a great day."
"I never do anything right. I am a complete and total failure."	"I can do anything I set my mind to do."

2. SEPARATE TRUTH FROM FICTION

With all the information that comes our way, from magazines, radio, television, books, and our friends, it is no wonder that we may feel uncertain about what's true and what's pure fiction (or simply a partial truth). When fictions or half-truths turn into self-talk, as they often do, they can become stumbling blocks on our path to positive change. As you progress in the Right Bite Program, you may find fictions arising from the past that seem to be in conflict with things you have been learning in this book. As these ambiguities or moments of doubt come up for you, address them very directly.

As before, turn to your journals and, on the left page, make a list of erroneous beliefs you have previously held regarding diets or food. Then, parallel to each statement, and on the right-hand side, write down a self-talk phrase that will correct that misinformation.

The greatest deception men suffer is from their own opinions.
—Leonardo Da Vinci

Self-talk fiction:	Self-talk truth:
You tell yourself:	You tell yourself:
"Potatoes are fattening."	"Potatoes are not fattening. It is what we put on them that is fattening. They have a high satiety index and will fill me up and not out."
"I will get fat if I eat more than 600 calories a day."	"A 600-calorie-a-day diet is unhealthy and will set in motion internal body changes that will eventually make me fat. Better that I eat in the neighborhood of 1500 calories."

Self-talk fiction:
You tell yourself:

"Avoid carbohydrates. Eat high-protein foods because they are lower in calories and more slimming."

Self-talk truth:
You tell yourself:

"Eat carbohydrates for balanced nutrition, a sense of satisfying fullness. Gram for gram protein and carbohydrates have the same calories."

3. CONFRONT YOUR FEARS

Anyone who has struggled with his or her weight over time will have developed fears, anxieties, or uneasiness about a variety of subjects associated with weight management. For example, you might be afraid that if you get into a physical exercise program your appetite will be stimulated, you will eat more, and you will end up gaining weight instead of losing it. To get the full benefits of the Right Bite Program, you need to be careful that these discomforts or fears don't get in your way, producing self-talk that brings doubts or causes you to lose confidence in what the Right Bite Program can do for you. When you conquer these fears and doubts by correcting your self-talk, you can allow yourself to integrate more and more of the program into your life. And as you do, you will reap the positive results. Along these same lines, I have always been inspired by something that Eleanor Roosevelt said: "I believe that anyone can conquer fear by doing the things he fears to do, provided he keeps doing them until he gets a record of successful experiences behind him."

As before, turn to your journal and, using the left-hand page, write down the negative self-talk statements that come to mind that have to do with fears, uneasiness or anxieties around weight loss and weight management. On the right hand page, write statements that counteract those fears or anxieties.

Self-talk triggering fear:
You tell yourself:

"I am afraid that I will start gaining weight if I start a physical exercise program."

Self-talk correction:
You tell yourself:

"I know that if I combine a healthy diet with a healthy physical exercise program I will be gaining lean body mass, and so will be gaining greater fat-burning abilities. Even though my scale weight may go up a bit, I will be toning my body and losing blubbery body fat."

Self-talk triggering fear:	Self-talk correction:
You tell yourself:	You tell yourself:
"I am afraid that when I feel a full stomach it means that I am getting fat or that I already am fat."	"Fullness is not fatness on the Core Diet. To feel full is normal and desirable."
"I am afraid to try because I might fail again and that would make me very disappointed and depressed."	"I am positive I will succeed if I commit myself to the Right Bite Program because I have determination. I realize that success is rarely achieved without challenges or hardships to overcome."

Change Your Mind, Change Your Life

The intent of these self-talk corrections, as well as the other mental calisthenics that follow, is to help you reeducate your brain and liberate yourself from fattitudes and diet myths that presently control your eating behavior. Each time that you repeat accurate weight-loss concepts and refute erroneous ones, you are helping to retrain your brain and nervous system. Olympic athletic trainers speak of using repetition to create new neuronal pathways that can teach an athlete to perform more effectively. This repetition—sometimes called *regrooving*—helps people unlearn old limitations and relearn better ways of executing a particular set of actions to be more successful at their chosen activity. It is the same with our mental training; we are creating new grooves to become Olympic champions in weight management. So make sure that you champion rational thoughts and reassert your newfound truths about how to manage your weight until the correct information is so deeply ingrained that all of your self-talk brings you closer and closer to your goals. And be patient with yourself in this process. Reeducating yourself requires tenacity and faith, whether it involves weight loss or learning tennis or golf.

Nix Excuses—Be a Winner

Ninety-nine percent of the failures come from people who practice the habit of making excuses.
—George Washington Carver,
American scientist, educator, author.

Because so many weight-management programs focus almost exclusively on weight loss without taking the full needs of the human body and mind into account, it is virtually impossible to stay on such limiting diets for long. The human body will instinctively rebel. Any reasons you might give to abandon such diets are probably valid, and your body is likely quite grateful that you did. However, it is important to face the fact that we humans are great excuse makers, so I always caution my clients against making excuses when it comes to the Right Bite Program. Without personal commitment at the outset, no program, no matter how good, is going to get results.

Mental calisthenics will help you maintain your commitment throughout the program. Being human, we all have a slight tendency to backslide, indulge ourselves, and then make excuses for our behavior. For this reason, be prepared to correct your course on those rare times when you stray from your path. One of the best defenses against backsliding is being aware of the more common excuses. Then, when you are tempted to use them, you will do so knowing what you are doing. Here is a list of common excuses I hear, along with my responses and suggestions for nixing them:

Excuse:	Response:
"I was hungry all the time, so I gave up."	"If you were hungry on the Right Bite Core Diet, you were not following the instructions that you are to eat when hungry."
"There wasn't anything for me to eat at the restaurant, so I went off my diet."	"Plan ahead whenever you eat out. Make a simple phone call to the restaurant where you are planning to go and check to see what they have on their menu that will fit the Right Bite Program. Also, if you order restaurant food creatively, there is always something you can eat."
"I never have time to exercise," or "I am always too tired to exercise."	"The Right Bite Program only requires twelve to fifteen minutes a day. You can easily fit that short period into your schedule."

Excuse	Response:
"I was afraid of what my friends would think. I didn't want to be different, so I went off my diet."	"If your friends really do object to your doing your own thing, then maybe you should look for new friends."
"I forgot."	"This is the world's worst excuse. The number of times that we actually do forget are rare; the number of times that we *say* we forgot is a different matter. Be totally honest with yourself and you'll know that you did not forget at all."
"I didn't know."	"This is a close runner up for the world's worst excuse. If you really didn't know, then go back and read the information you forgot one more time. Next time, you won't need an excuse."
"I felt sorry for myself, so went off my diet."	"There is no reason for feeling sorry for yourself if you are really following the program. The variety of foods available on this plan, plus the quantities that are demanded allow for a high level of satisfaction—even when we are going through difficult times and want a treat."
"I ate a little something I shouldn't have so I figured that since I'd blown it I might as well go the whole hog and eat as much junk food as I wanted."	"It is not the *little something* but the *really blowing it* that undermines you. Next time you eat that little something, do a realistic damage assessment. Chances are that if you stop there instead of really blowing it, it will be easy to repair the damage over the next couple meals. You only blow it if you quit. To quote an old homily, 'Quitters never win. Winners never quit.'"

Excuse:	Response:
"I'll start tomorrow or after my daughter's birthday party or . . ."	"There is no better time to start than *now*. The uncommitted person will always postpone a designated start day."
"This looks too hard—I just can't do it."	"Franklin Roosevelt once advised, 'When you get to the end of your rope, tie a knot and hang on.' In the case of the Right Bite Program, that translates into looking at how badly you really want to learn how to manage your weight. Any difficulties you perceive evaporate whenever you want something bad enough."

Belief in a Presence Greater Than Yourself

*Wisdom is knowledge of things human and divine
and the causes by which those things are controlled.*
—Cicero

This section may seem to you to belong more in a book about religion than a book about weight management. But I promise you that I won't proselytize. I hasten to add that since weight management is an issue of significant change in one's life, I would be remiss if I neglected to mention that people who are most successful at negotiating major changes tend to have a personal belief in a power greater than themselves. It is tremendously helpful to have faith in yourself, but having faith in a higher power to which you can turn for spiritual support seems critical.

We humans resist change, even when we know it is a change for the better. Belief in a power greater than ourselves reminds us that truths exist that transcend our own limited perceptions. Knowing these higher truths are there allows us to let go of the limitations or self-sabotaging thoughts that we place on ourselves, and so achieve our most challenging goals. As A. J. Clarke, an American clergyman, writes in Understanding Ethics, "He who believes is strong; he who doubts is weak. Strong convictions precede great actions."

I believe that our greatest inherent power comes from our faith in things unseen. In my own life, this means my faith in God. Others may call it by different names. By developing a simple, unshakable faith in a higher being, we are more likely to establish a faith in ourselves and in what we can accomplish.

Although the focus of this book is obviously not religious, I can say in all honesty that faith has played a significant role in learning to successfully manage my weight and then putting together the Right Bite Program. That faith didn't come easily for me, either. I think I was influenced by my grandfather who, when asked if he believed in God, always answered, "Well, you're crazy if you do, and you're crazy if you don't."

Though I had a simple faith in God when I was a child, I began to question that faith when I learned that Santa Claus, the Tooth Fairy, and the Easter Bunny were just make-believe. I lumped God together with them because, after all, I had no physical proof for my beliefs. The day before Christmas just after I turned five, a neighborhood child, bursting with the big secret, gleefully whispered to me that there was no such thing as a Santa Claus. In shock I confronted my mother who reluctantly admitted the truth. With growing apprehension, and expecting the worst, I asked her about the Easter Bunny and the Tooth Fairy. She uncomfortably confirmed that they also were make-believe. Well, I logically deduced, if they are imaginary, then God must be make-believe, too. My mother tried valiantly to argue to the contrary, but no amount of reasoning on that Christmas Eve could change my mind. I went to bed angry and disillusioned and refused thereafter to go to church or even to discuss God with anyone.

As I matured, the niggling suspicion that I might have been hasty in dismissing God along with Santa and the lesser fairies ate away at me. By the time I was a young adult, I recognized my deep need for spiritual nourishment and began searching for a higher meaning by examining the writings of great philosophers and by talking to others who had already acquired faith. I attended different churches hoping to connect with God. I read, I prayed, I argued. When pastors asked unbelievers to open their hearts and accept Christ, I struggled to acquiesce. At night I knelt at my bedroom window, staring up into the heavens and prayed for a sign—but afterwards I always felt the same inside, empty, unbelieving, and frustrated.

Finally, one day I noted that after years of praying, solutions to my baffling weight-control problems were slowly being provided. I sensed that I was being guided in directions that were not only helpful to me, but to others as well. This insight gave me the incentive to keep searching for the faith that had somehow seemed just out of my grasp.

Throughout the ages, man has had a universal yearning for "proof positive" that God exists, and that is what I wanted—a voice from a burning bush, a pulsating light, or best of all a small personal miracle meant just for me. How could I believe in something or someone I couldn't see, hear, or touch? I was receptive and willing to believe, but I wanted total belief without doubts, without constant questionings. I wanted to let myself go, to feel warm and glowy, secure and positive. I yearned for a faith like that of a friend I met in graduate school who had been a monk for twenty-four years. He said he "went from believing there was a God to knowing there was a God." At that point he left the monastery because he had found the answers he had been seeking for most of his life. By then I had solved my own personal weight-control problems, and my fledgling treatment program was not only saving lives but had begun to help others control their weight for the first time. This should have been the proof positive in the God I had prayed for but I still craved a literal, true, hellfire and damnation miracle . . . well maybe not that extreme; I would have settled for a couple of harp-playing cherubim.

I am still not certain why my miracle took the form that it did. It was not, to quote Shakespeare, "such stuff as dreams are made on." It was unquestionably tangible and solid with an intense reality that has not disappeared over time.

I was married and had three small children when I developed pneumonia. My symptoms continued to worsen, and after almost six weeks of fever, I couldn't struggle on. I had no idea how dangerously ill I was, nor did my hard-working husband.

Late one night, I awakened suddenly, with the feeling of a powerful presence in my bedroom. I felt strangely uneasy as though I were being intently watched. A few moments later a deep authoritative voice commanded me to "Come!" My room seemed to become brighter, and I made out a figure leaning against the right post of my canopy bed, arms crossed, staring at me. All at once, it was as though I were not ill at all. I felt strong and clearheaded, my feverish chills ceased and I breathed easily. I scooted close to the post, not the least afraid of the figure and eager to see the face. When I got close enough I gasped in recognition and asked, "Are you who I think you are?" He made no reply as though it were self-evident who he was. Well he certainly was not God, nor was he some long-dead family relative. An animated conversation ensued between us and continued for the remainder of the night. I remember every word. When I spoke, I either clasped his face and looked into his eyes or held his hands in great awe. I was also aware of an aromatic "woody"sweet-smoky scent surrounding him. Suddenly exhausted, I told my visitor I must sleep and he left, assuring me he would be back.

Before I drifted into unconsciousness, I picked up the phone by my bed and dialed my mother who lives in another state. I somehow felt it was necessary to tell her that I was in great peace and wished to die. My parents had been extremely worried by my prolonged illness and rec-ognized at once that I was in serious trouble. Panicked, my mother long-distance called both my doctor and my husband. I was immedi-ately taken to the hospital. That same morning, my mother was on a plane to Cleveland.

I knew very clearly that I had just had a unique and deeply religious experience. I was desperately ill and could do no more than carry that vision of my encounter that night in my heart and mind. I wasn't ready to discuss it with others, however; first because I hadn't the strength, but also because I feared that no one would understand. Would I be thought crazy? Would this vision be attributed to my sickness? I knew absolutely that I had witnessed an astonishing miracle, and no one would ever con-vince me otherwise. So, I remained quiet, guarding my secret.

When my mother arrived in Cleveland, she came directly to the hos-pital and remained by my bedside for the rest of the day. That night, at my home, she dragged herself to the room where I had been sleeping and climbed into my rumpled unmade bed. The next morning she hur-ried to the hospital. She was motherly and cheerful, but seemed dis-tracted. When I asked how she had slept, she admitted that something strange had happened during the night. She described how shortly before dawn she had been jolted from a deep sleep by an explosion of energy that suddenly filled the room. "I couldn't move," she continued, "and then I heard a powerful voice tell me to . . ."

Before she could complete her sentence, I broke in and finished it for her. "The voice said *come*, didn't it?" The hospital room became deathly still as we stared at each other. I started to cry. I knew my miracle was safe, that I would be believed—that the wonder of my night of revela-tion could be shared. My mother had felt the same overwhelming pres-ence as I had. When the initial shock had lessened, she told me that she had not seen the owner of the voice and that when the imperious sum-mons had been issued, she had quickly sat up. At that point the highly charged aura had immediately died away, and the room changed back to normal. With some amusement she observed that it was as if this entity had seen her and was startled to find a different person in my bed.

After my mother left the hospital that night I wasn't surprised in the least when my nocturnal visitor found his way to the hospital. Our early morning conversations were even more wonderful and comprehensive than the first. He helped me to restore my faith. He showed me I had been witnessing miracles throughout my life that I had been too obtuse to see, and he also presented me with a gift—an amazing creative skill in a field that formerly was totally foreign to me.

After a slow recovery from pneumonia, I was able to make exciting use of my impressive new talents. As a "bonus miracle gift" it continues to bring pleasure, enrichment, and a deeper meaning to my life and the lives of others. My near death experience has given me a renewed optimism and the ability to more easily face tough challenges. Moreover, the insights I have gleaned through this experience have strengthened my determination to make solutions available to those who suffer from debilitating weight problems. I have learned to enjoy every moment I am alive, not to fear death, and to appreciate the remarkable daily miracles that can be ours for the taking.

If you don't have faith yet, begin the process of looking for it by keeping your heart and mind open. Never give up, for your searching in itself will bring you rewards greater than you ever believed possible. If you already have faith, strengthen it at every opportunity and be joyful and grateful for this blessing, whether you are facing the challenges of weight loss, a life-threatening illness, or learning to enjoy life more fully.

Your Personalized Mental Calisthenics Program

Once you have all the elements of the mental calisthenics program in your mind, set up a defined routine for yourself that will allow you to practice and develop your skills in this area. Here's what I recommend.

1. Find a quiet moment each day to meditate, pray, or otherwise take time to acknowledge the presence of a power greater than yourself. Do this even if it is for only a minute. Some people like to simply sit or walk in nature, where they can contemplate the mysteries of the Creator. Give thanks for the good things in your life and affirm that you are going to be the best that you can be. Be sure you tell your God or source of spiritual guidance that any help "from on high" will be greatly appreciated.

2. Those of you who are seriously committed to the principles in this book will most likely have established some significant weight and fitness goals by now. Each morning review your primary goal for that day and articulate the means by which you plan to achieve it.

3. Commit to entertaining only thoughts of success, holding in your mind a clear mental picture of your success. Hold this picture and surround it with clear, brilliant light and color. Say aloud to yourself that you are succeeding. Say it often.

4. Review the positive and truthful components of your self-talk as well as your perceptions about diet and foods. Whenever a negative or self-deceptive thought, misconception, or fear comes to your mind concerning your body or your diet deliberately and immediately counter it with a truthful assertion.

5. Constantly remind yourself that nothing can defeat you, that you will faithfully work toward your goals; that you trust yourself; that you possess the self-discipline, determination, and desire that are required to reach your goals; and that you do not deceive yourself that short-cuts can take the place of commitment and work. There are no short cuts to excellence.

6. Think positively. As Abraham Lincoln dryly observed: "Most people are about as happy as they want to be." Theologian Norman Vincent Peale says, "Positive thoughts create around you an atmosphere propitious to the development of positive outcomes. When you think in positive terms, you achieve positive results. An inflow of new right health-laden thoughts through the mind creatively affects the circumstances of life, for truth always produces right procedures and right results." So while getting ready to start your day, follow Dr. Peale's advice and see to it that you have a stimulating "inflow of health laden thoughts" coursing through your mind.

   Examples:

   " I know this will be a great day."
   " I know that I can successfully follow my diet, and I can solve any problem that may arise today."
   " I feel good physically, emotionally, and mentally."
   " It is wonderful to be alive."
   " I know I will succeed in my program."
   " I am interesting (or fun, or exciting, or intelligent, or all of these)."

7. Always anticipate and expect the best, and you will in all probability create the conditions that produce exactly those results. If you anticipate the worst, you may well get the worst. Even when you encounter tough challenges, think of them as creative opportunities.

8. Slow down and learn to relax. Develop a pace that is truly comfortable for you. Take a "breather" every once in a while. For instance there is no greater way to energize your thoughts than to take a walk in the countryside, through a nearby park, or perhaps just down a street in the city that you really love.

9. If you have a dieting setback don't emotionally beat yourself up about it. No one has ever mastered any skill except through intensive, persistent, and intelligent practice, so if you don't get it right the first time, correct your course and do it again.

10. Go out of your way to talk optimistically about everything. Just expressing optimistic thoughts aloud will reinforce attitudes that help to ensure success.

11. Do something nice for other people every day. Go to sleep each night knowing that you made at least one other person a little wiser, a little happier, or a little better. From a Right Bite perspective, I cannot emphasize this point enough. Give a compliment to someone who has never before been kind to you. If you have time, or can make time, volunteer at a hospital or retirement home where a helpful cheerful face can sometimes do more than medications. If you are a married woman, tell your husband how much you appreciate the hard work he does; if you are a husband tell your wife she's the most wonderful thing that ever happened to you. When you have a pleasant thought about someone, tell that person. Don't just keep it to your self. You will be astonished to see what happens. Not only will you become happier yourself but the other person will also expand, softening and becoming warmer. It is tremendously rewarding to make others feel they are appreciated and worthwhile. As Ralph Waldo Emerson said, "You cannot do a kindness too soon because you never know how soon it will be too late."

12. Several times a day go over your own personalized list of mind exercises. Write them down and keep them within arm's reach so you can review them before you go to sleep. Some exercises will be difficult to perform because your mind doesn't yet truly believe them. One woman confided to me that after years of always feeling

like "the bad seed" in her family, the hardest Right Bite exercise for her was to tell herself, "I am a wonderful and intelligent person."

As you become increasingly proficient with the program, you may wish to expand your repertoire of mind exercises. Some mind exercises you may never wish to abandon. As good dieting insurance you may want to continue them for years, simply because we live in a media-driven society that constantly inundates us with unsound, misguided, often unhealthy weight-control information. Keep in mind that with new advances in science and technology, certain mind exercises may need to be modified. What today is a concept held to be true, tomorrow might require alteration because of new scientific information. Keep your mind open. Remember, intelligent people once thought the world was flat.

Let these mind exercises become a part of your everyday life. They will not only help you with your weight program, they can get you through your darkest moments, for they have universal applications.

However, be judicious and discriminating even in these exercises. Don't wash away your interesting quirks and eccentricities. Both my father and husband have always maintained that they find neurotics infinitely more interesting than the run-of-the mill mortals. Lucky for me! After several years of marriage, I once asked my husband if my many passions, intense emotional responses, and other endearing quirks (well I think they are endearing) bothered him. His reply was, "I never wanted to marry a Donna Reed." So, when you are cleaning out your brain with mind exercises, get rid of the trash but keep the spice.

The success of the Right Bite Program depends on sustained, consistent, self-disciplined, and intelligent effort applied over an extended period of time. Of course any person can be loosely committed to excellence once in awhile, perhaps for minutes or days—but those who can maintain this dedication over a lifetime will ultimately enjoy success beyond even their own expectations. Henry Doherty, an American industrialist, in discussing the qualities he looked for in his management team, said, "Plenty of men can do good work for a spurt and with an immediate promotion in mind, but for promotion, you want a man in whom good work has become a habit."

The Magic of Mental Calisthenics

The magic of mind exercises is that they will begin to transform your weaknesses into strengths, and strengths you already have into invaluable assets that will ensure your success with the Right Bite Program. You will develop or strengthen the following:

FAITH

When you have faith in yourself and in a presence greater than yourself, you will find that your path to success goes much easier, even when you are confronted by obstacles that once would have stopped you in your tracks. Those who allow this greater force to be their partners find that this partnership helps them make quantum leaps toward attaining their dreams, reaching their goals, and perfecting their talents. If you truly want to achieve your weight-control goals—as well as any other goals in your life, give faith a central place in your life.

CHARACTER

Faith combined with your mental calisthenics will develop your character. Where character is concerned, I cannot do better than to offer the words of Abigail Adams in The Book of Abigail and John, which she wrote in a letter to her son, President John Quincy Adams, in 1780. She said:

> *It is not in the still calm of life, or the repose of a pacific station, that great characters are formed. . . . The habits of a vigorous mind are formed in contending with difficulties. All history will convince you of this, and that wisdom and penetration are the fruit of experience, not the lessons of retirement and leisure. Great necessities call out great virtues.*
>
> (From *Letters of Mrs. Adams*, 1848)

SELF-AWARENESS

A solid faith and illusion-destroying mental exercises will help you stand back and look at yourself with meticulous accuracy. It is sometimes painfully difficult to face sobering truths about ourselves, but in the long run, doing so can be an exhilarating and beneficial experience. Your body, for instance, will no longer be an enigma to you. You will be able to recognize your weight-gain triggers, making it possible for you to develop strategies to control or eliminate them.

Developing self-awareness will allow your rational brain to override the unhealthy impulses of your primitive brain. Self-awareness will enable you to apply the weight-control solutions found in the Right Bite. Awareness allows you to anticipate dieting trouble spots so that you can plan creatively. Awareness will help you discover what you cannot do, which is just as important as knowing what you can do. According to Havelock Ellis, a British writer, in *The Dance of Life*, "Men who know themselves are no longer fools; they stand on the threshold of the Door of Wisdom."

PERSEVERANCE, PERSISTENCE, AND COMMITMENT

The world is filled with people who are brilliant, talented, and supereducated, but who are dismal failures. Look around you. Haven't you ever commented about someone, "He had so much potential, yet look how he has wasted his life!"

Success is not guaranteed just because you managed to make straight A's in high school or got a higher degree. Winning is not a matter of luck and everything always going your way. Perseverance coupled with faith and logic-producing mental exercises are major ingredients in determining success no matter what obstacles you encounter. I am convinced that people who struggle up the ladder toward their goals despite countless obstacle, are the ones who will ultimately succeed. They are the ones who, when they reach one goal, reach higher for the next. These people see adversity and difficulties as challenges to meet—tests in life that sharpen their skills and improve their mastery.

Your faith and mental exercises will help you find the inner strength to remain committed to your goals—to persevere. Those who excel have done so through persistent commitment. As Thomas F. Buxton, an English philosopher affirms in *The Remedy*, "With ordinary talent and extraordinary perseverance, *all* things are attainable."

SELF-DISCIPLINE

Discipline, according to *The American Heritage Dictionary* is "training expected to produce a specific character or pattern of behavior, especially training that produces moral or mental improvement." An old Chinese proverb says, "He who conquers others is strong; he who conquers himself is mighty." Through discipline you will develop the important self-control that will become a part of you . . . you will rule the empire of your self and succeed in controlling and eliminating your triggers. You will follow your own direction and purpose.

Discipline *can* be developed or strengthened by repeating a desired behavioral pattern over and over. When you act as your own drill sergeant, you can instill permanent qualities that will ensure your success, not only in your weight control program but also in any of your life endeavors.

In the context of dieting, willpower and discipline are two distinctly different things. To stay on a poor nutritionless diet requires willpower. To follow a good diet requires discipline. Diet discipline is insisting that you do what is right for yourself even if you are tired or you find it inconvenient, difficult, or scary. The disciplined person can postpone an immediate gratification in order to obtain the greater reward of controlled eating and controlled weight. The undisciplined person grabs a bag of greasy chips and gobbles them down without worrying about the future consequences of hasty actions . . . until it is too late. A disciplined person plans ahead rather than leaving future events to chance.

Discipline is developed to some degree in all of us—some more than others—from the time we are small. We are developing discipline when we are able to brush our teeth daily without being dragged to the bathroom by the ear, or when we can put homework or violin practice ahead of a computer game; or save our allowance for a book rather than immediately spending the money on a yo-yo. For many of us, our parents instilled some basic discipline by telling us zillions of times how to do, or how not to do something before we could voluntarily do it ourselves.

If you are "self-aware" that you lack discipline, you can develop the dieting behavior you want by repeating the desired behavior—practicing—until that behavior becomes a habit. Be persistent. Keep going even when the initial excitement wears off. Don't ever take your eyes off your weight goal.

With discipline, you become your own boss—master of yourself. You will have the power within you to make decisions and take personal initiative. You will know what has to be done, when it should be done, and how well it can be done. As you develop discipline, you will feel its potent force throughout your body and mind. Then you can say, as Pietro Aretino did in 1537 in a letter to Agostino Ricchi, May 10, 1537, "I am, indeed, a king, because I know how to rule myself."

STRENGTH AND COURAGE

The unique significance of the Right Bite three-part program is that by following its format your metabolism will be changed from that of a fat person to that of a thin person. If this transformation is to be permanent, you must be patient while your new body is evolving. Effecting major changes in bodily processes cannot be rushed. The Right Bite's revolutionary weight-control plan is not always an easy one. Obstacles may be thrown in your path as you strive for your weight-control goals, but with determined commitment backed with a sustaining faith that you can climb over them you will be successful.

Obstacles can take the shape of well-meaning friends and opinionated family members who do not recognize your serious intent and knowingly or unknowingly encourage you to tamper with your weight-control triggers. Obstacles may manifest themselves as temptations when you are eating at restaurants or traveling. When you hit a weight-loss plateau and your scale weight doesn't budge, or when you observe frustrating minor weight fluctuations that cause you to despair of ever reaching your goal, it will take every ounce of patience and courage to soldier on. Keep in mind that your formally abused body is gradually and carefully adjusting itself to its new metabolism.

It takes courage—dare I say "guts"—to do what is right for yourself. Courage resists fear. Courage will prevent you from impulsively replacing the challenge with a fad diet or another single-strategy diet that promises faster, more spectacular results. The successful dieter courageously faces problems and solves them. Adversity is strengthening and will bring out the fight in you. When temptations arise, you will not be afraid to say "no." You will not be timid about making special dietary arrangements. The blossoming courage guarantees you will never succumb to peer pressure or to any pressure that threatens to keep you from reaching your weight-control goals. Winston Churchill believed that "courage is the first of human qualities because it is the quality which guarantees all others."

Mental calisthenics will ensure your success on the Right Bite Program, a program scientifically proven to work because it eliminates and controls the appetite/weight-triggering agents that have sabotaged your past dieting attempts. The Right Bite Program has given you the key that will ultimately empower you to win your weight-control battles. Insert it in the lock and open the door to your future happiness.

Looking Ahead

In the next chapter, I will discuss tips and strategies for fine-tuning the Right Bite program and for ironing out trouble spots. You will learn how to eat out or travel without adding pounds or detonating your weight gain triggers.

As Jean-Baptiste Rousseau said in *Émile* (1762), "Nature never deceives us; it is we who deceive ourselves."

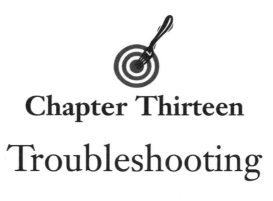

Chapter Thirteen

Troubleshooting

A smooth sea never made a skillful mariner.
—Hubert H. Humphrey

While I have made every effort to anticipate everything you will need for being successful with the Right Bite Program, I know there are questions and challenges that may come up along the way. For this reason, I've included the following list of challenges, questions and answers from my clinical consultations. By the end of this chapter, you will be able to anticipate and cope with a wide variety of issues ranging from how to order the Right Bite way when you dine in restaurants to why I recommend using flax seed oil.

Question: How do I stay on the Core Diet when I eat out at restaurants?
Answer: It is a fact that many restaurants prepare foods that are high in fat, calories, and salt. However, you will usually be able to find foods on the menu, or ask for special preparation to avoid these foods. Eating out is a skill you can polish and refine quickly. Many people feel so self-conscious when ordering the correct foods to maintain their diets that they decide it is less traumatic to break the rules "just this once" than to order carefully or make special demands on the cooks. What you need to realize is the whole world is not watching you make your food selections. It is highly unlikely that your waitress will stand at your elbow

smirking and guffawing behind her hand, or that the entire restaurant clientele will sidle to your table and peer over your shoulder at your menu choices. Relax! The worst they can accuse you of is caring for your own body and your own nutritional needs and choosing to eat a healthy and nutritious meal. I have found that most people these days express their admiration for those who make such choices. All you will need is the courage and confidence to apply the principles you have learned in the Right Bite Program, a little creativity, and determination to follow through.

During the first three months of the Core Diet, you should avoid almost all fast food restaurants, so if you are a fast food junkie, eating out will be a little more difficult for you. Fortunately, there are a few fast food restaurants that serve baked potatoes, or have salad bars with fresh vegetables, and grilled chicken sandwiches. In these eateries, choose the grilled chicken and discard the customary white bread served with it.

It is easy to eat at most full-service restaurants. Most offer standard entrees of grilled chicken or fish, baked potatoes, and salads and vegetables for a side dish. Here are some tips:

1. If you know the restaurant where you plan to go but you have never actually eaten there before, call ahead and ask what's on their menu. If the restaurant serves absolutely nothing you can eat (this would be exceedingly rare) then speak with the manager and find out if it would be a problem to have a meal prepared to your specifications. Even fast food restaurants are catering to the health conscious patron these days and will usually do their best to accommodate you.

2. If there are items on the menu that you would be able to enjoy with some minor changes, don't hesitate to tell the waitress how you want the meal prepared. If you don't want your food breaded, fried, or with sauces on it, say so. Also, don't be afraid to send your order back if it is not entirely satisfactory. One of my favorite restaurants serves a grilled fish with a very rich cream sauce. I simply request that the fish be grilled or poached without the sauce. Restaurants truly want your patronage and are very eager to please.

3. Order potatoes plain. No butter. No gravy. No sour cream. Bring along your calorieless butter-flavored spray, and use that if you like.

4. Order salads plain with oil and vinegar dressing on the side, or bring your own dressing in a small, inconspicuous bottle.

5. For a beverage, decaf coffee, decaf tea, herb tea, or water with a slice of lime or lemon is fine. I always carry a few decaffeinated tea bags or herb teas with me. All restaurants will provide hot water for tea.

6. After twelve weeks, when you are able to expand your menu, do so according to the guidelines of the Right Bite Program. Some restaurant selections you might consider are plain pasta with marinara sauce. Some restaurants are even carrying whole wheat pastas and steamed brown rice. Some popular franchised sandwich shops serve veggie sub sandwiches on whole wheat bread with no mayo or butter. If you enjoy eating Chinese food you will find a wide selection of seafood, chicken, and vegetable dishes. Ask that your meal be cooked without MSG or extra salt, and that it be served with steamed rice. The little bit of starch used to thicken Oriental sauces is acceptable.

7. If you can stand the excitement of a salad bar, you will probably find a wide variety of fresh vegetables to choose from and even some types of legumes. Plain, unmarinated chick peas or garbanzo beans are standard fare at most salad bars. Of course avoid all the dishes with mayonnaise or sauces

8. Always have at least two snacks with you if you will not be going home after dining out.

9. If you know you will be dining out, anticipate that your meal may be served much later than your usual dinner hour and eat a snack before leaving. Also always carry a snack with you. This extra snack has kept my diet on track more times than I can tell you.

Last year I went to my husband's twentieth high school reunion. Dinner was to be served at 8:00 p.m., which is two hours later than I am accustomed to eating. I ate a snack prior to going, but for some reason dinner was delayed until 10:00. Rather than diving headlong into the fattening appetizers I gobbled down my extra snack and remained in control throughout the evening. Had I not had a snack available when I became hungry, my cheeks would not only have been stuffed with pepperoni pinwheels but I probably also would have overeaten when the meal was finally served.

Question: How do I handle eating at the homes of friends or relatives?

Answer: The best way to handle eating at the home of friends or relatives is to let them know you are following a nutritious, health-promoting program that you would like to maintain. Let them know that this program is very important to you, especially because it will change one's metabolism from that of a fat person to that of a thin person.

Secondly, *always* check to see if the foods you will be needing for your program will be available to you. I have found that friends and family who learn about an individual's diet have positive reactions. Nearly always they are keenly interested, sometimes to the point of deciding to embark on the same program, but all are usually warmly supportive. Generally, you can expect friends and family members to be "on your side." It has been my experience that they will always prepare meals that are diet-acceptable. At the very least they will provide ingredients and foods you can eat, even if most of their guests look forward to grilled bratwurst on white buns with a scoop of white macaroni salad swimming in mayonnaise.

For the few friends and family members who honestly seem to forget your dieting needs, or who do not realize that you are serious about controlling your weight—after all, they do have their own lives—you will need to make a call before dining with them to find out what is being served. More thoughtful people, knowing you are following a special program, will automatically know to set aside, for example, a grilled chicken breast if they are serving fried chicken, or to leave butter or special sauces off your portion of a vegetable dish. Be happy when this happens but don't count on it.

Several years ago, my grandfather died unexpectedly in the middle of the winter, and the entire family—children, grandchildren, and great grandchildren—flew in to attend his funeral. After frightful snowstorm delays, I went directly from the airport to his home, where all the relatives were congregating for a prefuneral reunion and meal. I, of course, had my food neatly packed in my purse, never knowing what I'd be facing should my flight be snowbound. Also, there was no way for me to ascertain ahead of time who was in charge of the reunion menu. Therefore I was deeply touched when as soon as I walked through the door of my grandfather's home, one of my aunts put her arms around me in welcome and then led me to the table where a buffet had been spread. She mentioned that she was aware of how I ate so she had seen to it that the cooks prepared almost everything "á la Stephanie." I felt enormous appreciation for her thoughtfulness at a time when our hearts and minds were focused on the loss my grandfather. After a grueling day of travel, I was also grateful to have a hot meal rather than the nearly frozen contents of my snack food parcel.

The worst mistake you can make is not calling ahead and planning. I myself learned the hard way. Several years ago, my husband and I were invited to a large formal dinner given by a Chinese couple with whom we occasionally dined. I knew Ling was aware that I practice what I preach, so I assumed that the meal would have numerous items I could eat. I took for granted that Ling would have her usual assortment of steamed rice, fresh seafood or chicken, and wonderfully cooked vegetables as in days past. I did not call ahead, nor did I anticipate that she was going to prepare what she described as "a very special American-style dinner."

You can imagine my shock and dismay when the salads arrived. They looked like bowls of mayonnaise with a couple decorative green leaves on top. I poked around my bowl of mayonnaise, pretending to eat. Finally, the entrée arrived—a large fatty ham. No one dislikes ham more than I do, except maybe my husband. We exchanged glances and tried to hide our grimaces. Next came a molded gelatin salad that looked like a milky, lavender-colored breast, followed by a bowl of transparent rice noodles that resembled shredded Saran wrap. My husband's lips froze into a polite smile while he cut his ham slice into smaller and smaller pieces and attempted to conceal them under his jello salad. It was a disastrous social situation, but perhaps all was not lost. In the past Ling had always served steamed rice. Although it might be white, not my preferred nutritious brown, it would help to sustain us until we could escape from this horrible predicament. Well, our agony was to be prolonged. Ling announced that the climax of her meal was a special rice dish that she had worked on all day with her sister. My husband and I breathed a mutual sigh of relief. At last our gnawing hunger would be gracefully appeased. Ling proudly produced a large platter loaded with wee steamed rice cakes, shaped into teeny circles each surrounded by a wettish green rim which the guests later learned was seaweed, not mold. There was some sort of intricate symbolic design in the center of each cake. The material on the platter emitted the nauseating smell of spoiled fish, and already light-headed I wondered if my face had turned as green as my spouse's. Somehow we found a way to excuse ourselves early. We recovered our appetites in the fresh air and ended the evening at our favorite restaurant where we ravenously devoured pasta. Since that day, I have never forgotten to call my hostess to see what foods are to be served.

If you are sure that there is nothing your family will be serving that your diet allows, or that you desire to eat, feed yourself beforehand or bring your own food. If there are a few prepared dishes you can eat, then supplement them with a light Core-approved snack. Also call ahead and volunteer to bring a tasty dish to pass, one that will complement the foods already on the menu. For example, I frequently bring a green salad or a fruit salad to share when I am invited out. A hostess usually welcomes additional attractive foods on the table.

Get accustomed to friends and family members asking about your program. Not only are they curious but some may want to improve their own health and appearance by solving specific weight problems. Their questions are not intended to make you uncomfortable. You will find that your health goals will attract the interest of others who agree that it is wise to keep in shape. I should know. My own husband, who is very athletic and health conscious, chose to share his life with someone similarly oriented—me!

Also, it is comforting to remember that as you progress on the Right Bite Program and are isolating your triggers and changing your metabolism, your diet will become much more flexible. You will be able to enjoy a wider variety of food at outings by following the guidelines in the program. When this moment arrives, if you really, really enjoy that mayonnaise-drenched white macaroni salad and grease-dripping bratwurst, I see no reason why, once in a while, you cannot indulge yourself. However, I predict that when it comes time for you to spear a bratwurst off the grill, you will no longer crave it as you once did. Healthy eating fosters healthy eating, and even when people on the Right Bite Program know they can have an occasional splurge, most choose to stick pretty close to the Right Bite foods.

Question: How can I travel and maintain my diet?

Answer: For the first three months when you are just learning the Right Bite program, I would certainly not embark on a three-week African safari or a hike up Mt. Everest. Once you leave familiar surroundings, you are at the mercy of whatever eating habits are customary in the country you are visiting.

In general, traveling to familiar areas, by car, train, or airplane is easy and just takes a little planning ahead.

1. Pack at least half of your large carry on bag with food. Because of the unpredictability of food offered in transit, and because of unexpected delays, your carry-on food could be critically important for maintaining your program.

2. Pack extra food for those traveling with you. It never fails that as soon as my family members see me take out my whole wheat bread sandwich, they all want a bite or expect me to magically produce sandwiches for them. In fact,

even before my food is visible, my children in particular are clamoring for food or drink. Traveling is stressful even when it's fun, and eating is one of the ways that people deal with that stress.

3. If the transportation of your choice serves healthy, delicious food, you may wish to reserve your carry-on snacks for later. I have been pleasantly surprised of late to note the improvement in food quality on some airlines. If the food is acceptable, then you will only need to use your reserve when necessary or to supplement your meal.

4. Call ahead. Many times during a travel itinerary dietary requests will be honored. For example, it is a little-known secret that most airlines will prepare vegetarian, no-salt, and even kosher meals if requested at the time you make your reservation. Both kosher and vegetarian, in most cases, will be close to Right Bite approved.

5. Carry plenty of edibles with you so that you still have food in your carrying bag when you arrive at your destination. If your travel schedule has been disrupted due to delays or missed connections, restaurants may be closed or inaccessible, and the only available food will be that which you have carried with you.

6. Traveling is fatiguing no matter how smoothly things go. Try to be well rested by going to bed early for two or three nights in a row just prior to your departure. If possible, lean back and close your eyes during your trip, and when you arrive at your destination try your best to schedule time for short naps. This is particularly important where you are crossing time zones. Disrupted sleep cycles and sleep deprivation are major sources of stress for travelers and therefore should be approached as weight-gain triggers.

Question: What do I do if I get hungry when I am out shopping or doing errands?
Answer: Always carry a snack with you.

Question: I work from eight to five every day and don't get home until six. Can you give me some tips on getting through a day like this?
Answer:
1. Eat a good healthy breakfast *á la Stephanie* before going to work. This will keep your blood sugar levels stable for the rest of the day and prevent temptations when one of your

colleagues passes around a box of sugared donuts or goose liver paté.

2. Pack at least two snacks: one for the customary work break with your friends, and the second one for your journey home. Many a person's best resolve has been ruined by arriving home ravenously hungry after a frustrating drive home in clogged freeway traffic. This second snack will tide you over as you prepare dinner.

3. If you opt to lunch at a restaurant, never assume that you will be able to order a meal that conforms to your program. Follow the suggestions I give on eating out at the beginning of this chapter.

4. If you choose to eat at work, pack your lunch the evening before and store it in one of those plastic containers made especially for people who travel around with their own meals. These handy containers have several pockets in which to put different foods. Also, you may just wish to carry several small plastic-lidded containers with your food. If your life is extremely hectic, prepare and freeze several meals on the weekend.

5. Remember that after three months, you will be expanding the Core Diet. Therefore every food-centered function, including eating out and traveling will become easier and easier as you isolate, understand, eliminate, or control your triggers.

Question: I've been on the Right Bite Diet for two weeks but have only lost two pounds. Am I doing something wrong?

Answer: Keep in mind that the Right Bite Program is not just about losing weight but also about the following: (1) It is designed to slowly change your metabolism from a fat person's to a thin person's; (2) it is intended to repair the damage from past unsuccessful dieting attempts; (3) it offers a food plan you will cheerfully want to follow for the rest of you life; (4) it does not make false or misleading promises about weight loss. I would love to tell you that you will lose ten pounds a week, every week for three months or more, and be wearing a string bikini by summer. But any program that promises this is bound to convert even a moderately fat person's metabolism into an enormous person's metabolism. I am not here to promote empty promises. That's not what my life's work is about. This program is dedicated to building healthy lifestyles so you can attain your ideal weight and maintain it comfortably forever.

That said, the most dramatic weight loss for most people takes place during the first seven days of being on the Right Bite Program. This is because some of the weight loss consists of water. It is not uncommon to lose five to twelve pounds that first week if you are severely overweight or have been overeating for several days prior to starting the program. After this period of time weight loss is unpredictable for many reasons: your fitness level, your age, your current weight, your percentage of lean body mass, your gender and the extent to which your metabolism has been damaged by previous dieting.

In *general*, after the first week, you can expect to lose from a quarter of a pound to two pounds per week, and this will vary. Some weeks you may hold with no loss, then the following week suddenly drop four to five pounds. Some weeks you may gain just to lose double the next week. If you could graph weight loss, it would look like a seismograph with its zig zagging line—up and down—but with a general trend downward. Don't look for a straight line down, because as your body repairs damage from past diets your metabolism will go through many changes. Be optimistic.

Above all, keep in mind that you will consistently be losing fat weight while replacing it with lean body mass, even if your scale does not always register a change. Remember, I weighed exactly the same for a whole year after I started an exercise program. At the end of the year I was much more slender but weighed the same. Why? Because my body's composition was completely transformed. I had lost seven pounds of fat and gained seven pounds of muscle tissue.

Your body needs time to heal and change its metabolism, build fat-burning enzymes, and shrink mammoth body systems that formerly supported your larger size. Your body also has to be convinced that you are no longer going to do something radical, such as fasting, skipping meals, binging, or taking diet pills. Losing weight slowly gives you time to make permanent changes in your eating behavior.

I have had a few clients who had slow starts their first week, but as their bodies adjusted to the Right Bite Program's delicious, health-promoting foods, their metabolisms speeded up and their weight dropped more quickly. The longer they were on the program, the more significant was their weight loss. Some people seem to lose the same amount of weight per week, and still others lose variable numbers of pounds each week. One thing is for certain, you will lose pounds and ounces until you arrive at your slimmest healthy weight.

If you have only a small amount of weight to lose, you may never see a change in your scale weight. Don't panic. What you will see is a dramatic difference in your body tone, size and your total appearance. The year I initiated the exercise I was not overweight to begin with but I went down one pant size while my scale weight remained the same. If you are slender, you may even gain scale weight when fat is exercised away and you gain a more toned and compact lean body. It is certain however, that you will not look fat.

Also, do not compare your weight loss to others: men typically lose weight faster because they generally have more lean body mass and weigh more to begin with. Many wives become frustrated when their husbands, on the same program, lose weight twice as fast as they do.

Don't forget that if you have been following an extremely radical diet prior to embarking on the Core Diet, such as ones that advocate very few calories, fasting, or high protein, or if you have abused diet pills, laxatives, or diuretics, you will most likely have an initial rebound water-weight gain. You will want to review the section on side effects in Chapter 8 if you fall into this category. Don't let this temporary water-weight gain frighten you. The side effects generally last only seven to ten days.

Researchers at Case Western University examined differences between groups of successful and unsuccessful dieters and compared both groups with those of a third group consisting of people who had always been thin. They found that successful dieters lost weight much more *slowly* than unsuccessful ones, and they adopted eating patterns they could live with permanently, even after they had reached their desired weight. Also, the successful group curtailed sweets.

Question: I am 5'4" and want to be a size three. What can I do to achieve my goal? Am I being realistic?

Answer: The Core Diet will reduce you to your slimmest healthy weight, and if you are destined to be a size three, you will be. If your bone structure and lean body mass are naturally stocky and thick (your genetic birthright), all the dieting in the world will not put you into a size three. At the start of the program, if you are large busted and over-weight, when you reduce, you will still be proportionally chesty but now you will be slim. I had an overweight client who was 5'3". After losing fifty pounds she had diminished to a size three for shirts and a seven to nine for her pant size. We humans come in a wide range of sizes and shapes. Regardless of how much you reduce and exercise you will still exhibit your own physical variations. Can you imagine if animals were as nutty as people? We would have giraffes trying to diet away their long necks, elephants starving to look like Chihuahuas, and bulldogs with robust muscular legs coveting the long slender legs of greyhounds. Be content to be your slimmest healthy weight and accept your physical variation. I guarantee that you will not be fat at this weight. You will be lean and well toned and you will feel so much better physically and emotionally that conforming to somebody else's ideas of body size will be the furthest thing from your mind.

Question: I have always gone off diets because I get too hungry. How can I stay on this diet if I become hungry?

Answer: If you have read your Core Diet instructions carefully, you will recall that a major rule is to *eat when hungry; stop when full!* Now, tell me, if you can always eat when hungry, how can you go off your diet? This rule is important because it gives your body a flexible caloric range within which to function as well as to accommodate periods of increased energy expenditure, stress, preperiod needs, and illness. This caloric range also provides a guilt-free leeway for you during such occasions as vacations and holidays or other times when it is desirable and normal to eat a bit more. In my opinion, it is better to eat more of Core Diet foods at this time than risk splurging on foods that will just add extra pounds. There is nothing wrong with maintaining your weight at the same level for a few days to get through a challenging situation. Your body does not always need to be in a negative caloric balance —that is, taking in fewer calories than your body needs.

Question: I've never been a person who eats breakfast. Is this really something that I have to learn how to do?

Answer: Yes. Breakfast is essential to help maintain stable blood sugar levels. It prevents the see-saw swings that cause feelings of hunger. It will also keep you feeling fortified the rest of the day. Breakfast will also speed up your metabolism. If you do not eat breakfast, your body may interpret this omission to mean you are in a "fasting mode," and it will set into motion your metabolic processes to conserve calories, resist the burning of fat, and to store anything eaten as fat.

Question: My children are all overweight, too. Is it OK to include them when my husband and I go on the Right Bite Program?

Answer: First of all, always check with your doctor before embarking on any diet and exercise program. In my clinical experience, children do very well on the program, but because they are rapidly growing they eat proportionately more than adults and can still lose weight or at least grow out of their overweight proportions without putting on additional pounds.

You can greatly aid your child's weight loss and fitness efforts by throwing out or seriously restricting their TV and electronic games. More than 60 percent of overweight children and adolescents spend excessive time watching television. The percentage of obese children has doubled in the last ten years. Also, adults who watch three or more hours of television a day double their risk of becoming obese.

Getting rid of soft drinks can greatly help your child. Soft drink consumption leads to excessive energy-related intake and inadequate intake of calcium and other nutrients.

Question: Why do I seem to like sweets more than my husband?

Answer: Studies have shown that there is a gender difference in our craving for and response to sweets. Unfortunately, women, whether dieting or not, crave and respond to sweets generally more than males do. Researchers believe this is due to our hormones.

Question: I love potato chips. Will I ever be able to eat them again?

Answer: Yes, but eat the fat-free chips on the market. Also, I would consider even "fat-free" chips a high-pleasure food, so follow the instructions for incorporating these foods appropriately. Researchers have found that substitution of fat-free chips for regular chips can help reduce fat and energy-related intakes for some individuals.

Question: My colleagues are always asking me to go out to eat but I am afraid that I will ruin my diet. Should I ever go?

Answer: Yes, follow the guidelines and tips for eating at restaurants, keeping the rules and instructions of the Core Diet firmly in mind, and you will have no trouble eating out. To build self-confidence, choose the restaurant where you want to go and would feel most comfortable. If you have done your homework carefully, you will already know what is on the menu and will know exactly what to order. There will be no surprises. Studies have shown that a person will actually consume less when dining with four coworkers than with four family members! And, of course, a person eating alone tends to consume less than she will eating with coworkers or family members.

Question: I work from eight to five and get home at six. Then I have to make dinner and take care of my family. I am too exhausted to get up in the early morning to exercise and too tired by the time everyone is in bed. What should I do?

Answer: Exercise over your lunch break and other breaks during the day. Studies have shown that overweight women who exercised for fifteen minute three times a day tallied at least an extra thirty-five minutes of exercise per week more than people exercising for twenty to thirty minute periods. In a study from the University of Nebraska, walkers who split their workouts into two fifteen minute strolls five days a week doubled their weekly mileage compared to those who walked thirty minutes three times a week. If you have an hour lunch break, it should not take you any more than fifteen minutes to eat a packed lunch. That leaves you forty-five minutes to walk briskly or find stairs to climb. If you have other breaks during the day, you will find walking more energizing and relaxing than slurping down some coffee and chatting with coworkers. Also, most people just beginning exercise programs find it is easier to stick to a schedule of short workouts than long ones.

Question: All my friends are on high-protein diets and say their weight loss is phenomenal. They are pressuring me to quit my Right Bite Program and start a high-protein diet. I am losing weight but not as fast as my friends. What should I do?

Answer: While you can have dramatic weight loss on high-protein diets they are not good prescriptions for long-term success. Eighty thousand Americans were surveyed in the *American Journal of Public Health* in 1982 and ten years after that. Guess what? The people who were most likely to gain weight were the high-protein meat eaters. Among your friends, you will be the one person who maintains your weight loss, so stick with the Core Diet Program.

Question: My friends tell me that if I eat a balanced diet I won't need supplements. Why do you recommend them on your program?

Answer: I recommend supplements for several reasons. First of all, to correct damaged metabolisms and help restore bodies formerly malnourished from past dieting programs or malnourished from careless "hit-or-miss" eating. Studies show that few if any persons ever eat a balanced diet on any one day. According to a recent study by the U.S. Department of Agriculture's Continuing Survey of Food Intakes by Individuals, just 1 percent of Americans meet minimum standards for dietary adequacy. Another sobering fact is that even if you eat the balanced diet prescribed by the USDA, you still will not be meeting all your nutritional requirements. It is absolutely impossible to fulfill your entire vitamin and mineral requirements on anything less than 2000 calories a day. Unless you are as active as an athlete and every day deliberately see to it you have a totally sufficient diet, you cannot be sure that your nutrient needs are being taken care of. For example, just to get 100 IUs of vitamin E you would have to eat eight cups of almonds or sixty-two cups of spinach. Women of childbearing years average only ten milligrams of iron a day when they need eighteen milligrams. To meet the RDA, you would have to eat at least 2500 nutrient-dense calories, which is 500–1200 calories more than the average woman consumes now.

Research also shows that those who take supplements are more health conscious, tend to eat more judiciously, and generally maintain better health. They also have stronger immune systems and lower risks for heart disease, cancer, osteoporosis, hypertension, memory loss, and giving birth to babies with birth defects.

By the time you consume a commercial food, many nutrients have been lost in handling, processing, shipping, and cooking. When you buy produce in a store, you have no idea how long it has been sitting on the shelves. I have been in grocery stores where the produce looked like it had been retrieved from the Titanic.

Always select a high-quality supplement with a broad range of vitamins and minerals. Make sure the supplement you choose includes vitamins A, D, K, E, and C; beta carotene; all the B vitamins (B1, B2, B6, biotin, pantothenic acid, niacin, and folic acid); and trace minerals such as selenium, manganese, copper, iron, chromium, and boron. Make sure that your supplement provides 100 percent of the Daily Value and is balanced. By that I mean don't get a vitamin that has 25 percent of the minimum daily requirement for one vitamin and 300 percent of another. Women will also need a calcium-magnesium supplement. A regular vitamin-mineral supplement will not provide all you need. Also, don't take your calcium supplement with your multiple-with-iron supplement since the two compete for absorption. Take them at least two hours apart, or take one with breakfast, the other with lunch or your evening meal.

The bottom line is that you can't get all the nutrients you need from supplements or food—you need them both. No one can follow a perfect diet all the time, and illness, stress, growth, and increased activity all cause our needs to vary daily.

Question: Do we really consume too many sugars?

Answer: Yes! People living in the modern world consume an average of 328 calories of refined carbohydrates a day from sugar, fructose, and sucrose. This adds up to a whopping 16 percent of the total energy-related intake, which is quickly converted to excess body fat.

Question: My daughter runs competitively at school, and she wants to go on the diet with me. Would this be wise?

Answer: She would do quite well on this diet. The best meal to eat before exercising is one that has a low glycemic index. In a research study two groups of subjects were given a low-glycemic meal and a high-glycemic meal respectively, with the same number of calories and carbohydrate grams. They were then told to cycle on a stationary bike until exhaustion. Time to exhaustion was 59 percent longer after subjects ate the meal with a low GI. The foods in the Basic Core program are perfect for pre-exercise meals.

Questions: I am really confused about what I should have as my goal. Is there such thing as a perfect body. If there is, what is it anyway?

Answer: Ideally, according to Victor Katch, Ph.D. and other physiologists and anatomists, a 5'5" woman with an average frame should weigh 125 pounds and have the following dimensions:

wrists	6.0"	neck	12.9"
forearms	9.5"	relaxed biceps	10.5"
flexed biceps	11.0"	shoulders	38.0"
chest	32.5"	waist	25.8"
abdomen	30.7"	buttocks (hips)	37.1"
thighs	22.0"	calves	13.4"
ankles	8.1"		

Her body composition should be:

fat, 30 lbs. (24%)—storage fat, 18.7 lbs., essential fat, 11.3 lbs.
muscle, 48.9 lbs. (39%)
bone, 15 lbs. (18.75%)
remainder, 31.2 lbs. (25%)
lean body weight, 95 pounds

The anatomist's perfect female has considerably more flesh on her bones than the models we see in womens magazines. The average measurements of a contemporary fashion model are 33-23-33. Projected measurements of a Barbie doll, in inches, if she were a full-sized human being are 36-18-33. The models you see today in magazines and on TV are 83 percent of their ideal body weight. We define anorexia as being 85 percent of your ideal body weight, so it is no wonder most women are confused. What does it mean to be 83 percent of your ideal body weight? If you are 115 pounds and wanted to be model thin at 83 percent of that, you would need to weigh 95 pounds. The question always remains how can we satisfy our yearnings to keep in step with the times—to conform to society's transitory concept of physical perfection—when nature has intended something else for us? My answer to this dilemma is that you should attain your slimmest healthy (fittest) weight using the Right Bite Program and you will become your *own* most perfect body.

Question: Which exercise burns the most calories?
Answer: Cross-country skiing. There are also machines that mimic cross-country skiing.

Question: A friend has been telling me about phytochemicals and why they are important in our diet. Does your diet include these?
Answer: Phytochemicals are non-nutritive substances in plants that possess health-protective effects. They consist of phenolic compounds, terpenoids, pigments, and other natural antioxidants. There are almost 2000 known plant pigments, including over 800 flavonoids, 450 carotenoids, and 150 anthocyanins. These pigments not only provide eye appeal, they protect us from disease. Grains, fruits, and vegetables contain an abundance of phenolic compounds, terpenoids, pigments, and other natural antioxidants that have been associated with protection from and/or treatment of chronic diseases such as heart disease, cancer, diabetes, and hypertension as well as other medical conditions. For example, in a single orange there are more than 170 phytochemicals. It is very important to eat foods as close to their natural state as possible because refining causes a loss of phytochemicals. Refining wheat, for example, causes a 300-fold loss in phytochemical content. I put together the Right Bite program with phytochemicals in mind. Whenever you shop, choose the least-refined and freshest foods you can find.

Question: I notice that you mention flax seed oil a lot in your menus and also list it as an oil of choice. Why is this such an important oil?
Answer: Flax seed oil can lower both blood cholesterol and LDL cholesterol levels. It is also one of the richest sources of n-3 fat, which provides flax with its anti-inflammatory effect and the ability to boost the immune system. Flax is also an extremely rich source of lignans, which are converted to mammalian lignans (enterolactone and entero-diol) by bacterial fermentation in the colon. These mammalian lignans appear to be anticarcinogenic. The lignan metabolites bear a structural similarity to estrogens and can bind to estrogen receptors and inhibit growth of estrogen-stimulated breast cancer.

Most of the questions you will have can be answered quickly by turning to the index and then looking for the general themes you are interested in. If you need further assistance, email me at: RIGHTBITE@aol.com.

Chapter Fourteen

Taking the Plan into Your Future

A windmill is eternally at work to accomplish one end,
although it shifts with every variation of the weathercock,
and assumes ten different positions in a day.
—Charles Caleb Colton, *Lacon (1825)*

There will come a time when you have reached your goal weight and have determined that it is your true set point weight. At that point you will be asking a slightly different kind of question: "How do I easily maintain this weight?" I suspect that by this time you will have a pretty good idea about how to answer this for yourself, having completed the Right Bite Program, with its Phase I: Basic Core, Standard-Pleasure Plan, and successfully expanded your diet with medium-pleasure foods, high-pleasure foods, and occasional deviation foods. You have discovered the weight-gain triggers that are your nemeses, and you know how to control and/or eliminate them. You've learned what to do to get back on track in the event of a trigger sneak attack. You exercise regularly and have developed an optimistic "can do it" mental attitude. The answer to how you might maintain your set point weight really is the sum total of what you *already* know from your Right Bite experience and insights.

Rules for Maintaining Your Slimmest Healthy Weight

1. Follow the Right Bite Program and all the guidelines that are relevant to you for avoiding and maintaining control of your personal weight-gain triggers.

2. Select most of your foods from standard-pleasure and medium-pleasure foods categories. Only a fraction of your menu should include high-pleasure foods or deviation foods. When you add medium- or high-pleasure or deviation foods, follow the instructions for their safe inclusion.

3. Weigh yourself once a week, at the same time of day, under the same conditions.

4. If your weight climbs a bit, then eliminate deviation and high-pleasure foods until you reduce to your set point weight. I have observed that it is deviation and high-pleasure foods that cause an increase in weight, not basic or medium-pleasure Core foods. So, as logic would have it, if you gain weight, it is usually only deviation and high-pleasure foods that you will need to reduce and learn to manage better.

5. If you have a slip, don't panic; return immediately to the Right Bite Program's Basic Core eating plan, and the weight will melt right off.

6. If you drop below your slimmest healthy weight, eat more Core diet foods. Don't use deviation foods to increase your weight.

As you continue to experience success with the Right Bite Program, you'll start to notice changes not only in your weight but also in your general health. You'll find that you have more energy, more stamina, more overall strength, and a brighter outlook on your life. The psychological benefits are so broad that I hesitate to even begin listing them, but certainly greater self-esteem and confidence are high on the list.

The Right Bite Program is a program for life. By now you will have begun to understand why this is so and why it is infinitely more effective than quick-fix, fad diets you may have tried in the past. The tools it provides you allows you to ultimately make food judgments on your own, and monitor your eating as well as your exercise and behavioral habits so that you need never have to struggle with weight again.

Sharing this program with others has been one of the greatest delights of my life. What has motivated me throughout the writing of this book is the thought that this plan might touch thousands more people than I will ever be able to reach counseling one private client or even giving one workshop at a time.

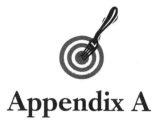

Appendix A

Core Calculations— What to Do If You Can't Be Sure When You Are Full

Unless you are among the 1 percent of readers who have lost their ability to tell when they are full and when they are hungry, this appendix will be of no interest to you. If you are among that 1 percent, or if you do not feel confident about trusting your feelings of fullness and hunger, the following material will help you feel much more secure about what, when, and how much to eat.

In the beginning, you will be making food choices in your diet according to a simple set of calculations, ultimately moving toward learning how to better trust your bodily feelings to moderate your caloric intake. I have found that it is important to have this system of checks and balances to avoid either overeating or undereating in a manner that would act as a trigger. This section provides complete instructions for following the Right Bite Program using calculations to precisely fine-tune your diet.

This section is also beneficial for those who would like to add high-pleasure or deviation foods to a meal and not exceed their caloric range. By knowing how to estimate your caloric needs, you will be able to make food selections wisely and not overeat.

Phase I: Calculated Core

Here you will achieve the same goals as I discussed in Chapter 8, not just by monitoring your feelings of fullness but also by paying attention to your caloric intake. This is accomplished by (1) familiarizing yourself with the caloric values of foods in that chapter, and then (2) calculating your caloric intake according to the simple calculations that follow.

BASAL METABOLIC RATE

We start with a calculation of how many calories you burn when you are totally at rest. While you'd have to be vegetating to burn that few calories, the estimations you'll get with this formula are useful for determining how many calories you should be taking in to either lose weight or maintain your present weight. The formula looks like this:

For women: BMR = 655 + 9.6(W) + 1.8(H) - 4.7(A)

For men: BMR = 66 +13.7(W) + 5(H) - 6.8(A)

Here's what the letters in brackets mean:

BMR = Basal metabolic rate

W = current weight in kilograms

H = height in centimeters

A = Age

The first thing you probably noted about the formula is that weight is in kilograms and height is in centimeters. Unless you are familiar with metric measurements you'll probably want to convert the numbers to pounds and feet. So here's how to do that:

To obtain weight in kilograms: weight in pounds divided by 2.2

To obtain height in centimeters: height in inches times 2.54

Let's take an example.

Mary is 48 years old. She weighs 125 pounds. Divide that by 2.2 and you get 57 kilograms. (125 ÷ 2.2 = 57)

Mary's height is 5' 4" which is 64 inches. Multiply the 64 inches by 2.54 and you get 163 centimeters. (64 x 2.54 = 163)

Now insert these numbers in the Harris-Benedict formula, like this:

655 + (9.6 x 57) + (1.8 x 163) - (4.7 x 48) = BMR

655 + 547 + 293 -226 = 1269

So that's it! The energy you need to take in to maintain your body in its at-rest (no activity) state can be provided with a total intake of 1269 calories.

MAXIMUM CALORIC LEVEL (MxCL)

Now that you have your basal metabolic rate, that is, the calories you'd need if you were just vegetating, you'll want to figure out how many calories you'll need in reality. After all, it's virtually impossible to stay in a vegetative state unless, of course, you are in a coma. Any activity beyond this is going to burn some calories. You'll want to know the total number of calories you will ideally eat to maintain your present weight in a way that won't trigger a weight gain. I call this the maximum caloric level, or MxCL for short. Here's how to calculate your MxCL:

First, determine your level of activity. This will be somewhat subjective, but that's okay. Think in terms of light activity as being most sitting and standing activities, typing, sewing, playing cards, or driving your car under relaxing conditions. Exceptional activity would be an athlete training for world-class competition. Most of us are in the very light to moderate activity range.

Women: very light activity (1.3), light (1.5), moderate (1.6), heavy (1.9) exceptional (2.2).

Men: very light activity (1.3), light (1.6), moderate (1.7), heavy (2.1) exceptional (2.4).

Using the above factors, we determine that Mary is very sedentary. So we would use the activity factor of 1.3:

Maximum caloric level = 1.3 x 1269 = 1649 calories

That final number is Mary's current maximum caloric level. But keep in mind that this may vary, for example, spring comes and she adds gardening to her daily schedule. She finds that she now goes up to the moderate activity level, that is 1.6, sending her possible MxCL up to 2030.

But there's another factor to consider, too. If your metabolism has been affected by past dieting, it may be very sluggish. Until you've been on the Right Bite Core Diet for three months or so, to give your body a chance to repair and heal, you may want to reduce your activity factor by .2.

As she started out on the Right Bite Program, Mary decided that her activity level was light and she had a sluggish metabolism. So to calculate her MxCL she first reduced her activity factor (1.3) by .2, which gave her 1.1. Thus, her MxCL would be: 1.1 x 1269 = 1396 calories. That's the maximum number of calories she should eat if she is going to maintain her present weight.

But what if Mary wants to lose some weight? She'd need to do another calculation, for her weight-loss caloric level, or WLCL.

WEIGHT-LOSS CALORIC LEVEL (WLCL)

To lose weight, Mary will need to take in fewer calories than she'll need to maintain her basic energy needs. To do this, she'd take the number she got above (her MCL) and edge her calorie intake downward, in small increments, every four days. The calorie level at which she began to lose weight would be her weight-loss caloric level. This is the healthiest caloric level to eat in order to lose weight. It represents a moderate decrease in calories so that her body will not respond as though she were going into starvation mode. Don't forget, that starvation mode can set off powerful appetite and weight-gain triggers. So that you do not inadvertently undereat and go into starvation mode, you will want to know your minimum caloric level (MCL), which you can find as follows.

MINIMUM CALORIC LEVEL

To determine your minimum caloric level edge your calories down from your Weight-Loss Caloric Level until you experience your first undesirable symptoms associated with insufficient calories. Add fifty calories to that level and you have your minimum caloric level.

In Mary's case, she felt that she was experiencing the symptoms of insufficient calories at 1300.

CALORIC RANGE

You need to know two numbers to calculate your food intake: your MxCL and your MCL, that is, your maximum and minimum calorie levels. As you've seen above, Mary's caloric range is from 1300 calories to 1649 calories.

PUTTING IT ALL TOGETHER

Now you've got all the information you'll need to keep your calorie intake at a level where you can maintain your ideal weight or lose weight without triggering your appetite or a weight gain. Here's how you put all this together (use your food journal for this):

1. Follow the instructions for Phase I of the Core Diet (Chapter 8) for twelve weeks exactly.

2. Record all the food and beverages you eat, their calories, the totals for every meal, and your total daily caloric level.

3. Record how you are feeling physically and emotionally.

4. Record your weekly caloric range, by averaging your daily caloric levels.

5. Determine your minimum caloric level, as we did in the previous pages.

6. Determine your maximum caloric level, (MxCL)

7. Determine your weight-loss caloric Level (WLCL)

8. Structure your diet to fit within your minimum caloric level and your maximum caloric level (your caloric range) and adjust it as you lose weight and your caloric needs change.

Guidelines for Structuring Your Diet to Fit within Your Caloric Range

It's useful to keep the following guidelines in mind. You may wish to make a photocopy of the following and post it in a prominent place where you can refer to it from time to time as a reminder:

A. Meet your minimum caloric level without exceeding your maximum caloric level. Make sure your total calories for the day add up to at least your minimum caloric level, and preferably to your weight-loss caloric level. There are three ways to do this:

1. Design a menu: Design a menu each night with caloric totals that are between your MCL and your WLCL. If you have met your MCL menu by the end of the day and feel that symptoms you are experiencing indicate you are still hungry, edge your calories up by adding snacks or meals—but do not exceed your maximum calorie level. Your goal is to match or come as close as you can to your weight-loss caloric level.

2. Eat when hungry, stop when full. You may feel that you have only partially lost your ability to tell when you are hungry and full and do not want to rely exclusively on these calculations. Therefore, eat when you believe you are hungry, stop when you believe you feel full, and toward the end of the day total up your calories.

✓ If your calories fall short of your minimum caloric level add additional snacks or meals to make up the caloric difference.

✓ If your calories exceed your minimum caloric level and you are still hungry, add additional calories but do not exceed your maximum caloric level. Of course, if you are not hungry, congratulate yourself. You've estimated your calorie intake and need to add no further calories.

✓ If your calories exceed your maximum caloric level for a day (this is rare), do not panic. You may have needed the extra calories. Or maybe you miscalculated your maximum caloric level and need to recalculate it. Or you may have been influenced by a weight-gain trigger. The most common scenario is that people tend to undereat and have to add calories to meet their minimum caloric level.

3. Combination method: Use a combination of the above methods; that is, plan your menu the night before, but the next day try to eat when hungry and stop when full, keeping the menu you designed the night before in mind, but not pressuring yourself to follow it rigidly. Just do your best to make your calories for the day end up being at least your minimum caloric level.

   By practicing eating when you are hungry and stopping when you are full, then double-checking where you are toward the end of the day, you will build confidence in your ability to read your body's signals and eventually not have to count calories.

B. Fine-tune. Fine-tuning is easy:

1. If your weight begins to increase over the week(s), and you are sure your weight fluctuation is not due to factors such as increased lean body mass, water retention, stress, and so on, gradually edge your Maximum Caloric Level downward every few days until you stop gaining weight. The caloric level at which you stop gaining weight is now your maximum caloric level.

   Continue to gradually edge your calorie intake downward every few days until you begin to lose weight. This is your weight-loss caloric level and the level you will return to when you want to lose weight. Continue to edge your calories downward until you note your first uncomfortable symptoms associated with insufficient calories. Add fifty calories to this level to obtain your new minimum caloric level. You may now eat within your new range.

2. If your weight stays the same for several weeks, and you feel physically and mentally comfortable, then do nothing but enjoy eating within your range if you are happy with your new slimmer weight. If your weight stays the same for two weeks and you still need to lose weight or think

you have not yet gotten down to your true set point weight, then follow the guidelines above to again determine your maximum caloric level, weight-loss caloric level, and minimum caloric level.

Fine-tuning is necessary because your minimum caloric level, maximum caloric level and weight-loss caloric level will constantly change as you lose weight and become healthier and more physically fit. These caloric levels will also change during periods of stress, increased activity, decreased activity, a change in routine, illness, and surgery, so it is important that you be aware of these times and modify your diet accordingly.

Phase II and Beyond

Follow Phase II for the Right Bite Program delineated in Chapter 9 for the remainder of the program, with the exception that you will be calorie conscious and continue the calculations and modifications begun in Phase I.

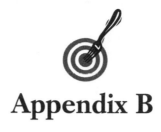

Appendix B

Lives of Quiet Desperation— Recognizing and Healing Serious Eating Disorders

Recovery was not to be seen as a smooth slope,
but as a series of radical steps, each inconceivable,
impossible, from the step below.
—Oliver Sacks

Most of us who have weight issues are aware of others who have them, and it is not unusual for us to trade stories and information about our experiences. I have noticed over the years that many clients who are developing weight-management skills through the Right Bite Program bring up questions about friends, relatives, or even family members who are bulimic or even anorexic. Since I always try to answer any questions my clients have, I have found that sharing what I know about bulimia and anorexia has often led to getting help for people who otherwise might have ended up with serious health problems. For these reasons, I felt it was important to include the following information in this book, starting with this letter from a grateful mother:

> Dear Stephanie,
> This is a simple letter with a very complex message. I thank you for saving my daughter's life. The transformation that you brought her through has truly been a miracle.

When I think of the years and lost adolescence that most anorexic/bulimics experience through psychotherapy and realize that because of you my daughter avoided all of that and is now happy and well, I lose my breath. My eyes well with tears. I thank you ever so much.

I don't mean to sound dramatic; however Sonja's recovery and this whole experience with your therapy has been nothing short of dramatic and miraculous.

We inform people at every opportunity about your approach and treatment. I know that you have unlocked the key to anorexia and bulimia treatment. I pray for you and the families stricken by this ever-so-frightening illness that soon the medical-psychological world will acknowledge that there is another way to treat this illness.

Stephanie, keep up your wonderful work. Just treating one or two patients at a time will gradually build numbers. Eventually doctors will have to acknowledge your efforts and results. I just want to hurry them so. I'm so concerned for the thousands of young women wasting precious young years and some even losing their lives so needlessly, not to mention the exorbitant costs of this treatment.

I am enclosing some recent photos of Sonja. I thought you may enjoy seeing the results of your love and commitment. We now have a very happy, very lovely emerging 16-year-old in our midst. What an incredible difference in one year's time. You should feel such pride Stephanie. You are doing beautiful things. Sonja and I love you.

Love,
Allison

Anorexia and bulimia are extremely serious eating disorders that occur at the end of the vast spectrum of diet and weight-related problems. They are also weight-gain triggers in and of themselves, which makes treatment very difficult. My views on the causes and treatments of eating disorders differ from the majority of those who treat these conditions. My conclusions concerning these illnesses have been formed from my own struggle and eventual victory over weight problems, from my education and research, and from my clinical work with clients on both ends of the weight spectrum, from the thinnest to the fattest.

The Causes and Development of Eating Disorders

Although anorexia and bulimia are commonly believed to be psychological disorders, with current treatment emphasizing psychotherapy, I believe that in the majority of cases they are physiological disorders that are camouflaged or concealed by the conspicuous psychological problems they create. I believe that the person's food choices and habits preceding the onset of the eating disorder, as well as the choices they make while the disorder is developing, are themselves triggering factors in anorexia and bulimia.

In almost every instance, clients I have counseled for these disorders had decided to diet prior to the onset of their anorexic/bulimic symptoms. Their reasons for losing weight were personal and diverse. They included the onset of uncontrolled eating, which was causing alarming weight gain; the presence of a lifelong weight problem; the dictates of current fashion; the urgings of a spouse; the desire to shed post pregnancy pounds; concern over gradual weight gain due to a less active life style; a response to an insensitive comment made about one's figure; uncontrolled weight gain in the absence of overeating; and the recommendations of doctors. After they made a valid decision to lose weight, preanorexic and bulimic clients innocently engaged in some sort of "harmless" dieting before noticeable symptoms of their eating disorders appeared.

The seeds of anorexia and bulimia are planted well before a person has naively embarked upon a diet that turns into a recognizable eating disorder. The eating problem arises from an inadequate diet that at first subtly and then increasingly less subtly disturbs the body chemistry, causing the eventual personality and behavioral changes associated with eating disorders. Maladaptive behavior follows closely on the heels of peculiar eating habits before actual uncontrolled binging and other abnormal symptoms become a part of the pattern.

Dieting, and even fasting, have become all too common with children, even with girls in the fourth, fifth, and sixth grades. Research indicates that 50 percent of nine-year-olds have dieted! Teachers of my clients noted that with the onset of dieting, formerly cheerful, conscientious students, though not yet bulimic or anorexic, began to exhibit the behavioral traits that characterize these illnesses. Clearly, inadequate diets had preceded what was later to be diagnosed as "emotional problems." Not only teachers but also parents and clients themselves indicated that the psychological manifestations common to eating disorders arose soon after they started dieting and as a direct result of the dieting. At the time they never dreamed that their behavior posed any danger to them. For example, it is a common practice for girls in grade school and above to skip breakfast, lunch, or both. Such behavior provides the first giant step toward the development of eating disorders and their corresponding behavioral changes.

I strongly believe that as soon as a parent, teacher, or medical practitioner is aware that a young person is practicing any type of dieting, it should be perceived as a red flag. From that moment on this child should be considered in a possible preanorexic or prebulimic state. I further contend that doctors who prescribe diets of fewer than 1400–1500 calories for overweight youngsters and adolescents, especially girls, are themselves creating future bulimics and anorexics.

Although the determined and inflexible manner in which those with eating disorders pursue thinness and weight loss may seem irrational to others, their behavior can easily be explained: Victims of these disorders are terrified that they will become obese. They may see obesity as a threat to their social standing—which is extremely important to most adolescents—or to their self-esteem. This precipitating fear in the development of anorexia and bulimia is directly related to one or more physical and emotional events with which the young person has had to deal. The observation that a family member is grossly overweight is enough to instill in a child the fear that if she herself eats with a healthy appetite she will become misshapen and "different," or that she might die of heart trouble or diabetes, like "fat Aunt Madge." Some of my clients afflicted with eating disorders were trying to emulate models or teen stars. To tease a young girl approaching puberty about her weight or her maturing figure can create apprehension, as can benign remarks about weight such as, "You are really becoming quite the young lady, now that you are *filling out*." Will "filling out" continue indefinitely and uncontrollably? To budding adolescents, any bodily change they don't understand can elicit fear or concern. Fear or concern can become a motivation for dieting, and if it is not carefully guided by a professional, dieting precipitates and perpetuates bizarre eating behavior.

As developing young girls become sexually aware of their bodies for the first time, it is not uncommon for them to be drawn to the fascinating adult world of cosmetics and emaciated fashion models. It is no surprise that twelve and thirteen year olds, particularly those alarmed by an increasing appetite due to a normal growth spurt they do not understand, begin experimenting with diets. I view it as a natural consequence that impressionable boys and girls and young men and women will try to define acceptable body shape and beauty by society's standards. Women strive be thin, a goal that requires dietary restriction, and men strive to be big, strong, and powerful, a goal that requires ample food.

The very fact that in grade school vulnerable adolescent girls are given the message that femininity means "thin," and boys, that masculinity means "large," is enough to explain why many more young females than males become anorexic or bulimic. To meet unrealistic standards of the day, girls often deliberately try to retard their bodies' growth, while boys, who have been given different, perhaps healthier goals, are more concerned with the acceleration of their bodies' development.

I do not translate young girls' desire to look like beanpole fashion models or svelte movie stars as evidence of disturbed personalities. What I do see is immature adolescents, at an age when they must begin their biologically normal struggle for independence from parents, being enticed by the glamorous but warped values of Madison Avenue and the media. And it is a rare parent who can convince their children not to buy into those values but to be themselves. What begins as normal emulative behavior can rapidly deteriorate into emotional illness when the metabolism of the young person's body, through its owner's bizarre eating habits, goes out of whack.

Many who treat eating disorders will point to studies indicating significantly increased frequencies of familial alcoholism associated with anorexia and bulimia. When I learn from a client that there is alcoholism in her family, it alerts me to the probability that the client herself cannot tolerate alcohol and that her responses to certain foods will also be abnormal. To me, familial alcoholism signifies only that the client may have inherited an abnormal carbohydrate metabolism predisposing her to improper handling of her food. Many studies show that alcoholism is largely a physical disease, and that the alcoholic's unsteady metabolism can be passed to his or her children, where it may manifest itself in several ways including alcoholism, drug addiction, and eating disorders.

This is not to deny that alcoholism produces deep psychological disturbances and grievous family trauma or that there are metabolically sound persons who turn to alcohol for psychological reasons alone. However, I believe that within families, there is much more of a physical correlation between alcoholism and eating disorders than an emotional one.

I have divided eating disorder victims into two categories:

1. Those whose uncontrolled weight gain, binges, or psychological symptoms first occurred after embarking upon a diet. Please refer to the Chapters 2 and 3.

2. Those who have a history of sudden "inexplicable" and uncontrolled eating and weight gain, regardless of whether or not they are dieting or have just completed a diet (most of the triggers discussed in this book are relevant).

The symptoms of people in first group are precipitated largely by inadequate reducing diets, which cause marginal malnutrition, clinical malnutrition, and other metabolic abnormalities. Symptoms of people in the second group result from known or suspected weight-gain or binge-triggering agents, which can alter blood sugar and/or insulin, levels as well as from other precipitants discussed in the chapters on triggers. Of course, there is overlap between these two categories, especially as the eating disorder progresses, and the dieter feels compelled to employ more and more severe methods to control his or her weight.

Malnutrition or marginal malnutrition (defined as inadequate calories, nutrients, or both) appears to make people in the first group more susceptible to destabilizing weight-gain triggers, which might not have affected them at a higher, more nutritious caloric level and/or weight. Conversely, if people who are particularly sensitive to specific destabilizing agents, such as cigarette smoke, caffeine, menstrual changes, or medications, choose to diet, or to exert control over their food intake, the result may be malnutrition or marginal malnutrition. These can become added factors, intensifying the effects of the triggers and making the weight problems more severe. In both groups, there is usually an eventual combination of malnutrition and weight-gain triggers that encourage binging that locks such people into a downward spiraling pattern of overeating and futile efforts to gain control of their eating through ever more stringent dieting and purging methods.

I am further convinced that diets or behaviors that deprive the person of nutritional requirements and adequate calories themselves create and reinforce the abnormal physiological and psychological manifestations we see with people suffering from these severe eating disorders. Malnutrition and marginal malnutrition, which are both known to cause psychological changes, not only can create the depression, anxiety, guilt, low self-esteem, and nonreactive shallow personalities found in eating disorder victims but intensify them as well. Many people I have counseled originally believed that 1000–1200 calorie diets were sufficient to maintain good health. Others erroneously thought that they could eat between 500–800 calories a day and still meet nutritional needs. I have observed that any diet under 1400 calories (except under certain conditions such as having a sluggish metabolism caused from past dieting, biochemical individuality, being very small in stature and thus not needing many calories, etc.) will cause physical and mental problems.

These less than optimal diets also trigger overeating and a rapid weight increase. Once uncontrolled eating and weight gain occur, the fear of obesity is magnified tremendously especially when periods of overeating begin to exceed periods of conscious food restriction, or when scale weight leaps overnight or refuses to budge, even when the client is not overeating.

Young people especially become bewildered and frightened at the thought of losing control of their weight and their eating. Despondent over their unsuccessful attempts at weight loss, and fearing further weight gain, they restrict calories, exercise furiously, and/or panic-purge by fasting or taking laxatives, diuretics, or diet pills. The deleterious effects of the purge (electrolyte imbalance, glycogen depletion, blood sugar alteration, dehydration, and further loss of nutrients and calories) plus the damage produced by other triggering agents discussed in this book, act synergistically with the inadequate diet to trigger further metabolic and mental abnormalities, weight gain, and binging. A vicious cycle is established. This person's eating and behavior have created exactly what she has been trying to avoid: a metabolism that favors rapid fat deposition, even if she is literally starving herself to death. Because anorexics and bulimics recognize that eating like a normal person causes a rapid weight gain, they continue to undereat or purge, which only worsens their condition. As overeating, uncontrolled weight gain, or inability to lose weight become unmanageable, their terror of becoming obese grows to phobic proportions. The anorexic's fear that she will become immense if she should try to eat normally again pervades her being and traps her into self-imposed starvation. Despite her dangerously low weight, the anorexic tries to create as much leeway as she can, losing more and more weight as a "buffer" should she begin to gain weight uncontrollably.

Not only are the bodies of anorexics and bulimics severely affected, but so are their brains. The brain subjected to fasting, nutrient deficiencies, low blood sugar, and chemical and hormonal imbalances can no longer function well. The sufferer will manifest some or all of the following symptoms: depression, manic or hyper states, obsession, inflexibility, phobic behavior, suicidal tendencies, inability to reason, hostility, shallow nonreactive personality, perfectionist tendencies, and more. In most cases, any psychotherapist who believes that these are the "normal" personality traits of anorexics and bulimics is sadly mistaken. These traits are psychophysiological consequences of their eating disorders. Having known a great many anorexics and bulimics before, during, and after their recovery from their disorders, I can assure you that these symptoms go away as soon as the metabolism is normalized with a healthy diet. There are, of course, people with chronic depression or other personality disorders who also adopt anorexic or bulimic behavior. Behaviors associated with these conditions obviously won't disappear simply by eating a more healthy diet, but reason tells us that these people will have a better quality of life when they return to a healthy diet.

I am not recommending you actually take this action, but if you want to gain a glimmer of what it feels like to be anorexic or bulimic, try to imagine what it would be like to stop eating and to drink nothing but water for days at a time. Imagine what it feels like to follow a 500-calorie, unbalanced diet for several weeks, punctuated by fasts in which you only drink caffeinated beverages. How do you think this behavior would affect you physically—mentally? Weigh yourself at the end of this period. Later, follow this by a huge ingestion of concentrated refined carbohydrates such as sweets and pastry. Eat as though you had to accumulate enough calories in your stomach to sustain you during the journey over Donner's Pass in the dead of winter. How do you think you would feel after eating? Now weigh yourself and imagine that your scale registers five to ten pounds higher than usual. Imagine your panic. Imagine giving yourself twelve hours to get rid of the weight because if you don't, you believe a great deal of it will turn to fat. How will you do it? How will you feel after you vomit, overexercise, take laxatives, or fast? Well, the chances are pretty good, I'd say, that you are not going to feel serene and content. Like anyone else on such a diet, you will manifest a shallow, nonreactive, depressed, personality. The old adage, "don't judge a man until you have walked in his shoes" is very true when it comes to explaining eating disorder behavior.

Anorexia and Bulimia as Self-Perpetuating Triggers

Once anorexic and bulimic patterns are established they become self-perpetuating triggers. Here is why.

1. Basal metabolic rate decreases, making it difficult to resume normal eating without rapid weight gain. Therefore, victims keep dieting radically to prevent the inevitable weight gain.

2. Lean body mass has shrunk, augmenting the decreased basal metabolic rate.

3. Lipoprotein lipase, the fat-depositing enzyme, increases, making weight gain easier than usual.

4. Anorexics and bulimics usually overexercise or perform the wrong kinds of exercises, while undereating. This contributes to the loss of lean body mass and a decreased metabolic rate.

5. Bulimics tend to have hyperinsulinemic and hypoglycemic responses to the large quantities of sweets and carbohydrates they usually consume. Binges actually "train" one's pancreas to overreact to carbohydrate consumption, even when the amount is small. As you will recall, high insulin and low blood sugar create ravenous hunger and a craving for sweets.

6. Anorexics and bulimics suffer from malnutrition or marginal malnutrition that makes them *think* and *behave* irrationally. Also, malnutrition and marginal malnutrition magnify fears and anxieties out of proportion. The eating disorder victim's irrational thinking, once established, tenaciously perpetuates the behaviors that are causing her to feel irrational in the first place from suboptimal eating to overexercising.

7. Mindset. Whereas some obese people may not truly want to lose weight badly enough to maintain a weight-loss program, the anorexic and bulimic have just the opposite mindset—they want to lose weight more than anything in their lives and will do whatever they must to accomplish this goal. The problem is that they think that undereating, unbalanced dieting, and other radical methods are the most effective ways to achieve weight control and weight loss. When I convince anorexics and bulimics that they can be both very slim and healthy by following the Right Bite Program, they are extremely enthusiastic and successful in its implementation.

8. Studies have shown that in clients with bulimia, repeated binge eating increases gastric capacity. This delays gastric emptying and blunts cholecystokinin (CCK) release, a hormone that helps to tell us when we are full. The ability to hold more than the normal amount of food, coupled with not feeling full, helps to perpetuate bulimia.

9. Chronic radical dieting makes it impossible for the bulimic and anorexic to distinguish true hunger and satiety, which further perpetuates the disease.

10. Hyperinsulinemic or hypoglycemic responses to food also perpetuate anorexia and bulimia.

Treatment Requires Close Monitoring

For almost two decades, I have successfully used the Right Bite Program to solve weight control problems. The only significant difference between the program described in this book and the one I have structured for clients with eating disorders, such as anorexia and bulimia, is the addition of a fourth component—daily monitoring. If you or your physician wishes to obtain my complete methodology for treating these eating disorders, please consult References, where my complete methodology is listed.

Daily monitoring of a person through recovery is essential because of the potentially life-threatening nature of the disease. Monitoring is intense, time consuming, and rigorous during the first three months. There's a five-day, residential orientation period that introduces clients to the program and gets them started with around-the-clock monitoring. After that, contact is usually maintained by telephone at scheduled times. In case the client encounters problems or has questions, she is also allowed unlimited calls any time of day or night as well. It has been my experience that few clients ever abuse this privilege, and they enjoy a great sense of security knowing that help is only a "dial away" twenty-four hours a day.

Three Phases of Recovery

There are three sequential stages of recovery for people with eating disorders, and I don't consider a person well until they have successfully passed through all three. These phases are not always entirely distinct and often overlap. My complete methodology describes in detail the physical and emotional/behavioral characteristics that define each phase, answers common questions of clients, addresses problems that may arise and calms clients' fears. It further discusses typical therapist assignments that help the client move toward recovery.

Passing through each of the three phases of recovery is like peeling the leaves off an artichoke. Each leaf removed represents progress made—a pound gained (if anorexic) or lost (if overweight), a weight-fear conquered, a misconception straightened out, a binge that does not occur or one that does not end in a purge. The leaves vary in size and thickness—with the larger tougher ones generally being on the outside and the softer smaller ones on the inside. The most serious problems and fears usually manifest themselves during Phase I, and as one moves toward recovery, the problems and fears gradually diminish—the leaves become smaller, more tender, and easier to remove. The client has the greatest difficulty in the first four weeks, after which, recovery moves rather quickly and with little turbulence thereafter.

FUNDAMENTAL FEAR

Somewhere during the second and third phases, many clients who have been making outstanding progress will suddenly plateau and have great difficulty moving forward. At first it may appear that they have valid reasons for not overcoming a certain hurdle, when in the past handling challenges seemed increasingly easy. They may say in response to the same assignment, "I forgot," "I was too busy," "My sister got sick and I was too worried to do it," and the list of excuses goes on. When an assignment has been postponed for a prolonged period of time, I suspect that the client has come up against her basic fundamental fear—the originating fear that is hidden in the heart of the artichoke.

For some clients this fundamental fear seems to be the driving force from which all the other weight problems have sprung. For example, one young anorexic, who had always had heavier legs in proportion to the rest of her body (even as an anorexic), had trouble allowing her body to gain the last few necessary pounds because of her fundamental fear—"My legs are too big." To rid herself of large legs is the reason she dieted in the first place. This client finally had to come to terms with the fact that she would never have ballerina legs and that to try to have such legs meant that her upper body would become so emaciated that she would appear to be skeletal. Other clients may not be dissatisfied with any specific body part but instead have a preconceived scale weight number over or under which they refuse to go. Weighing more than this "magic" number causes them to feel fat, even though they do not look any different at 110 or 115 pounds.

One young bulimic woman was 5' 6" and weighed 125 pounds when she came into the program. At the conclusion of the program, her weight had settled at 133, yet her measurements had decreased. At first the number 133 was difficult for her to accept. After doing her mind exercises and receiving numerous compliments about her new toned, well-muscled body, I knew she had conquered her fundamental fear when she said "I would rather be a size eight and weigh 133 like I do now, than weigh 125 and be a size ten."

SUCCESSFUL RECOVERY

For almost two decades, I have employed the three-pronged Right Bite Program and its fourth component described in this book for treating anorexia and bulimia. Its outstanding success in normalizing the weight of almost every client can be attributed to the fact that the Core Diet is nutrient dense and structured to prevent people from eating fewer than 1400 calories a day. It also removes from clients' paths triggering destabilizing agents that are guilty of initiating and perpetuating the anorexic-bulimic condition.

As part of the treatment program, I help clients scrutinize each trigger discussed in this book. I give them comprehensive explanations to demonstrate how uncontrolled weight gain, orgiastic eating, and general metabolic havoc (including the anorexic and bulimic distorted perceptions of body) occur. When examining the diets of eating-disorder victims, one finds they are riddled with destabilizing triggers and that their caloric content comes mainly from nutrient-sparse foods. When eating-disorder victims are empowered with this knowledge, they voluntarily follow the treatment plan and are eager to get well.

Unless you have been an anorexic or bulimic, you cannot imagine the terror of not knowing why, or when, you might suddenly lose all control of food intake. The Right Bite treatment program, with its in-depth discussions of weight-gain triggers, teaches dieters how to avoid foods, substances, or acts that precipitate uncontrolled eating or weight gain. This information eliminates many unhealthy obsessions and fears, and gives the client the incentive to eat healthily. As physical health and biochemical equilibrium are restored, clients' abnormal mental symptoms dissipate.

It is my opinion that the anorexic or bulimic person's "morbid preoccupation with weight" is less centered on a desire to be abnormally thin, than it is on an underlying and legitimately based panic at becoming uncontrollably obese. My program eliminates this fear because clients are given facts and a plan of action: valid physical reasons for their weight problems and a scientific program to control their weight. I find that unhealthy concerns with weight persist in individuals on other programs because they have not been given positive proof that their problems are physically, not emotionally induced, and their wild eating episodes and abnormal weight fluctuations have not been brought under permanent control. My program removes clients' fears by putting the client in firm control of her weight and eating so that she is no longer a victim.

However, like "recovered" alcoholics, who spend the rest of their lives not drinking but ever vigilant, or diabetics, who must always be aware of insulin levels and dietary restrictions, "recovered" bulimics or anorexics must of necessity be equally on guard during their lifetimes about their own metabolic limitations. I would not label this careful attention to diet a "morbid preoccupation with food," any more than a diabetic could be accused of having a "morbid preoccupation with food."

Exercise is also an important component of treatment because those suffering from eating disorders have grown skilled at detecting the difference between "fat" and "lean" body weight. My program takes advantage of this ability and teaches clients how to increase lean body weight via a sound scientific knowledge of good nutrition along with specific kinds of exercise. The client, now on a diet that eliminates uncontrolled *fat* weight gain and binging is able to observe her body in the process of building healthy lean tissue, and consequently her fears of becoming obese steadily recede. Any weight gain that is unaccompanied by proper exercise will be predominantly adipose on a suboptimal musculature. This unacceptable kind of weight gain only intensifies the anorexic's and bulimic's fears of becoming fat.

Another component of my program is designed to help erase a pervasive fear that haunts many who suffer from eating disorders—the suspicion that they might be mentally unstable, or have deep, incurable emotional problems. This portion of the program also shows clients how to rid themselves of unhealthy attitudes, negativisms, and physiological and nutritional fallacies. After embarking on my program, fears begin to subside as these individuals realize that their strange eating problems are physical, that they have lost their frightening compulsion to overeat, and that they are no longer gaining unwanted pounds. They rapidly come to realize that their previous biochemical instability induced their abnormal mental and emotional state. I also continue to reaffirm what the client discovers herself: that she is not mentally ill, that her concerns about weight are legitimate, and that although her family troubles may be real they did not precipitate her eating disorder.

I realize that in the course of living, all human beings must cope with draining emotional problems, but most of us do not binge or starve ourselves as we attempt to solve them. Because I believe that bulimia and anorexia are physically induced diseases, I feel that probing for emotional causes for these eating disorders is futile, time-consuming, and expensive, and can create and exacerbate emotional problems for the client. Further, I feel that before a bulimic or anorexic can obtain help from psychotherapy, uncontrolled binging and weight gain must be brought under control by correcting the diet so that one can more clearly see what, if any, legitimate emotional problems exist.

When the fear of uncontrolled eating and weight gain diminishes, most of the psychological problems alleged to be causing the individual's illness evaporate as well. For ones that don't, at least the client is able to put them into a normal perspective. If emotional problems still exist, the client, now eating properly and no longer purging or starving, may elect to get psychiatric help, but her condition will be uncomplicated by an ongoing eating disorder.

A particularly satisfying bonus from the Right Bite's physical approach to treating eating disorders is the tremendous relief experienced by parents. All too frequently they have been unjustly blamed for creating the emotional climate "responsible" for their children's disorders, and when they discover they are innocent of this crime, a heavy blanket of undeserved guilt is lifted from their shoulders.

Last, I would like to express my point of view about the strong personality characteristics associated with anorexics, such as a driving perfectionism. I believe that these traits are an integral and beneficial part of the whole personality and should not be tampered with. I applaud the unique qualities of my clients and encourage each person to consider her neurotic and idiosyncratic traits as part of having a spicy and healthy personality. It is my conviction that these qualities should be cultivated, because, along with high intelligence, they make recovered anorexics and bulimics intensely interesting and successful people!

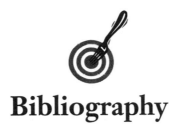

Bibliography

Albrink, M. J., Newman, T., Davidson, P. D. Effect of high-and low fiber diets on plasma lipids and insulin. *American Journal of Clinical Nutrition* 1979; 32: 1486–1491.

Abdallah, L. Cephalic phase responses to sweet taste. *Am. J. Clin. Nutr.* 1997; 65: 737–743.

Amery, A., Bulpitt, C., Scharpdryver, A., et al. Glucose intolerance during diuretic therapy. *Lancet* April 1, 1978; 681–683

Ammon, H. P. Biochemical mechanism of caffeine tolerance. *Arch. Pharm.* 1991; 324(5): 261–267.

Anronow, W. S., Cassidy, J., Vangrow, J., March, T., Kern, J. C., Goldsmith, J. R., Kehmka, M., Pagano, J, Vawter, M., Effect of cigarette smoking and breathing carbon monoxide on cardiovascular hemocynamics. *Circulation* 1974; 50: 340–347.

Bailey, C. *Fit or Fat.* 1978; Boston: Houghton Mifflin Company.

Bailey, C. *The New Fit or Fat.* 1991; Boston: Houghton Mifflin Company.

Bailey, C. *The Ultimate Fit or Fat.* 1999; Boston: Houghton Mifflin Company.

Ball, M. F., Canary, J. J., and Kyle, L. H. Comparative effects of caloric restriction and total starvation on body composition of obesity. *Annals of Internal Medicine* 1967; 67: 60–67.

Barnard, N. D., Nicholson, A., Howard, J. L. The medical costs attributable to meat consumption. *Preventive Medicine* 1995; 24: 646–655.

Bertiere, M. C., Sy, T. M., Baigts, F., Mandenoff, A. K and Apfelbaum, J. Stress and sucrose hyperphagia: role of endogenous opiates. *Pharmacol Biochem. Behav.* May 1984; 20(5): 675–679.

Bornemisza, P. and Suciu, I. Effect of cigarette smoking on the blood glucose levels of normals and diabetics. *Rev. Roum. Med—Med. Int.* 1980; 18(4) 353–356.

Blackburn, G. L., Kanders, B. S., Lavin, P. T., Keller, S. D., and Whatley, J. The effect of aspartame as part of a multidisciplinary weight-control program on short- and long-term control of body weight. *Am. J. Clin. Nutr.* 1997; 65: 409–418.

Blundell, J. E. and Greenough, A. Pharmacological aspects of appetite implications for the treatment of obesity. *Biomed. & Pharmaacother.* 1994; 48: 119–125.

Bray, G. and Delany, J. Opinions of obesity experts on the causes and treatment of obesity—a new survey. *Obesity Research* November 1995; 3(Suppl 4): 419S–423S.

Bruner, A. B., Joffe, A., Duggan, A. K., Casella, J. F., and Brandt, J. Randomized study of cognitive effect of iron supplementation in non-anaemic iron-deficient adolescent girls. *Lancet*; 1996; 348: 926–928.

Bulik, C. Abuse of drugs associated with eating disorders. *J. Substance Abuse* 1992; 4: 69–90.

Cahill, G. H. Starvation in man. *New Engl. J. Med.* 1979; 282: 668–75.

Cameron, D. P., Cutbush, L., and Opat, F. Effects of monosodium glutamate induced obesity in mice on carbohydrate metabolism in insulin secretion. *Clinical and Experimental Pharmacology and Physiology* 1978; 5: 41–51.

Carlsson, S., Perrsson, P., Alvarsson, M., Efendic, S., Norman, A., Svanstrom, L., Ostenson, C., Grill, V. Weight history, glucose intolerance, and insulin levels in middle-aged Swedish men. *Am. J. Epidemiology* September 15, 1998; 148: 539–545.

Cashman, L. *Pharmacology for the Dietitian* 1997; Escondido, CA: Nutrition Dimension.

Coleman, E. *Diet Exercise and Fitness* 1990; Escondido, CA: Nutrition Dimension.

Craig, W. J. Phytochemicals: guardians of our health. *J. Am. Diet. Assoc.* 1997; 97 (suppl. 2): S199–S204.

Dager, S. R., Layton, J., Strauss, W., Richards, T., Heide, A., Friedman S., Artru, A. Hayes, C., and Posse, S. Human brain metabolic response to caffeine and the effects to tolerance. *Am. J. Psychiatry* 1999; 156(2): 229–237.

Dalvit, S.P. The effect of the menstrual cycle on patterns of food intake. *American Journal of Clinical Nutrition.* 1981; 34; 1811–1815.

Dalvit-McPhillips, S. A dietary approach to bulimia treatment. *Physiology and Behavior* 1983; 31:209–212.

Dalvit-McPhillips, S.P. The effect of the human menstrual cycle on nutrient intake. *Physiology and Behavior* 1984; 33: 769–775.

Dalvit-McPhillips, S. *A Physiologically-based Methodology for Treating Anorexia, Bulimia, and Bulimic-Anorexia on a One-to-One Basis* 1989; Ann Arbor, MI: U.M.I.

DeMarco, H. M., Sucher, K. P., Cisar, C. J., Butterfield, G. E. *Medicine and Science in Sports and Exercise* 1998; 31(1) 164–170.

Devlin, J. J., Walsh, B. T., Guss, J. L., Kissileff, H. R., Liddle, R. A., and Petkova, E. Postprandial cholecystokinin release and gastric emptying in patients with bulilmia nervosa. *Am. J. Clin. Nutr.* 1997; 65(1): 114–120.

Driscoll, R. J. RN. Food addiction. *N.J. Nurse* 1995; 25(1): 4.

Dulloo, A., Jacquet, J., and Girardier, L. Poststarvation hyperphagia and body fat over-shooting in humans: a role for feedback signals from lean and fat tissues. *Am. J. Clin. Nutr.* 1997; 65: 717–23.

Facchini, F. S., Hollenbeck, C., Jeppesen, J., and Chen, Y., Reaven, G. Insulin resistance and cigarette smoking. *Lancet* 1992; May 9: 1128–1130.

Ferguson, H.E. *The Edge.* 1982; Cleveland, OH: Howard Ferguson.

Feunekes, G., Graaf, C., Meyboom, S., and Staveren, W. Food choice and fat intake of adolescents and adults: associations of intakes within social networks. *Preventive Medicine* 27: 645–656.

Flatt, J. P. The different storage capacities for carbohydrate and for fat, and its implications in the regulation of body weight. *Ann NY Acad Sci* 1987; 499: 104–123.

Foster, C., Costill, E. L., and Fink, W. J. Effects of preexercise feedings on endurance performance. *Medicine and Science in Sports* 1979; 11(1): 1–5.

Foster-Powell, K. and Miller, J. B. International tables of glycemic index. *Am. J. Clin. Nutr.* 1995; 62: 871S–893S.

French, S. and Jeffery, R. Consequences of dieting to lose weight: effects on physical and mental health. *Health Psychology* 1994; 13(3); 195–212.

Friedman, J. L. and Stricker, E. M. The physiological psychology of hunger: a physiological perspective. *Psychol. Rev.* 1976; 83: 404–431.

Freinkel, N., Singer, D. L.; Bleicher, S. J., Anderson, J. B., and Silber, C.K. Alcohol hypoglycemia. Carbohydrate metabolism of patients with clinical alcohol hypoglycemia and the experimental reproduction of the syndrome with pure ethanol. *J. Clin. Invest.* 1963; 42: 1112–1133.

Fullerton, D. T., Getto, C. J., Swift, W. J., and Carlson, I. H. Sugar, opiates and binge eating. *Brain Res Bull* June 1985; 14(6) 673–680.

Geiselman, P. Sugar-induced hyperphagia. *Appetite* 1988; 11 (Suppl) 26–34.

Goldstein, D. J., Potvin, J. H. Long-term weight loss: the effect of pharmacologic agents. *Am. J. Clin. Nutr.* 1994; 60: 647–657.

Grant, A. *Nutritional Assessment.* Second Edition 1979; Seattle, WA: Ann Grant.

Green, T. L. Reactive hypoglycemia: current diagnosis and treatment. *Journal of AOA* 1981; 80(12) 827–830.

Greeno, C. G. and Wing, R. R. Stress-induced eating. *Psychol. Bull.* 1994; 115(3): 444–464.

Guthrie, J. and Morton, J. R. Food sources of added sweeteners in the diets of Americans. *Am. J. Clin. Nutrition* 2000; 100(1): 43–48.

Hall, J. B. and Brown, D. A. Plasma glucose and lactic acid alterations in response to a stressful exam. *Biological Psychology* 1979; 8: 179–188.

Hanson, M. Lower extremity blood flow in intermittent claudication—the role of the glucose tolerance test. *J. Vascular Diseases* 1987; October: 756–759.

Hansten, P. Glucose. In: *Drug Interactions.* Philadelphia: Lea and Febiger 1979: 349–357.

Harnack, L., Stang, J., and Story, M. Soft drink consumption among U.S. children and adolescents: nutritional consequences. *Am. J. Clin. Nutr.* 1999; 99(4): 436–441.

Hawkins, A., Biebuyck, J. F. Ketone bodies are selectively used by individual brain regions. *Science* 1979; 205: 325–327.

Herbert, V. The five possible causes of all nutrient deficiencies: illustrated by deficiencies of B12 and folic acid. *Am. J. Clin. Nutr.* 1973; 26: 77–88.

Hetherington, M. and Macriarmid, J. Chocolate Addition: a preliminary study of its description and its relationship to problem eating. *Appetite* 1993; 21: 233–246.

Holt, S., Miller and J. C., Petocz. Interrelationships among postprandial satiety, glucose and insulin responses and changes in subsequent food intake. *European J. of Clinical Nutr.* 1996; 50: 788–797.

Holt, S. and Miller J. C. Increased insulin responses to ingested foods are associated with lessoned satiety. *Appetite* 1995; 24(1): 43–54.

Holt, S. Miller, J. C., Petocz, P., and Farmakalidis, E. *Europeean J. of Clinical Nutr.* 1995; 49: 675–690.

Huber, G. B. Heaton, K. W. and Murphy, D. Depletion and disruption of dietary fiber. Effects on satiety, plasma glucose and serum insulin. *Lancet* 1977; 2: 679.

Hudspeth, W. J. Sugar and a fad disease: a case of mistaken identity. *Psychology Today* 1980; October: 120.

Jaravi, A. E., Karlstrom, R., Granfeldt, I., Bjorck, I., and Asp, N. Improved glycemic control and lipid profile and normalized fibrinolytic activity on a low glycemic index diet in type 2 diabetic patients. *Diabetes Care* 1999; 22(1): 10–18.

Jenkins, D., Jenkins, A., Wolever, T. A., Vuksan, V., Rao, A.; Thompson, L. and Jossee, R. G. low glycemic index: lente carbohydrates and physiological effects of altered food frequency. *AM. J. Clin. Nutr.* 1994; 59 (suppl): 706S–709S.

Johnson, W. G., Jarrell, M. P., Cupurdia, K. M., and Williamson, D. A. Repeated binge/purge cycles in bulimia nervosa: role of glucose and insulin. *Int. J. Eat. Disord.* 1994; 15(4): 331–41.

Jung, R. C.; Khurana, D. G., Corredor, A. Hastillo, R. F., Lain, D., Patrick, P., Tunketaub, P., and Dunowski, T. S. Reactive hypoglycemia in women: results of a health survey, *Diabetes* 1971; 20: 428–434.

Jung, T. T., Shetty, P. S., James, W. P., Barrand, M. A., and Callingham, B. A. Caffeine: its effect on catecholamines and metabolism in lean and obese humans. *Clinical Science* 1981; 60: 527–535.

Kern, P. A. The effects of weight loss on the activity and expression of adipose-tissue lipoprotein lipase in very obese humans. *New Engl. J. Med.* 1990; 322: 1053–1059.

Kerr, D., Sherwin, R., Pavalkis, F., Pierre, F., Sikorski, L., Rife, F., Tamborlane, W. and During, M. Effect of caffeine on the recognition of and responses to hypoglycemia in humans. *Ann. Intern. Med.* 1993; 119: 799–804.

Koivisto, V., Soman, V., Nadel, E., Tamborland, W. V., and Felig, P. Exercise and insulin. *Federation Proceedings* 1980, 39(5)0: 1481–1486.

Konner, M. *The Tangled Wing: Biological Constraints on the Human Spirit.* 1982, New York: Harper and Row.

Kronhaber, A. The stuffing syndrome. *Psychosomatics* 1970; 11: 580–584.

Lacey, J. J., and Gibson, E. Controlling weight by purgation and vomiting. *J. Psychiatric Research* 1985; 19: 337–341.

Lambert, M. Drug and diet interactions. *Am. J. Nursing* 1975; 75: 103.

Lemon, P. E., Nagle, F. J. Effects of exercise on protein and amino acid metabolism. *Medicine and Science in Sports and Exercise* 1981; 13(3): 141–149.

Levine, A. S. Effect of breakfast cereals on short-term food intake. *Am. J. Clin. Nutr.* 1989; 50: 1303–1307.

Levine, A. S., Billington, C.A. Why do we eat? A neural systems approach. *Annu. Rev. Nutr.* 1997; 17: 597–619.

Liegel, R. L. K. Behavioral and biochemical correlates of iron deficiency. *J. Am. Diet. Assoc.* 1977; 398–403.

Linder, M. C. (ed) *Nutritional Biochemistry and Metabolism* 1991; New York: Elservier.

Lisner, L. Dietary fat and the regulation of energy intake in human subjects. *Am. J. Clin. Nutr.* 1987; 46: 415–424.

Long, W. A. and Ireland, T. A. *Insulin Secretion and the Development of Human Obesity.* 1988.

Looker, A. C., Dallman, P. R., Carroll, M., Gunter, E., and Johnson, C. L. Prevalence of iron deficiency in the United States. *J. Am. Med. Assoc.* 1997; 277: 973–976.

Lorro, A. D., Jr. and T. A. Binge eating in obesity *Addict Behavi.* 1981; 6(2): 155–66.

Lucas, A. R. Pigging out. *JAMA* 1982; 242: 82.

Lukaski, H. C., Hall, C. B., and Siders, W. A. Altered metabolic response of iron-deficient women during graded, maximal exercise. *Eur. J. Appl. Physiol* 1991; 63: 140–145.

Macht, M. Effects of high- and low-energy meals on hunger, physiological processes and reactions to emotional stress. *Appetite* 1996; 26(1): 71–88.

Madison, L. L. Ethanol-induced hypoglycemia. In *Advances in Metabolism* Vol. III. Levine, R., Luft, R., Eds. 1968; New York: Academic Press, 85–109.

Mandell, M. The diagnostic value of therapeutic fasting and food ingestion tests in a controlled environment: chronic multiple system cerebro-viscerosomatic ailments demonstrated to be unsuspected and unrecognized food allergies. *J. Int. Acad. of Metabiology* 1975; IV: 31-35.

Marcus, M. D. Wing, R. R. Lamparski, D. M. Binge eating and dietary restraint in obese patients. *Addict. Behav.* 1985; 10(2): 163–168.

Marks, V. Alcohol and carbohydrate metabolism. *Clinics in Endocrinology and Metabolism* 1978; 7(2): 333–349.

Marsoobian, V., Grosvenor, M., Jacob, M., and Ipp, E. Very low energy diets alter the counterregulatory response to fall plasma glucose concentrations. *Am. J. Clin. Nutr.* 1995: 61: 373–378.

Martini, M., Lampe, J., Slvin, J., and Kurtzer, M. Effect of the menstrual cycle on energy and nutrient intake. *Am. J. Clin. Nutri.* 1994; 60: 895–899.

Mattes, R. D., Engelman, E., Elsohly, M. A., and Shaw, L. M. Cannabinoids and appetite stimulation. *Pharmacol. Biochem. Behav.* 1994; 49(1): 187–95.

McBean, L. D., and Miller, G. Allaying fears and fallacies about lactose intolerance. *Am. J. Clinical Nutrition* 1998; 98(6): 671–677.

Meisler, J., St. Jeor, S., Shapiro, A., and Wynder, I. American Health Foundation rountable on healthy weight: Proceedings of an expert panel discussion held in New York, N.Y. *Am.J. Clin. Nutr.* 1996; 63 (Supplement 3): 409S–477S.

Michell, A. R. What is the importance of salt appetite? *Perspectives in Biology and Medicine* 1994; 37 (4): 473–485.

Millen, B. E., Quatromoni, P. A., Gagnon, D. R. Cupples, L. A., Franz, M. M., and D'Agostino, R. B. Dietary patterns of men and women suggest target for health promotions: The Framingham nutrition studies. *Am. J. Health Promotion* 1996; 11: 42–53.

Miller, D. L., Castellanos, V. H., Shide, D. J., Peters, J. C., and Rolls, B. J. Effect of fat-free potato chips with and without nutrition labels on fat and energy intakes. *Am.J.Clinical Nutrition* 1998; 68(8): 282–290.

Miller, J. B. International tables of glycemic index. *Am. J. Clin. Nutr.* 1995; 62: 871S–893S.

Miller, W. C. Oscai, L. B., Arnall, D. A. Effects of dietary sugar and of dietary fat on food intake and body fat content in rats. *Growth* 1987; 51(1): 64–73.

Miller, W. C. Diet composition, energy intake and exercise in relation to body fat in men and women. *Am.J. Clin. Nutr.* 1990; 52: 426–430.

Miller, W. C., Niederpruem, M., Wallace, J., and Lindeman, A. Dietary fat, sugar, and fiber predict body fat content. *J. Am. Diet. Assoc.* 1994; 94: 612–615.

Milner, R. D. G., Protein-calorie malnutrition. In: Hegsted, D. M., Chichester, D. O., Darby, W. J., McNutt, K. W., Stalvery, R. M., and Stotz, E. H., (eds.) *Present Knowledge in Nutrition* 1976; New York: The Nutrition Foundation, Inc. 428–436.

Mitchell, S. L., and Epstein, L. H. Changes in tastes and satiety in dietary-restrained women following stress. *Physiol. Behav.* 1996; 60(2): 495–499.

Monsen, E. R.; Hunger and Satiety. *Am. J.Clinical Nutrition* 1998; 10(98): 1111.

Morley, J. E., Levine, A. S. and Rowland, N. E. Stress-induced eating. *Life Sci.* May 9, 1983; 32(19): 2169–2182.

Morley, J. E., Levine, A. S., Yim, G. K., and Lowy, M. T. Opioid modulation of appetite. *Neurosci. Biobeha. Rev* 1983; 7(2): 281–305.

Moss, R. A., Jennings, G., McFarland, J. J., Carter, P. Binge Eating, vomiting, and weight fear in female high school population. *J. Fam. Pract.* February 1984; 18(2): 313–320.

Munro, J. F. and Cantley, P. The management of obesity. *International J. of Obesity* 1992; 16 (Suppl. 2): S53–S57.

National Heart, Lung, and Blood Institute Expert Panel on the Identification, Evaluation and Treatment of Overweight and Obesity in Adults. Executive summary of the clinical guidelines on the identification, evaluation, and treatment of overweight and obesity in Adults *Am. J. Clinical Nutrition* 1998; 10(98:) 1178–1191.

Nelson, L. and Tucker, L. Diet composition related to body fat in a multivariate study of 203 men. *J. Am. Diet. Assoc.* 1996; 96(8): 771–777.

Netzer, Coninne T. *The Complete Book of Food Counts* 1997; New York: Dell.

Newsholme, E. A. The glucose fatty-acid cycle and physical exhaustion. *Ciba Found Symp.* 1981; 89–101.

NIH Technology Assessment Conference Panel. Methods for voluntary weight loss and control. *Ann. Inter. Med.* 1993; 119(7 pt 2): 764–770.

Nikkila, E. and Taskinen, M., Ethonol-induced alterations of glucose tolerance, postglucose hypoglycemia, and insulin secretion in normal, obese, and diabetic subjects. *Diabetes* 1975; 24(10): 933–943.

Nisbett, R. E. and Storms, M. D. Hunger, obesity and the ventromedial hypothalamus. *Psychological Review* 1972; 79: 443–453.

Nursing 94 Drug Handbook 1994; Springhouse, PA: Springhouse Corporation.

Nutrition Task Force on Prevention and Treatment of Obesity. Long-term pharmacotherapy in the management of obesity. *J. Am. Med. Assoc.* 1996; 276(12): 1907–1915.

O'Keefe, S., Marks, V. Lunchtime gin and tonic a cause of reactive hypoglycemia. *Lancet* 1977; June 18: 1286–1288.

Palmer, R. L. The dietary chaos syndrome: a useful term. *Br. J. Med. Psychol.* 1979; 52: 187–190.

Peale, N.V. *The Power of Positive Thinking* 1952; New York: Prentice Hall, Inc.

Pera, V., Clark, M. and Abrams, D. Current treatment of obesity: a behavioral medicine approach. *Rhode Island Medicine* 1992; 75 (October): 477–481.

Permutt, M. A., Delmex, J., and Stenson, W. Effects of carbohydrate restriction on the hypoglycemic phase of a glucose tolerance test. *J. Clin. Endocrinol. Metab.* 1976; 43: 1088.

Physician's Desk Reference 1998; Oradell, NJ: Medical Economics Company 1998.

Poehlman, E. T., Toth, M. J., Gardner, A.W. Changes in energy balance and body composition at menopause: A controlled longitudinal study. *Annals of Internal Med.* 1995; 123: 673–675.

Powers, D. E. and Moore, A. O., *Food Medication Interaction* Eighth ed. 1993; Phoenix, AZ: Food Medication Interactions.

Raiten, D. J., Talbot, J. M., and Fisher, K. D. Executive summary from the report: Analysis of adverse reactions to monosodium glutamate. *J. Nutr.* 1995; 125: 2892A–2906S.

Rajaram, S., Weaver, C., Lyle, R., Sedlock, D., Martin, B., Templin, T., Beard, J., and Percival, S. Effects of long-term moderate exercise on iron status in young women. *Medicine and Science in Sports and Exercise* 1995; 27: 1105–1110.

Rau, J. H., Mitchell, J. E., Eckert, E. E., et al. Neurological correlates of compulsive eating. *J. Nerv. Ment. Dis* 1978; 166: 435–437.

Rodin, J. Insulin levels, hunger, and food intake: an example of feedback loops in body weight regulation. *Health Psychol.* 1985; 4(1): 1–24.

Rodin, J., Wack, J. Ferrannini, E., and DeFronzo, R. Effect of insulin and glucose on feeding behavior. *Metabolism* 1985; 34(9): 826–831.

Rodin, J. Weight change following smoking cessation: the role of food intake and exercise. *Addictive Behaviors* 1987; 12: 303–317.

Rodin, J. Effects of pure sugar vs mixed starch fructose loads on food intake. *Appetite* 1991; 17: 213–219.

Rodin, J., Raidke-Sharpe, N., Rebuffe-Scrive, M., and Greenwood, M. Weight cycling and fat distribution. *International J. Obesity* 1990; 14: 303–310.

Rodin, J., Mancuso, J., Granger, J., and Nelbach, E. Food cravings in relation to body mass index, restraint and estradiol levels: a repeated measures study in healthy women. *Appetite* 1991; 17: 177–185.

Rolls, B., Effects of intense sweeteners on hunger, food intake, and body weight: a review. *Am. J. Clin. Nutr.* 1991; 53: 872–878.

Rolls, B. J., Castellanos, V. H., Shide, D. J., Miller, D. L., Pelkman, Thorwart, M.L., and Peters, J. C. Sensory properties of a nonabsorbable fat substitute did not affect regulation of energy intake. *Am. J. Clin. Nutr.* 1997; 65: 1375–1383.

Romicu, I. Energy intake and other determinants of relative weight, *Am. J. Clin. Nutr.* 1988; 47: 406–412.

Rutledge, T. and Linden, W. To eat or not to eat: affective and physiological mechanisms in the stress-eating relationship. *J. Behav. Med.* 1998; 21(3): 221–240.

Sayegh, R, Schiff, I., Wurtman, J., Piers, P., McDermott, J., Wurtman, R. J. The effect of a carbohydrate-rich beverage on mood, appetite, and cognitive function in women with premenstrual syndrome. *Obstetrics and Gynecology* 1995; 86: 520–528.

Schwartz, R. S. and Brunzell, J. D. Increase of adipose lipoprotein lipase activity with weight loss. *J. Clin. Invest.* 1981; 67: 1425–1430.

Selye, H. Stress and aging. *J.Am. Ger. Soc.* 1970; 16(9): 669–680.

Selye, H. Hormones and resistance. *J. Pharmaco. Sci.* 1971; 60(1): 1–27.

Selye, H., Stress and the reduction of distress. *J. South Carolina Med. Assoc.* 1979; November: 562–567.

Selye, H., The nature of stress. *Basal Facts* 1979; 7(1): 3–11.

Simonson, D. C. Hyperinsulinemia and its sequelae. *Horm. Metab. Res. Suppl.* 1990; 22: 17–25.

Soh, N. L., and Brand-Miller, J. *European J. Clin Nutr.* 1999; (53): 249–254.

Smith, S. and Sauder, C. Food cravings, depression, and premenstrual problems. *Psychosomatic Med.* 1969; 31: 281–271.

Stellar, E. Salt appetite: its neuroendocrine basis. *Acta. Neurobiol. Exp.* 1993; 53: 475–484.

Stunkard, A. J. Eating patterns and obesity. *Psychatric Quarterly* 1959; 33: 284–292.

Sutton, J. R. Hormonal and metabolic responses to exercise in subjects of high and low work capacities. *Medicine and Science in Sports* 1978; 10(1): 1–6.

Thomas, D. E., Brotherhood, J. R., and Brand, J. C. Carbohydrate feeding before exercise: effect of glycemic index. *Int. J. Sports Med.* 1991; 12: 180–186.

Thurnham, E. I., Red cell enzyme tests of vitamin status: do marginal deficiencies have any physiological significance? *Pro. Nutr. Soc.* 1981; 40: 150–160.

Tordoff, M. and Alleva, A. Oral stimulation with aspartame increases hunger. *Physiol. Behav.* 1990; 47: 555–559.

Tremblay, A. Impact of dietary fat content and fat oxidation on energy intake in humans. *Am. J. Clin. Nutr.* 1989; 49: 799–805.

Tremblay, A., Wouters, E., Wenker, M., St.-Pierre, Bouchard, C., Despres, J. Alcohol and a high-fat diet: a combination favoring overfeeding. *Am. J. Clin. Nutr.* 1995; 62: 506–511.

Tremblay, A. and St-Pierre, S. The hyperphagic effect of a high-fat diet and alcohol intake persists after control for energy density. *Am. J. Clin. Nutr.* 1996; 63; 479–482.

Trout, D. L., Behall, K. M. and Odutala, O. Prediction of glycemic index for starchy foods. *Am. J. Clin. Nutr.* 1993; 58: 873–878.

Tuomisto, R., Hetherington, M., Morris, M., Tuomisto, M., Turjanmaa, V., and Lappalainen, R. Psychological and physiological characteristics of sweet food addiction. *Int. J. Eat. Disord.* 1999; 25: 169–175.

Udassin, R., Yehuda, S, Shapiro, Y., Birenfeld, C., and Sohar, E. Serum glucose and lactic acid concentrations during prolonged and strenuous exercise in man. *Am. J. Physical. Med.* 1977; 56(5): 249–256.

Vliet, Elizabeth Lee, M. D. *Screaming to be Heard: Hormonal Connections Women Suspect . . . and Doctors Ignore.* 1995; New York: M. Evans and Company.

Wahren, J., Felig, P., and Jorfeldt, L. Glucose metabolism during leg exercise in man. *J. Clin.Invest.* 1971; 50: 2725–2750.

Walsh, C. H., Wright, A. D., Allbutt, E., Pollock, A.,The effect of cigarette smoking on blood sugar, serum insulin and nonesterfied fatty acids in diabetic and non-diabetic subjects. *Diabetologia* 1977; 13: 491–494.

Walton, R., Hudak, R., and Green-Waite, R. Adverse reactions to aspartame: double-blind challenge in patients from a vulnerable population. *Society of Biol.Psychiatry* 1993; 34: 13–17.

Ward, R. M., Maisels, J. J. Metabolic effect of methylxanthines. *Seminars in Perinatology* 1981; 5(4): 383–88.

Weserterp-Plantenga, M. S., and Verwegan, C. R. T. The appetizing effect of an aperitif in overweight and normal-weight humans. *Am .J. Clin. Nutr.* 1999; 69(2): 205–212.

Westerterp, K. R., Wilson, S., and Rolland, V. *Int. J. Obesity and Related Metabolic Disorders* 1999; 23(3): 287–292.

Woelver, T., Jenkings, D., Alexandra, L., Josse, R. G. The glycemic index: methodology and clinical implications. *Am. Society for Clinical Nutr.* 1991; 54: 846–854.

Wolever, T., Nguyen, Phu-My; Chiasson, J. L., Hunt, J. A., Josse, R. G., Palmason, C., Rodger, N. W., Ross, S. A., Ryan, E., and Tan, M. H. Determinants of diet glycemic index calculated retrospectively from diet records of 342 individuals with non-insulin-dependent diabetes mellitus. *Am.J. Clin.Nutr.* 1994; 59; 1265–1269.

Wolraich, M Sugar intolerance: is there evidence for its effects on the behavior in children. *Annal of Allergy* 1988; 61(12): 58–62.

Whitney, E. N., Cataldo, C. B. *Understanding Normal and Clinical Nutrition* 1983; New York: West Publishing Company.

Whitney, E. N. and Hamilton, E. M. N. *Understanding Nutrition* 1987; New York: West Publishing Company.

William-Olsson, L. Smoking and platelet stickiness. *Lancet* 1965; October 30: 18–22.

Williform, H., Scharaff-Olson, M., and Blessings, D. Exercise prescription for women. *Sports Medicine* 1993; 15(5): 299–311.

Wright, J. and Marks, V. *Alcohol-Induced Hypoglycemia.* 1978; Guildford, Surrey, U.K: Departments of Clinical Biochemistry, St. Luke's Hospital and University of Surrey.

Wurtman, J. J. Wurtman, R. J., Gowdon, J. H., Henry, P., Lipscomb, A., and Zeisel, S. H. Carbohydrate craving in obese people: suppression by treatments affecting serotinergic transmission. *Int'L J. Eating Disorders* 1981; Autumn: 2–25.

Wurtman, R. J. Effects of their nutrient precursors on the synthesis and release of serotonin, the catecholamines, and acetylcholine: implications for behavioral disorders. *Clinical Neuropharmacology* 1988; 11 (Suppl. 1): S187–S193.

Wurtman, R. J. Ways that food can affect the brain. *Nutrition Reviews* 1986; May (Suppl.): 2S–7S.

Wurtman, R. J., and Wurtman, J. Brain serotonin, carbohydrate-craving, obesity and depression. *Obesity Research* 1995; 3 (Suppl.4): 477S–480S.

Yanovski, S. Z., Hubbard, V. S., Heymsfield, S. B., and Kukaski, H. C. Bioelectrical impedance analysis in body composition measurement: National Institutes of Health technology assessment conference statement. *Am.J. Clin. Nutr.* 1996; 64 (Supplement): 524S–532S.

Yanovski, S., Yanovski, K., Sovik. T., Nguyen, T., O'Neil, P., and Sebring, N. Holiday weight gain. *New Eng. J. Med.* 2000; 323, March 23: 861–867.

Yki-Jarvinen, H. and Nikkila, E. Ethanol decreases glucose utilization in healthy man. *J. Clin. Endocrin. Metab.* 1985; 61(5): 941–945.

Zeisel, S. H. Dietary influences on neurotransmission. *Adv. Pediatr.*1986; 33: 23–48.

Zimmerman, D., Hoerr, S. L. Use of questionable dieting practices among young women examined by weight history. *J. Women's Health* 1995; 4: 189–196.